PALLIATIVE CARE FOR ADVANCED ALZHEIMER'S AND DEMENTIA

GUIDELINES AND STANDARDS FOR EVIDENCE-BASED CARE

Gary A. Martin, PhD, is a licensed clinical psychologist and a geriatric and long-term care specialist who is an owner of Integrated Geriatrics Behavioral Health Associates, PA, an incorporated behavioral health provider group in Scottsdale, AZ. Dr. Martin is the clinical director of several retirement and assisted living communities in the Greater Phoenix area. In addition, he is the clinical director of 14 specialized behavior units, which are long-term care based, and 11 specialized dementia programs in the Greater Phoenix area. His areas of specialization include program development for dementia care programs and behavioral treatment programs for high-acuity patients in long-term care settings; staff training; palliative care; clinical oversight of persons with dementia; consultation with nursing homes, assisted-living facilities, families, and other caregivers on treating older adults; and the education and training of healthcare professionals, physicians, social service staff, and medical and gerontology students in the field of clinical gerontology. Dr. Martin is the recipient of numerous awards, including the Outstanding Community Service award from the Arizona Alzheimer's Consortium, the Provider of the Year award from the *Arizona Business Journal*, and several Best Practices awards from Arizona nursing home advocacy groups. Dr. Martin serves on the board of directors of the Alzheimer's Association, Desert Southwest Chapter, and is a member of the American Psychological Association (APA), the Gerontological Society of America (GSA), and Psychologist in Long-Term Care, Inc., (PLTC), where he was a founding member.

Marwan N. Sabbagh, MD, is a geriatric neurologist and dementia specialist. He is one of the leading experts in Alzheimer's disease research nationally. Dr. Sabbagh received his bachelor's degree in Physiology at the University of California, Berkeley (UCB) in 1987. He went on to the University of Arizona, College of Medicine in Tucson, AZ, where he received his MD in 1991. He completed a neurology residency at the prestigious Texas Medical Center and Baylor College of Medicine in Houston, TX, in 1995. From there, he underwent additional training in dementia/geriatric neurology at the University of California, San Diego (UCSD). Then, he served on the faculty at UCSD as assistant professor in the Department of Neurosciences. In 2000, he was recruited to the Banner Sun Health Research Institute to be the founding director for the Center for Clinical Research. Since becoming the director of the Cleo Roberts Center for Clinical Research at the Banner Sun Health Research Institute, Dr. Sabbagh has conducted more than 80 clinical trials and clinical research studies in Alzheimer's disease and other brain degenerative and medical conditions, including being the site principal investigator or national principal investigator for several prevention and treatment trials for Alzheimer's disease. He serves on the board of directors for the Desert Southwest Chapter of the Alzheimer's Association. Dr. Sabbagh has authored or coauthored more than 120 published articles, chapters, and abstracts in Alzheimer's disease research.

PALLIATIVE CARE FOR ADVANCED ALZHEIMER'S AND DEMENTIA

GUIDELINES AND STANDARDS FOR EVIDENCE-BASED CARE

Gary A. Martin, PhD
Marwan N. Sabbagh, MD

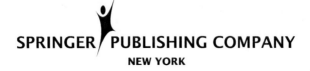

alzheimer's association
desert southwest chapter

SPRINGER PUBLISHING COMPANY
NEW YORK

Springer Publishing Company, LLC
11 West 42nd Street
New York, NY 10036
www.springerpub.com

Acquisitions Editor: Margaret Zuccarini
Project Editor: Peter Rocheleau
Project Manager: Gil Rafanan
Cover Design: Steve Pisano
Composition: Absolute Service, Inc.

ISBN: 978-0-8261-0675-9
E-book ISBN: 978-0-8261-0676-6

11 12 13/ 5 4 3 2

The author and the publisher of this work have made every effort to use sources believed to be reliable to provide information that is accurate and compatible with the standards generally accepted at the time of publication. Because medical science is continually advancing, our knowledge base continues to expand. Therefore, as new information becomes available, changes in procedures become necessary. We recommend that the reader always consult current research and specific institutional policies before performing any clinical procedure. The author and publisher shall not be liable for any special, consequential, or exemplary damages resulting, in whole or in part, from the readers' use of, or reliance on, the information contained in this book. The publisher has no responsibility for the persistence or accuracy of URLs for external or third-party Internet Web sites referred to in this publication and does not guarantee that any content on such Web sites is, or will remain, accurate or appropriate.

Library of Congress Cataloging-in-Publication Data

Palliative care for advanced Alzheimer's and dementia : guidelines and standards for evidence-based care / [edited by] Gary A. Martin, Marwan N. Sabbagh.
    p. ; cm.
  Includes bibliographical references and index.
  ISBN 978-0-8261-0675-9
  1. Presenile dementia—Patients—Care. 2. Alzheimer's disease—Patients—Care. 3. Presenile dementia—Palliative treatment. 4. Alzheimer's disease—Palliative treatment. 5. Palliative treatment—Standards. 6. Evidence-based medicine. I. Martin, Gary A. II. Sabbagh, Marwan Noel.
  [DNLM: 1. Dementia—therapy. 2. Advance Directive Adherence—standards. 3. Evidence-Based Medicine—standards. 4. Palliative Care—standards. WT 155 P167 2010]
  RC522.P35 2010
  618.97'6831029—dc22
                                                                    2010023683

Printed in the United States of America by The Hamilton Printing Company

*To the estimated one million people
in the United States today
with advanced dementia*

CONTENTS

FOREWORD

As a nationally syndicated talk show host, I have had the opportunity to converse with thousands of guests over a variety of topics. It is clear to me that passions run deep as people advocate for their individual cause. In that vein, I find a passion as an advocate and a caregiver for persons with Alzheimer's disease.

My father, our 40th president, was a great American. In many ways, he was larger than life. Knowing him as such a strong and energetic man made it even more tragic when he developed Alzheimer's disease. He showed his bravery and greatness when he announced to the world his final journey into Alzheimer's disease, thus, lifting the stigma that has surrounded this terrible condition. We, who loved and supported him, evolved into caregivers to care for him in the sunset of his life. For me, it was hard to see him have to give up things he enjoyed such as going to the ranch, horseback riding, chopping firewood, and entertaining. His communications devolved from playing games and reading children's books to, toward the end, simply responding to being hugged by the family he loved so much.

As a child and caregiver, along with Nancy, Ron, Patricia, and Maureen Reagan, I experienced the scope of *good caregiving* to a loved one with Alzheimer's. I deeply appreciate how the key elements of professional and lay caregiving can significantly and substantively improve the quality of life of a patient or resident with Alzheimer's disease.

This book, *Palliative Care for Advanced Alzheimer's and Dementia: Guidelines and Standards for Evidence-Based Care*, provides important information on best practices and appropriate ways to care for a person with advanced Alzheimer's and dementia. Dr. Martin and Dr. Sabbagh have assembled a team of experts to help craft recommendations that should ultimately become standards that all professional caregivers adopt. I commend their work and hope that we can work collectively to improve the outcome of this disease.

Michael Reagan
President
Reagan Legacy Foundation
Toluca Lake, CA

PREFACE

I have been working with people with Alzheimer's disease (AD) and other dementias for more than 30 years. Like most professionals in the field of geriatrics, for years, I focused my attention on those persons with mild and moderate levels of dementia, and I never gave much thought to those who suffer from advanced dementia. After all, people with advanced dementia are severely confused and often bedridden. They do not wander or get into trouble, and they do not make demands or complaints. In fact, for a long time, I erroneously assumed that they do not need special programs and their caregivers do not need special skills—that persons with advanced dementia only needed basic care (e.g., cleaning and feeding) as they decline through their final days, months, or years.

However, in the past decade, I learned that I was wrong. Through my work with the Alzheimer's Association, Desert Southwest Chapter, and its Palliative Care Project, as well as my work with quality dementia programs in the Greater Phoenix area, my colleagues and I have discovered that persons with advanced dementia indeed have unique caregiving needs that require specialized caregiving techniques and approaches. We are now convinced that these needs can only be met by caregivers who have very specific skills and training. Unfortunately, such skills and training are hard to find and rarely used.

Alzheimer's Disease and Other Dementias. AD is a progressive disorder that causes its victims to gradually decline over a long period of time. On average, it runs a course of 8–10 years or more and eventually lays waste to a person's personality, intellect, and ability to function. In the advanced stages, individuals lose the ability to walk, talk, and perform even the simplest self-care tasks. In other words, by the time individuals reach the advanced stages of their dementia, they are often immobile, completely helpless, and totally dependent on others for care.

According to the Alzheimer's Association, more than five million persons in the United States are affected by AD and related dementias, with 21% of those individuals in the late stages of their dementia. AD is the seventh leading cause of death in the United States, and it is estimated that we will see a 44% increase in the numbers of those with AD by 2025.

The caregiving and financial burdens are profound. The Alzheimer's Association and the National Institute on Aging report that direct and indirect annual costs of caring for individuals with AD in the United States are at least $148 billion. Annual costs of providing care to a person with AD are estimated to be more than $40,000 per year with families responsible for assuming one-half to two-thirds of the indirect costs of care. More than seven out of ten people with AD live at home, where almost 75% of their care is provided by family and friends. The remainder is paid care costing an average of $19,000 per year. Families pay out-of-pocket for care and many give up their jobs to care for family members at home.

Persons in the advanced stages of dementia consume more financial resources than those in the earlier stages. Although families provide 75% of the care in the early and middle stages of AD, by the advanced stage, almost 90% reside in long-term care settings. In the advanced stage of dementia, the cost often shifts to the federal and state governments because most families can no longer afford to pay for care that may span 3 years or more.

Caregiving Challenges. In nursing homes, persons with advanced dementia usually reside on traditional skilled-care units, side by side with persons who do not have dementia. The problem with this is that the caregivers in these programs are not trained or skilled in advanced dementia care. When asked, caregivers say that these individuals are the easiest to care for, because they often stay in bed and do not ask for help. Care consists of feeding them at mealtime, putting them to bed at bedtime, bathing them on bath day, and cleaning or changing them when they are incontinent. Virtually no other care is given, and very few (if any) recreational and social activities are available to them.

Persons with advanced dementia cannot tell others that they are hungry, thirsty, in pain, or that they are wet and need cleaning and changing. They do not ask for help and they do not use call lights to summon nurses. They cannot dress themselves, go to the bathroom on their own, or tell someone that they are tired. Common sense says that these individuals should need and receive *more* care than anyone else receives, and that they should be the *hardest* residents to care for (not the easiest!). After all, they rely entirely on caregivers for everything. Their care should take more time and energy, not less, which suggests that all their needs are not really being met. In other words, they are being neglected.

Think of newborn babies. Like persons with advanced dementia, newborns cannot do anything for themselves and cannot tell you what they need. However, in our society we would be viewed as abusive if we cared for newborns the same way we care for persons with advanced dementia. They are both helpless, and the philosophy, ethics, and standards of care should be the same for both populations. However they are not, and this needs to change.

Dementia Care Is Comfort Care. In my lectures and teachings over the years, I have frequently referred to dementia care as *comfort care*. This means that it is the caregiver's goal to get the job done while keeping the individual comfortable throughout any caregiving task. Persons with dementia who feel physically and emotionally comfortable tend to be at their best and do their best. They are less confused, exhibit fewer behavior problems, and function at a higher level. Pain will cause a person with dementia to become more confused and to potentially act out. So will virtually all other forms of physical discomfort, like being hungry or thirsty, hot or cold, sitting in uncomfortable positions, or wearing ill-fitted clothing (to name just a few). Because dementia care is comfort care, one of the most critical goals in dementia care at every level is to maximize comfort, and it is the job of caregivers to do everything possible to help persons with dementia be as comfortable as possible.

But achieving the goal of comfort with persons who have advanced dementia is challenging. There are a thousand different factors that go into making a person comfortable, and it is difficult to control all of them. Persons with advanced dementia do not have the wherewithal to address their own comfort needs and they cannot easily communicate those needs to their caregivers. It is therefore easy for pain and discomforts to go unrecognized and untended. Although fragile persons with advanced dementia are more likely to experience pain and other discomforts than anyone else, they are also the least likely to get help in alleviating those problems. Special attention needs to be given to issues of comfort when caring for persons with advanced dementia — comfort is everything to them.

Palliative Care Is Also Comfort Care. We also apply the concept of palliative care to the care we give to persons with advanced dementia. *Palliative care* is a philosophy and practice generally used with persons who suffer from irreversible terminal illnesses of any sort, and it further emphasizes the importance of individual comfort. But palliative care also suggests a deep holistic sense of awareness and respect for the individual. It focuses on maximizing the individual's quality of life (regardless of his or her condition), aggressively identifies and treats pain and other forms of discomfort, and includes sensitivity to each individual's emotional, social, and psychological well-being. Palliative care is an important overarching concept in advanced-dementia care and, as the title of this book suggests, the emphasis of this book is on applying palliative principles and practices to the advanced-dementia population.

As such, this book introduces palliative care programs and protocols for the treatment of people with advanced dementia. It proposes an interdisciplinary team working together to meet the highest standards of palliative care. The goals and objectives of any advanced-dementia care program are to:

- Address and enact measures that support the dimensions of quality of life: the physiological, psychological, social, and spiritual well-being of individuals and their families;
- Anticipate and meet basic comfort needs: hunger, thirst, body positioning, hygiene, continence, and management of pain;
- Provide person-centered care with attention to making meaningful connections;.
- Preserve dignity by individualizing care and promoting the tenets of personhood;
- Ensure that the milieu and surroundings are safe, comfortable, and homelike; and
- Address healthcare decisions that support the right to self-determination until the end of life.

"Forgotten Souls." It is interesting to note that out of the thousands of books written about AD and other dementias, only a handful have focused on the needs of persons with advanced dementia. Similarly, there are no accepted standards of care on how to best care for persons with advanced dementia, even though other stages of dementia have well-known and widely accepted standards of care.

People with advanced dementia are the "forgotten souls" in the dementia care continuum. They are the people who we think we know, but do not know at all. They are the people for whom we believe we are giving good care, but are not. They are the people who need the most but get the least. Moreover, it is time we recognize this problem and do something about it. We need greater awareness and public education. We need specialized training, improved skills, and better care for these highly vulnerable individuals. We need dedicated specialty programs and widely accepted effective standards of care. And we need policy changes and increased funding so that these forgotten souls can live the final days of their lives in greater dignity and comfort.

Guidelines and Standards. This book is designed both to steer professional care-givers in meeting the needs of those with advanced dementia and their families and to give insight into the philosophy, assessment, planning, implementation, and evaluation measures involved in palliative care. It offers guidelines and standards of care based on contributions from healthcare practitioners in many disciplines, state regulators, trade association members, and facility administrators. The guidelines and standards are, in many instances, extensive, but are not meant to overwhelm caregivers, whose professional life is, by nature, demanding. Instead, they are meant to serve as benchmarks and ideals. They are included here to help caregivers fully understand what people with advanced dementia should be able to expect from healthcare agencies, facilities, and providers—to express both the basic and optimal standards of care for a population who, to a large extent, cannot speak for themselves.

▪ REFERENCES

Alzheimer's Association. (2009). *Alzheimer's facts and figures* (full report). Retrieved January 23, 2010, from http://www.alz.org/alzheimer's disease facts figures.asp

Alzheimer's Association. (2009, March). *2009 Alzheimer's disease facts and figures* (topic sheet). Retrieved January 23, 2010, from http://www.alz.org/national/documents/topicsheet 2009 facts figures.pdf

Centers for Disease Control and Prevention. (2009, August 19). *Deaths: Preliminary data for 2007. National vital statistics reports.* Retrieved August 18, 2009, from http://www.cdc.gov/nchs/data/nvsr/nvsr58/nvsr58 01.pdf

Dougherty, J. (2004). *Late stage dementia care path.* Phoenix, AZ: Alzheimer's Association, Desert Southwest Chapter.

Ernst, R., & Hay, J. (1997). Economic research on Alzheimer's disease: A review of the literature. *Alzheimer's Disease and Associated Disorders, 11,* 135–145.

Evans, J. (2003). Advanced dementia mishandled in nursing homes. *Family Practice News, 33*(15), 24.

Field, M. J., & Cassel, C. K. (1997). *Approaching death: Improving care at the end of life* (Report of the Institute of Medicine Task Force). Washington, DC: National Academy Press.

Hancock, K., Chang, E., Johnson, A., Harrison, K., Daly, J., Easterbrook, S., et al. (2006). Pallia-tive care for people with advanced dementia: The need for a collaborative evidence-based approach. *Alzheimer's Care Quarterly, 7*(1), 49–57.

Hu, T. W., Huang, L. F., & Cartwright, W. S. (1986). Evaluation of the costs of caring for the senile demented elderly: A pilot study. *Gerontologist, 26*(2), 158–163.

Hughes, J. (2005). *Palliative care in severe dementia.* London: Quay Books.

Hughes, J. (2008, January). *What does palliative care mean and does dementia need it?* Paper pre-sented at the conference of the National Council for Palliative Care, London.

Hughes, J. C., Robinson, L., & Volicer, L. (2005). Specialist palliative care in dementia. *British Medical Journal, 330,* 57–58.

Koopman, R., Pasman, H., & Van der Steen, J. (2006). Palliative care in patients with severe demen-tia. In A. Burns & B. Winblad (Eds.), *Severe dementia* (pp. 193–204). Hoboken, NJ: John Wiley & Sons, Inc.

Kovach, C. R. (2007, April). Dying in nursing homes (editorial). *Journal of Gerontological Nursing, 33*(4), 3–4.

Long, C. O. (2009). Palliative care for advanced dementia. *Journal of Gerontological Nursing, 35*(11), 19–24.

Mitchell, S. L., Kiely, D. K., & Hamel, M. (2004). Dying with advanced dementia in the nursing home. *Archives of Internal Medicine, 164*(3), 321–326.

Phillips, L. R., Bursac, K., & Guo, G. (2005). Prevalence of Alzheimer's disease in Arizona: Future projections and implications. *Arizona Geriatrics Society, 10*(2), 19–24.

Sepúlveda, C., Marlin, A., Yoshida, T., & Ulrich, A. (2002). Palliative care: The World Health Organization's global perspective. *Journal of Pain and Symptom Management, 24*(2), 91–96.

Shega, J. W., Levin, A., Hougham, G.W., Cox-Hayley, D., Luchins, D., Hanrahan, P., et al. (2003). Palliative excellence in Alzheimer's care efforts (PEACE): A program description. *Journal of Palliative Medicine, 6*(2), 315–320.

Small, N., Froggatt, K., & Downs, M. (2007). Living and dying with dementia: Dialogues about palliative care. Oxford, England: Oxford University Press.

Volicer, L., & Hurley, A. (1998). *Hospice care for patients with advanced dementia.* New York: Springer Publishing Company.

World Health Organization (2002). *National Cancer Control Programmes: Policies and Managerial Guidelines* (2nd ed.). Geneva, Switzerland: Author.

Gary A. Martin

ACKNOWLEDGMENTS

It is an honor and a privilege to thank the many people who contributed to this book, on behalf of the Alzheimer's Association, the Desert Southwest Chapter Board of Directors, staff and volunteers, and, most importantly, the families impacted by Alzheimer's who have benefited from their work.

Our chapter's focus on advanced dementia was originally championed by Gary A. Martin, PhD, and Jan Dougherty, MS, RN, together with the multidisciplinary team of healthcare professionals who volunteered their time and expertise on our Advanced Dementia Task Force:

Tena Alonzo, MA

Melissa Beardsley, MSW

Rosemarie Bosch, MSW, LCSW

Hong Chartrand, MPA, MA

Ruth M. Cohen, Family Caregiver

Anna de Jesus, MBA, RD

Noemi de Vera, PhD, RN

Kathleen Deyo, ADC, ALF/MC

Jan Dougherty, MS, RN

Linda Duke, PT

Lori Eddings, RD

Kathryn Elliott-Hudson, MEd, NCC, LISAC

Paul Fredericks, BA, MAR

Maribeth Gallagher, MS, RN

Leslie Goin, MS, CTRS

Geri R. Hall, PhD, ARNP, CNS, FAAN

Paul Harrington, MSW, LCSW

Deborah Hollawell, RN

Antonia Horton, BA, NHA

Minnie Jim, BSW

Marialorna Kerl, MSN, RN

Mika Kondo, MSW

Kathy Kramer-Howe, MSW, LCSW

Dan Lawler, BA

Kathryn B. Lindstrom, MSW, FNP

Susana Marquez, BSW

Bianca Martinez, BSW

Marianne McCarthy, PhD, RN, ANP

Diane Mockbee, BS, ADC

Yen Nguyen, MPH

Jill Preston, BA, GCM

Pat Priniski, BSN, RN

Niela Redford, BSN, RN, MAOM

Onetta Revere, Ombudsman

Dawn Savattone, LMSW

Judith Sgrillo, BSN, RN

A. Elizabeth Swan, MBA, BSN, RN

Veronica Villafranca, MSN, RN

Barbara Volk-Craft, PhD, MBA, RN

Mary W. Voytek, MC, OTR/L

Jennifer Westlund, MSW

David Wilsterman, Pastor

Hank Zaremba, Former Caregiver

We are grateful to the support of the Nina Mason Pulliam Charitable Trust that enabled us to develop training and our original guidelines and standards for palliative care. I would also like to recognize the outstanding staff of the Alzheimer's Association, Desert Southwest Chapter—and of all Alzheimer's Association chapters across the country—for the help they give to families struggling with advanced dementia everyday. Dan Lawler, in his continued behind-the-scenes support of moving this book forward, also has our appreciation and respect. We thank Kathy Rich for her expert copyediting. She helped transform the book into a more readable and user-friendly product. Also, we wish to thank Jamie Hewlett for her critical reading and thoughtful comments and suggestions, and to Jennifer Leigh Jones, CPM and nursing graduate student at New York University, for updating references throughout the manuscript. Lastly, we are sincerely grateful to Gary A. Martin, PhD, and Marwan N. Sabbagh, MD, who volunteered their significant talents and skills to become our volunteer editors.

Deborah B. Schaus, MSW
Executive Director
Alzheimer's Association
Desert Southwest Chapter

PALLIATIVE CARE FOR ADVANCED ALZHEIMER'S AND DEMENTIA

GUIDELINES AND STANDARDS FOR EVIDENCE-BASED CARE

INTRODUCTION TO PROFESSIONAL MANAGEMENT OF ADVANCED DEMENTIA

1

DETERMINING AND DEFINING ADVANCED DEMENTIA

Marwan N. Sabbagh, Marianne McCarthy, and Gary A. Martin

DEFINING ADVANCED DEMENTIA

There are many types of chronic, progressive (frequently termed degenerative), irreversible dementias, all of which are presently regarded as terminal illnesses. All dementias are characterized by cognitive decline (such as memory, orientation, and executive function) that impacts daily life, but each type of dementia has different features that distinguish one from the other. The most common are Alzheimer's disease, frontotemporal lobe dementia, Lewy body dementia, vascular dementia, and Parkinson's dementia. During the early stages, the different types of dementias are associated with different clinical features. With milder *Alzheimer's disease* (AD), these include short-term memory loss, disorientation or confusion, some loss of independence in activities of daily living (ADLs), and some difficulty finding words. This progresses to impact remote memory, ADLs, continence, and sense of direction. As the Alzheimer's dementia advances, behavioral issues such as delusions start to emerge (discussed in later chapters). *Dementia with Lewy Bodies* (DLB) is characterized by progressive slowness of movements and Parkinson's-like features, well-described hallucinations (particularly visual hallucinations), very rapidly progressing dementia, fluctuations of clarity followed by confusion, and sensitivity to medication. Lewy bodies are changes seen in brain cells, most commonly associated with Parkinson's disease. What distinguishes DLB from Parkinson's is that Lewy bodies are concentrated in one part of the brain in Parkinson's, but widely distributed in DLB. *Vascular dementia* is caused by strokes if they are large enough or affect areas associated with cognition. The memory loss and cognitive decline can even start fairly abruptly following a stroke. Vascular dementia can be diagnosed by changes on a brain scan, an abnormal result of a neurological examination, and a clearly identified history of stroke. This type of dementia may not progress and can even improve with the right type of treatment. Often, vascular dementia is mixed with AD. In fact, most individuals with vascular dementia have enough biological changes in their brains to fulfill the pathologic criteria for Alzheimer's. Pure vascular dementia is far less common than the mixture between Alzheimer's disease and stroke-induced vascular dementia.

Another type of dementia, *frontotemporal dementia* (FTD) or *Pick's disease*, is relatively uncommon with an earlier age of onset (40–65 years of age). Many FTDs are linked to genetic mutations (scientists call these "the tau-opathies" or programulinopathies). Symptoms include prominent language changes, like anomia, aphasia, echolalia, and perseverative speech (a tendency to repeat a word or phrase in an obsessive manner, as if they are stuck on it [broken record]). Many patients suffering from this type of dementia lose social skills and display inappropriate behavior, judgment, and lack of insight.

Parkinson's disease (PD) is often associated with dementia (termed Parkinson's disease dementia [PDD]) in its later stages. Parkinson's disease initially begins with movement problems and is clinically characterized by the presence of tremor, cogwheel rigidity (stiff joints and limbs), and bradykinesia (slowness of movement). Parkinson's patients commonly have problems walking. Dementia is common in advanced cases, though estimates of dementia prevalence vary widely—anywhere from 27%–78% in some studies, but more recent data suggests that it approaches 50% of all people suffering from PD. Parkinson's dementia is different from Alzheimer's in that Parkinson's patients have slower recall, whereas Alzheimer's patients do not remember the same items at all.

From a clinical perspective, the phase of severe dementia can be defined as, "the portion of the dementia disease process in which cognitive deficits are of sufficient magnitude as to compromise an otherwise healthy person's capacities to independently perform basic activities of daily life, such as dressing, bathing, and toileting" (Reisberg et al., 2006). From this clinical perspective, the phase of severe dementia is enormously important because this is clearly the portion of the disease in which both caregivers, individually, and society, more generally, are most burdened, principally because of the increased burden of care. It is equally important to note that the severe dementia phase is the portion of dementia in which patients suffer most. Nevertheless, it is also a portion of dementia in which interventions can be most meaningful in alleviating distress and suffering for patients. For the most part, such interventions require an understanding of the clinical process of the severe dementia phase.

With advanced or late-stage Alzheimer's and other dementias, the person experiences significant losses, including the loss of ability to communicate, to execute independent ADLs, to meet personal care needs, and to achieve personal and social comfort. As independence is compromised, persons with advanced or late-stage Alzheimer's become less capable of caring for themselves. They suffer from increasing deficits in all aspects of their life while gradually losing touch with the world around them. Their inability to communicate can sometimes result in their needs being overlooked as they become increasingly reliant on caregivers to meet all their physiological, psychological, spiritual, social, and comfort needs.

The progression through the stages of AD is depicted in Figure 1.1.

As dementia progresses, all afflicted persons, regardless of underlying pathology, will enter into the later stages. These guidelines are provided to help in the assessment of individuals with dementia and to determine when they have progressed to an advanced stage. From the standpoint of the disease course, the severe dementia phase, encompassing both the moderately severe AD and severe AD stages, is

FIGURE 1.1

Progressive Decline Observed in Alzheimer's Disease

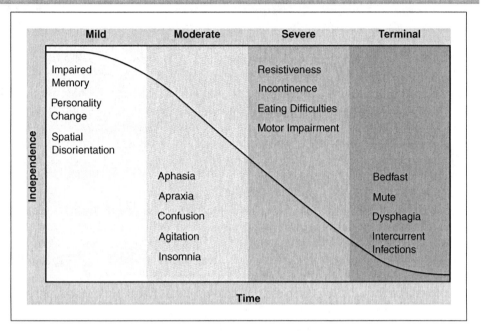

the major portion of AD. The clinically observed potential duration of the severe dementia phase in AD in patients who survive into the final substage of the disease is potentially 10 years, and some AD patients will survive for even longer periods in this phase of the disease. If the current usual time of demise in AD is used in calculating the typical time course of the severe dementia phase in AD, patients, on average, range from 1–3 years in the severe phase of AD. By comparison, the total duration of mild-to-moderate AD combined is approximately 3.5 years.

◼ ASSESSMENT SCALES

A variety of clinical or functional rating scales are used to classify the stages of dementia, including the following:

The Global Deterioration Scale (GDS) has seven ordinal stages (1–7) on a scale starting with Stage 1 (*no cognitive decline*) and ending with Stage 7 (*very severe cognitive decline*). The GDS incorporates both cognitive and functional aspects of aging and dementia using the AD trajectory. This scale is usually administered by a clinician.

The Functional Assessment Staging Tool (FAST) is used to assess functional decline in AD. Patients who are more impaired functionally also show continuing increments in cognitive loss. The FAST contains 16 stages. Stage 1 marks no difficulties for the patient, whereas Stage 7(f) describes the patient who is unable to hold his/her head up. The latter 11 stages subdivide the FAST in the late stages of 6 and 7. It is typically administered by a clinician (nurse or physician). The severe AD dementia phase is marked by a succession of dramatic and characteristic losses in functional abilities. These losses occur in a relatively characteristic pattern in the dementia of AD. The FAST stages have been enumerated to be optimally concordant with the corresponding GDS stages in AD (hence, the GDS/ FAST staging system). There is a strong correlation between the FAST stages and the GDS stages in AD patients who are free of non-AD related physical or mental disabilities. Despite this very strong relationship between the GDS and the FAST, there remains some variability, even in subjects with uncomplicated probable AD. The GDS and FAST may not capture some of the non-AD dementias such as FTD. Because these tools are often used to qualify patients with advanced dementia for hospice care, using these tools only may limit non-AD patients from qualifying for this important benefit.

The Mini-Mental State Exam (MMSE) is a 30-point cognitive screening tool that tests orientation, attention, memory, visuospatial construction, and language. It takes between 5 and 10 minutes to administer and is a clinical tool to estimate progression and sometimes medication effects. Prescription benefit coverage is often tied to the MMSE score for use of Alzheimer's specific medications. The maximum score is 30, with ≥26 considered normal, depending on age, education, and complaints; 24–26 indicates mild cognitive impairment; 20–24 indicates mild dementia; 10–19, moderate dementia; 1–9, severe dementia; and 0 profound impairment. A score of <10 is associated with advanced dementia. Many persons with advanced AD have scores of 0.

The Clinical Dementia Rating (CDR) is a clinical staging instrument for dementia. It characterizes six domains of cognitive and functional performance: memory, orientation, judgment and problem solving, community affairs, home and hobbies, and personal care. The information necessary to make each rating is obtained through a structured interview of the person and someone close to him or her, such as a family member. The CDR table provides descriptive domains that guide the clinician in making ratings based on interview data and clinical judgment. These domains include memory, orientation, judgment and problem solving, community affairs, home and hobbies, and personal care. Ratings in all but one category are on a 5-point scale; personal care uses 4 points). An overall score is derived by standard algorithm. This score is useful for staging the level of impairment: 0 (*no impairment*), 0.5 (*very mild*), 1 (*mild*), 2 (*moderate*), and 3 (*severe dementia*). CDR 3 is severe dementia. All the domains listed are severely affected. For memory, only highly learned material retained with new material rapidly lost and only fragments remain. Orientation is usually disoriented in time, and often to place and, in many cases, the orientation is only to person. Judgment and problem solving is severely impaired in handling problems, similarities and differences, and in social judgment. With community affairs, there is no pretence of independent function outside the house. For home and hobbies, there is no significant function in home or outside of one's own room. For personal care, the patient requires assistance in dressing, hygiene, and keeping of personal effects, and is often incontinent.

There are several assessment tools to measure behavioral changes in the dementia setting. These include the Neuropsychiatric Inventory (NPI) and its abbreviated version, NPI-Questionnaire (NPI-Q), the Behavioral Pathology in Alzheimer's Disease (BEHAVE-AD) Rating Scale, the Cohen-Mansfield Agitation Inventory (CMAI), and others. Either they are intended to screen for behavioral disturbance (e.g., the NPI-Q), or they are intended to quantify the extent of behavioral disturbance by domain (e.g., hallucinations, anxiety, delusions, etc.)

▨ GUIDELINES FOR DEFINING A PERSON WITH ADVANCED DEMENTIA

1. *The person must have a chronic, progressive, irreversible dementing disorder.*
   It is important to first establish a diagnosis of dementia. To determine that a person has advanced dementia, a formal diagnosis by a neurologist, psychiatrist, or geriatrician is advised. The person's condition must meet the definition of and diagnostic criteria for dementia contained in the *Diagnostic and Statistical Manual of Mental Disorders, Text Revision* (*DSM-IV-TR*; American Psychiatric Association, 2000). Criteria include impairment of attention, orientation, memory, judgment, language, motor and spatial skills, and function. By definition, dementia is not caused by major depression or schizophrenia. There should not be reversible metabolic, structural, or endocrinological disturbances. There is a gradual onset and continuing decline. Deficits should not occur exclusively during delirium, a state that may accompany advanced Alzheimer's. If medical evaluation is not available, there must be a clear indication of a true dementing disease process as shown on cognitive testing as well as through a history of chronic progressive cognitive–functional decline consistent with progressive dementia.

2. *The person must exhibit severe cognitive impairment.*
   With cognitive impairment, orientation is affected. People with advanced dementia are only oriented to self. They generally:
   ▨ Are unaware of surroundings
   ▨ Are unable to distinguish familiar people from unfamiliar ones
   ▨ Have very limited or no recognition of significant people, places, or personal items
   ▨ Exhibit severely impaired short- and long-term memory
   ▨ Are largely unaware of recent events
   ▨ Have no clear recollection of past events
   ▨ Exhibit decreased language capabilities
   ▨ Lack meaningful communication skills
   ▨ Have severely impaired ability to verbally express thoughts or needs
   ▨ Have a vocabulary consisting of severely limited number of intelligible words
   ▨ Have extremely limited verbal comprehension and cannot follow simple verbal instructions

3. *The person must exhibit severe functional impairment.*
With functional impairment, motor skills are affected. People with advanced dementia lose basic motor skills such as the ability to walk or use objects. The brain is no longer able to tell the body what to do. As dementia progresses, ambulation becomes affected. These individuals show obvious signs of unsteady and deteriorating gait and are at a high risk for falls and eventually are unable to walk independently. To be transferred from one surface to another, they require two or more people and often require assistive devices, particularly wheelchairs. People in an advanced stage lack the ability to carry out a purposeful course of action (cognitive abulia). They develop generalized rigidity and slowing of movement. Infantile neurological reflexes, such as grasp and snout reflexes, are frequently present. ADLs are lost, including grooming, hygiene skills, and self-help skills. People with AD require assistance with basic hygiene needs, such as grooming, bathing, and dressing. Eventually, they develop partial or total incontinence of bowel and bladder and require scheduled daily toileting. Essentially, they lose the ability to help themselves and require maximum staff intervention for personal safety.

In addition, their ability to eat will be affected as they become unable to feed themselves independently. They will require maximum assistance, including cueing and direction. Because they may be unable to swallow or chew food thoroughly, they may "pocket" the food in between their cheeks and gums and, ultimately, may be in constant danger of aspirating food and liquids.

Their diurnal rhythms also are disrupted. Their sleep patterns in the course of a 24-hour period can become excessive, or erratic and inconsistent. Disruptive sleep patterns are a frequent cause of placement into long-term care. Frequently, medication may be required to manage disruptive sleep, which is a major contributor to caregiver stress and burden.

Caregivers, both lay and professional, need to recognize the features of advanced dementia so they can implement strategies to handle the overall condition and promote palliation as well as some of the distinct features that are mentioned in this chapter.

▒ REFERENCES

Alzheimer's Association. (2009, February). *Alzheimer's disease and other related dementias fact sheet.* Retrieved January 23, 2009, from, http://www.alz.org/national/documents/topicsheet_relateddiseases.pdf

Alzheimer's Association, Desert Southwest Chapter. (2000). *Late-stage care path.* Phoenix, AZ: Author.

American Psychiatric Association. (2000). *Diagnostic and statistical manual of mental disorders* (4th ed., text rev.). Washington, DC: Author.

Folstein, M. F., Folstein, S. E., & McHugh, P. R. (1975). "Mini-mental state". A practical method for grading the state of patients for the clinician, *Journal of Psychiatric Research, 12,* 189–198.

Mitchell, S. L., Teno, J. M., Keily, D. K., Schaffer, M. L., Jones, R. N., Prigerson, H. G., et al. (2009). The clinical course of advanced dementia. *The New England Journal of Medicine, 361*(16), 1529–1538.

Morris, J. C. (1993). The Clinical Dementia Rating (CDR): Current version and scoring rules. *Neurology, 43*(24), 2412–2414.

Ozuna, J. M. (2004). Chronic neurologic problems. In S. M. Lewis, M. M. Heitkemper, & S. R. Dirksen (Eds.), *Medical-Surgical nursing: Assessment and management of clinical problems* (6th ed., pp. 1549–1580). St. Louis, MO: Mosby.

Reisberg, B. (1988). Functional assessment staging (FAST). *Psychopharmacology Bulletin, 24*(4), 653–659.

Reisberg, B., Ferris, S. H., de Leon, M. J., & Crook, T. (1982). The Global Deterioration Scale for assessment of primary degenerative dementia. *American Journal of Psychiatry, 139*(9), 1136–1139.

Reisberg, B., Weigel, J., Franssen, E., Kadiyala, S., Auer, S., Souren, L., et al. (2006). Clinical features of severe dementia-staging. In A. Burns & B. Winblad (Eds.), *Severe dementia* (pp. 15–127). Hoboken, NJ: John Wiley and Sons.

Rogan, S., & Lippa, C. (2002). Alzheimer's disease and other dementias: A review. *American Journal of Alzheimer's Disease and Other Dementias, 17*(1), 11–7.

2

THE CONTINUUM OF CARE

Kathryn B. Lindstrom, Rosie Bosch, Ruth M. Cohen, Paul Fredericks,
Geri R. Hall, Paul Harrington, Deborah Hollawell, Kathy Kramer-Howe,
Pat Priniski, Jennifer Williams, David Wilsterman, and Hank Zaremba

▓ INTRODUCTION

Persons with advanced dementia require a high level of care to meet basic needs for respect, dignity, and physical comfort. On average, individuals can be in the advanced stage of dementia from 1–3 years. Healthcare providers are obligated to provide exceptional end-of-life care to persons with advanced dementia and their families, although this is not always the case. The following information identifies the path that persons with advanced dementia may take as they progress through the continuum of care, beginning with living in the family home. Matching the most appropriate level of care or setting to the person depends on various factors, such as the person's finances, abilities, and family support. Dignity and comfort should be provided at all times, regardless of the setting, and optimized to meet the physiological, psychological, social, and spiritual needs of the person with advanced dementia.

Many professionals may be unfamiliar with the different levels of care for persons with advanced dementia. This chapter focuses on general information about various types of settings and care delivery models throughout the United States. However, readers should take into account different labels, terminologies, licensing requirements, and regulations from one state to the next and should contact their state health department or Area Agency on Aging (AAA) for details on local options and long-term care resources. Table 2.1 provides an overview of the long-term care options that are generally available in the United States.

▓ PROGRAMS AND FACILITIES

Home- and Community-Based Services (HCBS)

Caring for an older adult can be as challenging as it is rewarding. In many cases, families are the primary source of support for older adults who are no longer able to care for themselves. This responsibility can be demanding, not only on the family's time, but also on their personal energy, resources, and health.

TABLE 2.1

Long-Term Care Options

Categories	Common Names	Definitions[a]	Staffing	Services	Funding[b]
Home and community-based care	Independent living, senior housing, retirement centers adult day care, home health care, hospice	The person lives at home and receives care, or attends adult day care. Home care can be provided by family or by paid home care providers. Hospice care is reserved for individuals in the terminal stages of Alzheimer's disease or dementia.	Varies, based on services used.	Adult day health care companion, personal care, home health care, hospice	Private pay, long-term care insurance, AAA, Medicaid, VA, Medicare (only pays for skilled home health care and hospice)
Assisted-living facilities	Adult foster care	Provides room and board for at least one person and no more than four. Owner resides with residents and integrates them into his or her family. May offer dementia-specific care and programming. To do so requires a directed care license.	24-hour care required; staff may not be awake throughout the night	Meals, activities, activities of daily living, medication assistance	Private pay, long-term care insurance, Medicaid
	Assisted-living home	Provides rooms to 10 or fewer residents. May offer dementia-specific care and programming. To do so requires a directed care license.	24-hour care required; staff may not be awake throughout the night	Meals, activities, activities of daily living, medication assistance	Private pay, long-term care insurance, Medicaid

[a]Definition identifies what type of individual would be suitable for the level of care in that category.

[b]Funding refers to how the facility is paid for (i.e., the source of funding).

Categories	Common Names	Definitions	Staffing	Services	Funding
	Assisted-living center	Provides rooms or units to 11 or more residents. May offer dementia-specific care and programming. To do so requires a directed care license.	24-hour care required; staff may not be awake throughout the night	Meals, activities, activities of daily living, medication assistance	Private pay, long-term care insurance, Medicaid
Nursing care institution	Nursing home, skilled nursing facility, extended care facility	Provides inpatient or resident beds and nursing services to persons who need such services on a continual basis, but do not require hospital care or direct daily care from a physician. Some facilities offer dementia-specific care.	24-hour care required; 24-hour awake staff	Meals, activities, medication, personal care, nursing and rehabilitative services (Not all facilities provide dementia/ Alzheimer's services.)	Private pay, long-term care insurance, Medicaid, Medicare (limited— skilled only), VA (limited), Medicare, HMO

Abbreviations: AAA = Area Agency on Aging; HMO = Health Maintenance Organization; VA = Veteran's Administration.

Individuals with advanced dementia may need a combination of services when cared for at home.

HCBS is a general term for special programs delivered in noninstitutional settings. This level of care refers to care received in a person's place of residence, such as the home, an assisted-living facility, or at an adult day healthcare (ADHC) program. Informal in-home care is provided by family members and can be supplemented by professional caregivers for companionship, supervisory, or personal care services. Certified nursing assistants (CNAs) or caregivers can be hired by families for personal care services. Further, skilled home health care, or formal home care services, can be received at home or in an assisted-living facility when rehabilitative or restorative needs arise. These services are provided by licensed nursing, therapy, and social work staff who focus on the return of a person to a previous functioning level after an illness or injury. Sometimes families are able to access primary care providers, such as physicians and nurse practitioners who can come to the home to treat a person, thereby minimizing the increased agitation of traveling to an unfamiliar environment.

ADHC services are also considered a component of HCBS, providing respite and socialization away from the home for part of a day. In most states, ADHC programs are licensed for older and disabled adults who need socialization and hands-on care during the day. There is a licensed nurse on duty and qualified personnel to provide personal care, like bathing and incontinence care, from 7:00 A.M. to 5:00 P.M., and participants can enroll for half- or full-day sessions. These centers provide nutritious meals and snacks and are able to accommodate specialized diets as needed. They have age-appropriate and person-centered activities that meet the participant's individual activity level. Some ADHCs accommodate those persons in the advanced stages of dementia because they provide personal care services.

Caregiver respite programs offer individuals who care for older parents, spouses, grandparents, or friends a personal break from their role as caregiver by providing free time to shop, run errands, or simply see a movie. Ideally, in-home respite programs connect a primary family caregiver with a trained professional who will come to the person's residence and provide care while the primary caregiver attends to his or her own needs. In other situations, respite can also refer to care provided to a person in a facility for a short period of time (part of a day, evening, or overnight) to give temporary relief to a caregiver at home. This can be done on an occasional or regular basis. Funding may be available through the local AAA or families can pay privately for respite care.

Funding for most of the HCBS options is variable. For example, basic care may be considered custodial and not be paid for by Medicare or private health insurances. Skilled care, which is generally provided for a limited period, is typically paid for by a person's Medicare insurance coverage but requires individuals to have need of a skilled caregiver. Other times, private long-term care insurance may provide coverage for basic care services. Some facilities ask the family to pay privately whereas others are funded by the local AAA, the Veteran's Administration (VA), Medicare (home health care and hospice), and/or Medicaid (depending on the state). Some payer sources may have specific medical or financial eligibility requirements.

Assisted-Living Facilities

Assisted-living facilities can be divided into two types of residences: assisted-living homes and assisted-living centers. Assisted-living homes, also called group homes, provide services to a limited number of people—the maximum number of occupants varies from state to state but is often in the range of 10 residents per home. These are usually community-based houses situated in residential neighborhoods that are identical in structure to the other family homes in the neighborhood. In contrast, assisted-living centers house larger numbers of residents and are usually larger structures that might be more similar in appearance to apartment buildings or skilled care facilities. In some states, adult foster care is available as a licensed residential service that is similar to foster care services for other populations, where a household accommodates a limited number of persons to live there as part of their family and provides necessary care for them.

Some states license assisted-living facilities for different levels of care, depending on the needs of the population they are designated to serve under their license. Examples of these care levels include supervisory care, personal care, and dementia care. Each level has rules governing the types of services that must be provided, and a person may continue to reside there as long as the facility maintains the proper license and the resident meets the criteria specified by the license. For those states with licenses that specifically limit residents to those with dementia, only persons diagnosed with dementia can reside there, and programs and services must meet regulatory requirements for providing dementia-specific care. Although in past years, such programs tended to include only persons with mild-to-moderate dementia, in recent times there has been a rapidly growing population of persons with advanced dementia residing in assisted-living facilities.

Payment options are not as clear-cut as they are with nursing care institutions. Medicare does not cover any room and board expenses in assisted-living settings. Medicaid may cover such costs, but this varies from state to state. Some private long-term care insurance carriers provide coverage for assisted-living stays, but the coverage is spottier than for nursing care institutions. Coverage under hospice is similar to what is found in HCBS settings. Otherwise, the most common payment source for room and board in assisted-living facilities is private pay.

Nursing Care Institutions

Nursing care institutions (also called nursing homes, care centers, skilled nursing facilities, or subacute facilities) provide skilled and custodial services to its residents. Skilled services include physical, occupational, or speech therapy for persons who are able to show progress or for persons needing additional rehabilitative care after a hospital stay. Custodial care refers to basic personal care services geared toward meeting the person's activities of daily living. This setting provides meals, activities, medication administration, personal care, nursing, and rehabilitative services. A person can also receive targeted restorative therapies, when appropriate. More commonly, a resident may use CNA-provided ongoing restorative services to prevent further disability. These include strengthening exercises, range of motion, and assistance with food intake. Payer sources for nursing care institutions are private pay, long-term care insurance, Medicaid, Medicare (limited to a skilled need or rehabilitation), and the VA for qualified veterans.

Some individuals with cognitive impairment who require special assistance may reside in special care or dementia-specific units. Some facilities may have secure units for those who are wanderers or, on rare occasions, for those in the advanced stages of the disease. Such programs offer a segregated, low-stimulus environment and specially trained staff guide residents with special activity programming. In other settings, individuals of all stages are integrated throughout the facility.

Acute Care Facility or Hospital

Hospitals are generally inhospitable places for persons with advanced dementia who are unable to adjust to new and unfamiliar environments. Unfamiliar staff, routines, and people are confusing to persons with advanced dementia. Research indicates that acutely ill people with advanced dementia are at higher risk for hospitalization than less cognitively impaired people because of increased agitation and a sudden decrease in functional status related to acute infections or events. Use of hospitalization largely depends on the home or facility caring for the person with advanced dementia. In addition, hospitalizations for persons with advanced dementia are likely to be complex, costly, and last about 7 days longer than for persons without dementia. Some experts argue that persons with advanced dementia who have an acute illness are better cared for in skilled facilities than in hospitals. Research shows that when facilities use visiting healthcare providers who were more likely to treat acute conditions early, hospitalizations can be prevented.

However, the progression of dementia places individuals at higher risk for hospitalization. A person with advanced dementia will be prone to developing recurrent urinary tract infections as bladder function diminishes, and pneumonia, usually caused by aspiration, as their swallowing mechanism declines. Because many older individuals with infections do not present clinically in the normal way younger people do (e.g., burning, itching, urgency, temperature, elevated white blood count, presentation on x-rays), they may become delirious and severely agitated and be sent to the hospital. If the infection is caught early enough, a person would be more apt to remain in his or her familiar environment. It is for this reason that families and caregivers should report any slight change in behavior to the person's healthcare provider.

In the case of a fall and fractured hip, the family will be faced with the option of having surgery or not. It is important to understand that falling and recurrent falls can be common because of the declining nature of the brain. Usually, if the person is no longer ambulatory, physicians may not recommend surgery, as they would not be candidates for rehabilitation. If surgery is not indicated, pain control is of great importance for the person with advanced dementia who may not be able to verbalize how extensive the pain is.

Finally, the goal for all persons with advanced dementia is that they have completed advance directives prior to a diagnosis of dementia or behavior before they become incapacitated. Therefore, it is important for families to refer to the person's advance directives to understand and advocate for the person's expressed wishes related to hospitalizations and any medical or surgical interventions.

Hospice Services

As the health of a person with advanced dementia declines, the goals of care may become palliative, emphasizing comfort measures that optimize the person's quality of life at the end of life. This occurs when the person and family desire end-of-life care and elect a hospice benefit through their primary insurance carrier. This should be consistent with the person's expressed wishes. Hospice care is not setting-specific and can be provided wherever the person resides.

The Medicare Hospice Benefit, initiated in 1983, is covered under Medicare Part A (hospital insurance). Medicare beneficiaries who choose hospice care receive a full scope of noncurative medical and supportive services. The family is considered an integral part of care delivery. Medicare Hospice Benefit provides for the following:

- Physician services
- Nursing care
- Medications, durable medical equipment, and medical supplies that pertain to the terminal diagnosis
- Symptom management and pain relief
- Short-term inpatient and respite care
- Counseling
- Social work service
- Spiritual care
- Volunteer participation
- Bereavement services
- Physical, occupational, and speech therapy
- Homemaker and home health aid services

Medicare has three key eligibility criteria:

1. The person's physician *and* the hospice medical director use their best clinical judgment to certify that the person is terminally ill with a life expectancy of 6 months or less, if the disease runs its normal course.
2. The person or designated proxy chooses to focus on palliative and hospice care rather than curative treatments for their illness.
3. The person or designated proxy enrolls in a Medicare-certified hospice program, which is currently being proposed in the revised Medicare Hospice Conditions of Participation.

For persons who do not have Medicare, some commercial insurance carriers offer hospice care benefits to persons who are younger than 65 years of age.

Medicare has developed a list of general criteria that are used to determine a person's eligibility for hospice services with a diagnosis of advanced dementia (see Exhibit 2.1). When multiple comorbid conditions accompany dementia, a person may qualify for hospice care earlier in the course of dementia. Individual assessments are always necessary before a person is officially accepted into hospice services. It is not a prerequisite for a person to have advance directives completed before accepting hospice services. In addition, as the health of a person with advanced dementia declines, the hospice will document these changes and provide continuing comfort and care (see Table 2.2).

EXHIBIT 2.1

Eligibility Criteria for Hospice

General Guidelines for Eligibility for Hospice Admission

- The person has a life-limiting disease process with a prognosis of 6 months or less.
- The person and/or family have an awareness of the prognosis.
- The person and/or family are electing treatment directed toward relief of symptoms, rather than cure of the underlying disease.
- The person has a documented clinical progression of the disease.
- The person has had to have frequent physician office visits, emergency department visits, or hospitalizations in the previous 6 months.
- The person has impaired nutritional status as manifested by weight loss of greater than 10% over the last 6 months or a serum albumin count of less than 2.5 g/dL.

Dementia-Specific Guidelines

- A FAST (*Functional Assessment Staging Tool*) score of 7 (inability to dress independently, incontinence, speech limited to the use of a single intelligible word in interactions, ambulatory ability impossible without assistance, cannot sit up without assistance, fall over if no lateral arm rests are on a chair, loss of the ability to smile or hold up head independently) *AND*
- Person has had at least one of the following conditions within the past 12 months: aspiration pneumonia, urinary tract infection, septicemia, stage 3–4 pressure ulcer, fever, recurrent infections after antibiotics, significant change/decline in nutritional status (10% weight loss during previous 6 months), a low-serum albumin or significant dysphasia complicated by aspiration/choking/gagging with eating.

Hospices work collaboratively with each healthcare setting to meet an individual's needs. This could be the family home, assisted-living facility, or a skilled nursing facility. The plan of care is developed to address the terminal diagnosis— Medicare requires hospices to offer four levels of care to fully address the care needs of individuals and their families. These four levels of care are routine home care, continuous home care, inpatient respite care, and general inpatient care (see Exhibit 2.2). The most appropriate level of care used depends on the individual's needs. Hospices that are Medicare certified must offer all services required to palliate the terminal illness.

TABLE 2.2

Documenting Decline in Dementia

As individuals with advanced dementia progress in their disease state, documentation of physiological changes are necessary for the medical record. It is important to make changes to the care plan to reflect these changes. Accurate documentation of an individual's decline often is related to a facility and hospice program's ability to qualify for needed financial reimbursement. The following table identifies key behaviors to assess and notations on what to document as a dementia patient's progressive decline takes place.

Characteristics of Behavioral Changes Signifying Physiological Decline	
Behavior or Activity to Assess	**Notations on How to Document**
Difficulty eating	▦ No longer able to feed self ▦ Needs to be fed 100% of meal ▦ No longer able to sip from a straw ▦ Requires 60–90 minutes to eat or be fed ▦ Requires small or frequent amounts of food because of fatigue ▦ "Pockets" food
Decreased intake/poor appetite	▦ Change in usual amount of food taken—use specific measurements ☐ Declining percentage of each meal taken (compared with previous); be aware that most caregivers overestimate the amount of food taken ▦ Measure weekly weight of people who have had a significant change in food intake or for those with weights lower than 100 lbs; percentage of weight loss is significant (See chapter 9 for more information.)

Poor ambulation/ movement loss	▦ Crouching gait with head forward
	 ▦ Change in movement or transfer
	   ☐ Requires one-person assistance for ambulation/transfer, which can progress to requirement of two-person assistance for transfer
	 ▦ Loss of ambulation
	   ☐ No longer able to coordinate movement of feet
	   ☐ No longer able to walk in Merry Walker
	   ☐ No longer able to ambulate with assistance
	 ▦ Loss of ability to propel self in wheelchair, increased falls, and balance disturbance
	   ☐ Use of additional safety measures or equipment— adaptive devices for chairs (check with regulatory requirements): wedge cushion, Lap Buddy, lap belt, bed or chair alarms, low bed or mattress on floor, seating alternatives, bean bag, geriatric chair, Adirondack chair, recliner
	 ▦ No longer able to move independently
	 ▦ Developing contractures
	 (See chapter 12 for more information.)

Mood (may indicate depression)	▦ Increased sleep ▦ Increased weepiness ▦ Decreased participation in previously enjoyed activities ▦ Increase in social withdrawal ▦ Increased agitation

Continued

Table 2.2 *Continued*

Pain	▨ Note behaviors that may indicate pain, such as: 　☐ Grimacing 　☐ Guarding or resisting care 　☐ Tearfulness 　☐ Restlessness 　☐ Agitated behaviors, such as calling out 　☐ New expressions of pain related to activities of daily living (ADLs), transfers or ambulation ▨ Pain symptoms are generally reported as behavioral symptoms ▨ Use Pain Assessment in Advanced Dementia (PAINAD) if possible to quantify pain-related behaviors; document all changes in scores (See chapter 7 for more information.)
Other new or intensified behavioral symptoms	▨ Resistant to care—this is usually self-protective behavior and requires caregiver training to distract the person or to determine if a new behavior indicates pain ▨ Increased restlessness—generally caused by the need for repositioning or unmet pain need. Consider that akathesia (inability to sit still) may be a result of an antipsychotic medication ▨ Increase in vocalization (including calling out). Consider unmet basic needs, pain, and stimulation level ▨ Increased agitation; describe specific behavior that is increasing. Note that this is often a sign of delirium in persons with dementia. Consider possibility of an underlying cause such as infection, pain, or metabolic derangement ▨ Change in a person's sleep pattern ▨ Psychotic symptoms: paranoia, delusions, or hallucinations—usually indicate delirium (See chapter 6 for more information.)
Functional Assessment Staging Tool (FAST)	Consider documenting the FAST upon admission, and then reevaluate any functional change at recertification. Remember that FAST may not detect incremental declines that might be picked up with the indicators described above. (See chapter 1 for more information.)
Caregiver grief/ loss issues	Caregivers' grief experiences change over the course of dementia and vary depending on their relationship to the person with dementia. Generally in the late stage: ▨ Spouses experience increasing feelings of sadness, uncertainty, loneliness, and general emptiness. ▨ Spouses internally prepare for new experiences of grief to occur when the person dies. ▨ Adult children's expressed feelings of anger, resentment, and guilt soften to less obvious feelings of sadness, resignation, and regret. ▨ In response, some find new ways of interacting with the person whereas others distance themselves from the situation. ▨ Caregivers' feelings may not be readily apparent, even to themselves. Supportive listening from a group or a friend and use of the Marwit-Meuser Caregiver Grief Inventory can help them identify and express feelings. ▨ Following the death, family caregivers of people who were in institutions experience slower recovery from depressive symptoms compared to those who provided care at home and may particularly benefit from bereavement services. (See chapter 17 for more information.)

Source: Data from Jan Dougherty, *Documentation of Decline in Dementia* (unpublished manuscript).

EXHIBIT 2.2

Levels of Hospice Care

Routine Home Care

This care is provided to people on hospice services in their place of residence (a private house, an assisted-living home or facility, a nursing home, or a residential hospice home). The person or family remains responsible for paying room and board and the Medicare Hospice Benefit pays for all medical expenses pertaining to the hospice diagnosis. Some hospices charge co-pays for medications and services, whereas others do not. The person's primary insurance continues to pay for medical care pertaining to any other nonhospice diagnosis. Most hospice care is provided at the routine home care level of care.

Continuous Home Care

This level of care is provided when the person is experiencing acute symptoms requiring skilled nursing care. The hospice agency must provide a minimum of 8–9 hours of skilled care within a 24-hour period. A licensed nurse must provide more than half of the continuous care hours. A home health aide can provide the remainder of the hours. This level of care is intended only for brief periods of crisis with the goal of allowing the person to remain at home.

Inpatient Respite Care

Respite care is arranged by the hospice agency when the family or caregiver needs relief using inpatient facilities. It can be provided under contract in a Medicare-certified nursing home, hospital, or an inpatient hospice facility. Respite care is offered on a short-term basis, on average, no more than 5 days per episode. Medicare does not put a limit on number of admissions for respite care in hospice.

General Inpatient Care

This level of care is available for pain control or acute symptom management that cannot be managed in the person's place of residence. It must be provided on a short-term basis in a contracted Medicare-certified nursing home, hospital, or inpatient hospice facility.

CONCLUSION

Dementia is a condition that affects not only the person afflicted, but also the family and those close to him or her. There is an array of community-based programs and facilities that may care for the person with advanced dementia. Each state has the capability to assist caregivers and families in helping them to find the most appropriate level of care to meet the needs of a person with advanced dementia and the needs of the family caring for the person. It is recommended that professional or family caregivers begin with the AAA for local and state funded programs. For more specific information on state regulations for facilities, contact the Health Services Administration (or equivalent department, depending on the state). For Medicare information and eligibility guidelines, contact the Social Security Administration at http://www.Medicare.gov, and for Medicaid, contact the state's Medicaid office or provider. Those who successfully navigate the continuum of care can access multiple sources of support and thereby optimize the quality of life for persons with advanced dementia and their families.

▉ REFERENCES

AARP Public Policy Institute. (2007). *Valuing the invaluable: A new look at the economic value of family caregiving.* Retrieved January 23, 2010, from http://www.thefamilycaregiver.org/pdfs/NewLookattheEconomicValueofFamilyCaregivingIssueBrief.pdf

Ahronheim, J. C., Morrison, R. S., Morris, J., Baskin, S., & Meier, D. E. (2000). Palliative care in advanced dementia: A randomized controlled trial and descriptive analysis. *Journal of Palliative Medicine, 3*(3), 265–273.

Albert, S. M., Costa, R., Merchant, C., Small, S., Jenders, R. A., & Stern Y. (1999). Hospitalization and Alzheimer's disease: Results from a community-based study. *Journals of Gerontology. Series A, Biological Sciences and Medical Sciences, 54*(5), M267–M271.

Alzheimer's Association. (2003). *Partnering with your doctor: A guide for persons with memory problems and their partners.* Retrieved on January 23, 2010, from http://www.alz.org/national/documents/brochure_partneringwithyourdoctor.pdf

Alzheimer's Association. (2006). *2006 National public policy program to conquer Alzheimer's disease.* Retrieved January 23, 2010, from http://www.alz.org/advocacy/2006program/images/2006_Program.pdf

Alzheimer's Association. (2007). *Respite care guide.* Retrieved January 23, 2010, from http://www.alz.org/national/documents/brochure_respitecareguide.pdf

Alzheimer's Association. (2009a). *Alzheimer's facts and figures (full report).* Retrieved January 23, 2010, from http://www.alz.org/alzheimers_disease_facts_figures.asp

Alzheimer's Association. (2009b, March). *2009 Alzheimer's disease facts and figures (topic sheet).* Retrieved January 23, 2010 from, http://www.alz.org/national/documents/topicsheet_2009_facts_figures.pdf

Andrieu, S., Reynish, E., Nourhashemi, F., Shakespeare, A., Moulias, S., Ousset, P. J., et al. (2002). Predictive factors of acute hospitalization in 134 patients with Alzheimer's disease: A one year prospective study. *International Journal of Geriatric Psychiatry, 17*(5), 422–426.

Balardy, L., Voisin, T., Cantet, C., Vellas, B., & REAL.FR Group. (2005). Predictive factors of emergency hospitalization in Alzheimer's patients: Results of one-year follow-up in the REAL.FR Cohort. *Journal of Nutrition, Health & Aging, 9*(2), 112–116.

Berg, L. (1988). Clinical dementia rating. *Psychopharmacology Bulletin, 24,* 637– 639.

Bonsignore, M., & Heun R. (2003). Mortality in Alzheimer's disease. *Dementia & Geriatric Cognitive Disorders, 15*(4), 231–236.

Boss, P., Caron, W., Horbal, J., & Mortimer, J. (1990). Predictors of depression in caregivers of dementia patients: Boundary ambiguity and mastery. *Family Process, 29*(3), 245–254.

Centers for Medicare and Medicaid Services. (n.d.). *Medicare Hospice Benefits.* Retrieved January 23, 2010, from http://www.medicare.gov/Publications/Pubs/pdf/02154.pdf

Cortes, F., Gillette-Guyonnet, S., Nourhashemi, F., Andrieu, S., Cantet, C., Vellas, B., et al. (2005). Recent data on the natural history of Alzheimer's disease: results from the REAL.FR Study. *Journal of Nutrition, Health & Aging, 9*(2), 86–93.

Day, N., Musallam, K., & Wells, M. (1999). Observed behaviors of patients with probable Alzheimer's disease who are hospitalized for diagnostic tests. *Journal of Gerontological Nursing, 25*(11), 35–39.

Fillenbaum, G., Heyman, A., Peterson, B., Pieper, C. F., & Weiman, A. L. (2000). Frequency and duration of hospitalization of patients with AD based on Medicare data: CERAD XX. _Neurology, 54_ (3), 740–743.

Fillenbaum, G., Heyman, A., Peterson, B. L., Pieper, C. F., & Weiman, A. L. (2001). Use and cost of hospitalization of patients with AD by stage and living arrangement: CERAD XXI. _Neurology, 56_ (2), 201–206.

Freyne, A., Kidd, N., Coen, R., & Lawlor, B. A. (1999). Burden in carers of dementia patients: Higher levels in carers of younger sufferers. _International Journal of Geriatric Psychiatry, 14,_ 784–788.

Kovach, C. R., Wilson, S. A., & Noonan, P. E. (1996). The effects of hospice interventions on behaviors, discomfort, and physical complications of end-stage dementia nursing home residents. _American Journal of Alzheimer's Disease, 11_(4), 7–10.

Leibson, C., Owens, T., O'Brien, P., Waring, S., Tangalos, E., Hanson, V., et al. (1999). Use of physician and acute care services by persons with and without Alzheimer's disease: A population-based comparison. _Journal of the American Geriatrics Society, 47_(7), 864–869.

Long, C. O. (2004). Community-based nursing and home care. In S. M. Lewis, M. M. Heitkemper, & S. R. Dirksen (Eds.), _Medical-surgical nursing. Assessment and management of clinical problems_ (6th ed.). St. Louis, MO: Mosby.

Lucero, M. (2004). Enhancing the visits of loved ones of people in late stage dementia. _Alzheimer's Care Quarterly, 5_(2), 173–177.

Luscombe, G., Brodaty, H., & Freeth, S. (1998). Younger people with dementia: Diagnostic issues, effects on carers and use of services. _International Journal of Geriatric Psychiatry, 13,_ 323–330.

Mack, K., & Thompson, L. (2004). _A decade of informal caregiving: Are today's informal caregivers different than informal caregivers a decade ago?_ Caregivers of Older Persons Data Profile. Washington, DC: Center on an Aging Society. Retrieved October 16, 2005, from http://www.aging-society.org

National Family Caregiver Association. (2005). _Common bonds of caregiving._ Retrieved January 23, 2010, from http://www.thefamilycaregiver.org/who_are_family_caregivers/common_bonds_of_caregiving.cfm

Phillips, L., Brusac, K., & Guo, G. (2005). Prevalence of Alzheimer's disease in Arizona: Future projections and implications. _Arizona Geriatric Society Journal, 10_(2), 19–24.

Rabow, M. W., Hasuer, J. M., & Adams, J. (2004). Supporting family caregivers at the end of life. "They don't know what they don't know". _The Journal of the American Medical Association, 291_ (4), 483–491.

Schulz, R., & Beach, S. R. (1999). Caregiving as a risk factor for mortality: The Caregiver Health Effects Study. _The Journal of the American Medical Association, 282_(23), 2215–2219.

Schulz, R., Belle, S. H., Czaja, S. J., McGinnis, K. A., Stevens, A., & Zhang, S. (2004). Long-term care placement of dementia patients and caregiver health and well-being. _The Journal of the American Medical Association, 292_(8), 961–967.

Smith, G. E., Kokmen, E., O'Brien, P. C. (2000). Risk factors for nursing home placement in a population-based dementia cohort. _Journal of the American Geriatric Society, 48_(5), 519–525.

Wasow, M., & Coons, D. (1987). Widows and widowers of Alzheimer's victims: Their survival after spouses' death. _Journal of Independent Social Work, 2_(2), 21–23.

3

CAREGIVING

Kathryn B. Lindstrom, Rosie Bosch, Ruth M. Cohen, Paul Fredericks,
Geri R. Hall, Paul Harrington, Deborah Hollawell, Kathy Kramer-Howe,
Pat Priniski, Jennifer Williams, David Wilsterman, and Hank Zaremba

▨ INTRODUCTION

The term *caregiver* encompasses a wide variety of definitions. From family members to neighbors, friends to volunteers, or paid healthcare staff in various settings, a caregiver is someone who provides care from either a formal or an informal perspective. Informal care might include such things as phone calls to the person with dementia or to his or her caregiver, friendly visiting, monthly check-in visits, or other such activities. Formal caregiving suggests a more consistent, intense style whereby care may be provided several times a week or on a 24 hours a day, 7 days a week basis. The term *care partner* is now being used more liberally, suggesting that as partners, persons with dementia are still able to be involved in the care they receive and can voice their own concerns and assist with decision making. The term caregiver has come to suggest that the care recipients are no longer able to actively participate in the care they receive.

There are no limits to where caregiving may take place. From the individual's private home, to an assisted-living or skilled nursing facility, a hospice, or elsewhere, caregiving has no boundaries. The National Family Caregiver Association states the following:

> Although most caregiving goes on in the home, and most caregivers and recipients live under the same roof, talk to anyone whose parent is in a nursing home and you'll quickly learn that caregiving doesn't end when someone else is responsible for day to day care, or when caregiving takes place long distance. (2005)

Of people with Alzheimer's disease, 70% live at home, where 75% of the care is provided by family members and friends. The experience of the caregiver, often an elderly spouse, can be very stressful and is now a recognized risk factor for depression and mortality. Among other family caregivers, adult children are most likely to assume the role of primary caregiver. In 1999, adult children accounted for 44% of primary family caregivers for people age 65 or older who had limitations in performing basic everyday activities. The burdens of family caregiving can be problematic, related to time and logistical difficulties, the scope and demands of the physical tasks, significant financial costs, increased physical health risks, and the many emotional burdens and personal sacrifices.

Of the 5.3 million Americans with dementia, 90% will be institutionalized and cared for by professional caregivers before death. Professional caregivers also experience stress when caring for people with advanced dementia. Lack of training or support leads to caregiver frustration and job turnover. Families then need to adjust to new staff over and over, adding more stress to everyone. Education, training, and support, directed to both families and professional caregivers, are needed to meet the comfort needs in a dignified way for those with advanced dementia.

Persons with dementia will experience having someone care for their needs along their life journey. Although this process has been described as difficult, demanding, and exhausting, family members often express lessons learned during this time that allows them to make meaning of the experience. Professional caregivers may also become frustrated in not knowing how best to meet the needs of these individuals. Thus, it is important that all caregivers obtain the necessary information and support to help persons with advanced dementia attain the highest quality of life in the final years of their lives.

The purpose of this chapter is to provide information for professional caregivers to understand their role and how to best meet the physical, psychological, social, and spiritual needs of a person with advanced dementia. We provide information and advice to facility, community-based, and family caregivers on how to be effective caregivers. There are lists of information directed to professional caregivers and lists for professional caregivers to share with families. Copies can be made and shared with facility staffs and family caregivers. These lists do not include every possible helpful strategy but do give a beginning overview of the primary needs of each caregiver group. The chapter concludes with the section on the standards of care for healthcare facilities and personnel with caring for the person with advanced dementia.

ASSISTANCE FOR PROFESSIONAL CAREGIVERS

Regardless of the healthcare setting, professional caregivers play an integral role in meeting the ongoing needs of persons with advanced dementia. The workplace may be at a person's home, through a home health agency, group homes, assisted-living homes, or assisted-living centers. Professional caregivers may include hospital staff, hospice staff, certified nursing assistants, licensed nurses, therapists, activity staff, and any others who have direct contact with the person in the home or facility setting.

Professional caregivers provide comfortable, assistive, and insightful care for the person with memory loss who is no longer able to voice concerns, opinions, pain, or discomfort. They also can enhance family relationships by providing education and supportive care to family members. To provide an overview, facility or agency administrators may wish to share the following guidelines with their professional caregivers. Additional detailed information is located throughout other sections of this book.

Tips for Professional Caregivers in Healthcare Facilities and Agencies: Caring for Persons With Advanced Dementia

Professional caregivers can do several things to help ensure the best possible care for persons with advanced dementia. The following section lists the interventions for best outcomes in caregiving approaches.

1. *Shift the focus to palliative care.* Providing palliative care, or comfort care, that meets the quality of life needs of the person with advanced dementia is paramount. Palliative care is typically a paradigm shift for most professional caregivers. After all, the goal of nursing, medicine, therapy, and other disciplines is to treat and, above all, to cure! When curing is no longer an option, comfort and care are the primary objectives. It is not that caring is excluded at the onset, rather, the caring component takes on new and expanded meanings and challenges for professional caregivers. The emphasis shifts from length of life to *quality* of life. Palliative care is described as comfort care that is holistic in nature and includes interventions that address symptom control, psychological needs of individuals and families, quality of life, dignity, safety, respect for personhood, emphasis on the use of intact abilities, and manipulation of the environment.

   The principles of palliative care transcend all settings. No matter where the individual resides, professional caregivers can adopt, adapt, and implement successful caregiving strategies that focus on meeting comfort needs, regardless of the work setting.

2. *Get to really know the person.* When those with dementia are no longer able to verbally communicate their needs, they will seek other ways in which to tell professional caregivers when they are distressed, in pain, or have unmet needs. Often they will make their needs known by some outward expression of behavior that may be viewed as challenging or problematic. Professional caregivers have the responsibility to actively determine what is causing the distress or behavior and to provide a comforting intervention. Thus, there is a need to know the individual in all aspects: his or her history and current state of being, including, but not limited to, his or her religious or faith background; past employment status; birth order amongst their siblings; relationship with family; and ability to handle grief or loss. The life story or biosketch is a useful adjunct in getting to know the person. Include the family in every possible way to help know the person and to construct the plan of care. Consider the family as a joint partner in care, whether at home or in a facility setting.

   Person-centered care is directed toward meeting the individual's needs above those of the agency or facility. All aspects of caregiving, such as dressing and grooming activities, are tailored to the person's individual needs, comfort, and quality of life. Quality of life considerations include attention to the individual's physiological, psychological, spiritual, and social needs. It also assumes that the professional caregiver knows and upholds the individual's healthcare decision related to his or her advance directives. If this information is not readily known or available, secure the necessary details to be informed on the person's choices for health care. Thus, all aspects of care require knowing the person and crafting a plan of care that is person-centered.

3. *Make every activity a meaningful activity.* As the disease progresses in a person with advanced dementia, he or she will display more difficulty in performing activities of daily living. There will be a progressive inability to feed, toilet, bathe, dress, and groom himself or herself. The ability to walk will eventually be lost, requiring professional caregivers to sustain any purposeful movement for as long as possible while minimizing the risk of falls. It is important to incorporate as much independence for as long as possible. As the dementia robs the person of his or her capabilities, the professional caregiver will assume more of the actions related to the activities of daily living. Thus, the professional caregiver will assume more responsibility and provide more assistance to the individual as the dementia progresses.

Professional caregivers intervene for persons with advanced dementia by incorporating the philosophy that every activity is an opportunity for meaningful connections with the persons for whom they provide care and that anticipating needs is the best approach to care. Every activity of daily living should be considered purposeful and an opportunity to provide meaningful connections with the person (see chapter 14 on activity programming). Consult an activity professional for additional information on activity programs and how to incorporate meaningful connections into everyday routine activities of daily living.

Consider including spiritual activities to enhance meaningful connections. Like so many personal topics, spirituality is most often considered private. Even seasoned healthcare professionals are hesitant to assess a person's spiritual needs. Frequently, professionals report feeling inadequate to make an evaluation of another's spiritual condition as it may be outside their scope of expertise, even if the assessment is extremely simple. For example, does the person perceive a reality greater than him or her? Has the person had any religious formation in early years? Are there any community resources currently attending to the person's spiritual needs? What sensory experiences are meaningful spiritual connectors for the person with dementia? Was/is formal religion an important part of the person's life? Learn to incorporate spiritual components, such as reciting preferred or common Bible passages and hymns into the everyday caregiving routine when appropriate. Sometimes, when persons with advanced dementia can no longer talk sensibly, they can sing hymns or songs from their youth. It can be easy to think there is "no one inside" when the outward behaviors are gone, but caregivers must continually try new things to try to connect individuals with their environment.

4. *Be flexible.* Recognize that even with the best-made plans, there will be changes in the day-to-day experiences and care for a person with advanced dementia. What may work well one day may not work the next. It is important to go with the flow on a daily basis. Although this book gives general approaches to care, you may find other ways to maximize an individual's comfort and minimize distress. Find out what works best under most circumstances, document it in

the record, and use the intervention knowing that changes to the plan of care may need to be modified based on the individual's changing needs. Above all, be consistent yet flexible!

5. *Document what works and what does not.* Care plans are typically required for all medical records. Use the care plan as if there were no other means of communicating the care needs of the person with advanced dementia to other team members. When there are changes to the care plan, document discussions with family members. Track what interventions appear to get the best results in minimizing distress and providing comfort and quality of life.

6. *Be an active part of the team.* Professional caregivers provide significant input into the care plan for persons with advanced dementia and function as part of the interdisciplinary team. The team will include the individual's primary care provider, nurses, certified nursing assistants, direct caregivers, therapy staff, social service staff, and others. Notify key members or the primary contact of the interdisciplinary team if you notice the following:

    ▪ The person is having increased difficulties eating or swallowing, or is losing weight.

    ▪ Toileting efforts become more challenging or incontinence needs to be managed more effectively.

    ▪ The person becomes resistive to bathing in the shower or tub.

    ▪ Dressing and grooming activities become more difficult to manage.

    ▪ There is evidence of decreased upper- and lower-extremity mobility or there is a greater propensity for falling.

    ▪ There is evidence of pain or generalized discomfort.

    A discussion with family members or the responsible party is warranted to validate changing needs and to modify or adjust the care plan. Above all, be an active part of the team!

7. *Pursue ongoing training.* General orientation to dementia care is not enough when working with persons with advanced dementia. Although many of the fundamental dementia care principles apply, readiness to take on new challenges in the advanced stages of dementia requires additional knowledge and perhaps new or refined approaches to care. Continue to update yourself on the principles and practices of advanced dementia care at your place of employment, from books, journals, and other educational resources.

8. *Take care of yourself.* Professional caregivers often experience the same types of grief or frustrations that family members do. Taking care of oneself physically, mentally, and spiritually may sound trite, but it is not. Caregivers may become dissatisfied with their jobs and experience burnout if opportunities are not available to process their experiences, especially the deaths of long-time facility residents or aggravating factors in the work setting. Some examples of administrative assistance include active problem solving at the unit level, caregiver debriefing and bereavement support, recognition of professional caregivers that provide exemplary care, and innovative educational programming. Joint personal and management efforts to sustain positive advanced dementia programming require supportive care of and for the professional caregivers.

Tips for Professional Caregivers in the Hospital: Caring for Persons With Advanced Dementia

Professional caregivers can do several things to help ensure the best possible care for the persons with advanced dementia who are hospitalized. The following section lists the interventions for best outcomes when caring for a person with advanced dementia in an acute care setting.

1. *Make sure that all shifts of hospital staff know that the person has dementia,* including the etiology and stage of the dementing illness. This should include physicians, anesthesiologists, nurses, aides, housekeepers, respiratory therapists, physical therapists, dietitians, clergy, and even housekeepers.

2. *Encourage the family to provide an extra layer of supervision* and interpretation for the person with advanced dementia. In the emergency department (ED), and if admitted to the hospital, encourage family to stay with the person as much as possible. Provide for family to sleep in the room. Encourage family to rotate visitation responsibilities so the burden is not on one person, if possible. Keep the family informed as to when tests are being done so someone can accompany the person to these tests. The family caregiver provides familiarity, continuity, and reassurance during the times when the person with advanced dementia is most likely to be confused.

3. *Do not leave the person with advanced dementia alone or out of sight.* Organize all hospital staff to rotate duties so someone is around as much as possible. Although a person with advanced dementia does better with quiet, it may be helpful to have the person's room near the nurses' station. Persons with advanced dementia are unable to use call lights. They are also unable to inhibit behavior, so they are at high risk for falls, elopement, injury on equipment and side rails, and removal of IVs and tubes.

4. *Be careful in giving false reassurances to the family.* Review the disease process of advanced dementia and support the family in understanding this serious diagnosis. Ask for support from a palliative care team if your hospital has one.

5. *Develop an open relationship with families* so they feel free to ask questions and participate in the care as much as possible. They have been caring for their loved one for some time and they know what things will agitate or comfort them.

6. *Strive for quiet, calm, and continuity in the person's room* as much as possible. Ask the family to bring the person's robe and pillow from home to ensure continuity. Keep the television off when the person is in the room. If possible, use a private room. Limit visitors to only those who visit the person at home on a regular basis. If family members are coming from a distance, have them make multiple small visits instead of staying in the room for hours. Potentially-confusing pictures of people or animals should be taken down if they are within the person's line of sight. Ask physicians to hold rounds outside the room and keep phones and pagers on vibrate. Minimize equipment

noise while the person with advanced dementia is in the room, including floor polishers and other machinery. Provide continuity of staff whenever possible and give the staff directions on how to communicate with the person with advanced dementia.

7. *Ensure that basic care needs are addressed.* Advocate for regularly-scheduled pain medication because the person with advanced dementia is unable to ask for pain medication. Whenever possible, use a pain rating scale that is for persons with dementia (see chapter 7). Closely monitor bowel and bladder function, as this can further complicate the individual's medical progress. Assist during meals relative to the individual's dietary needs and abilities. If there are religious or faith convictions about diet or other rituals, be sure that the dietary department, chaplain, and other staff members know this at the time of admission and throughout the stay.

8. *Determine what kind of bathing is best for this person* (e.g., bed bath, bag bath, towel bath) by asking the family. Showers usually cause increased agitation.

9. *Determine what time of day is best for tests and higher-stimulation activities.* Advocate to the physician to discuss diagnostic tests with family to determine their plan of care based on the individual's desires.

10. *Make sure that copies of all advance directives are in the medical record,* including the Medical Healthcare Power of Attorney, living will, and guardianship papers.

11. *Start planning the discharge as soon as the person with advanced dementia is admitted.* Collaborate with the social worker, therapists, and family to provide optimum care for the individual. Assume that persons with advanced dementia will be less able to function and more confused at discharge than they were before admission. At the very minimum, family caregivers will need more in-home help, perhaps for a minimum of 1 week after discharge. If a person with advanced dementia requires nursing home placement for a rehabilitative (skilled) or restorative stay, have the family visit a couple of facilities and ask questions about the facility's ability to care for persons with advanced dementia.

12. *Post a simple biography* or life story of the person at the bedside so that care providers will know more about the person. Referring to familiar topics can help distract or engage him or her, if necessary.

ASSISTANCE FOR FAMILY CAREGIVERS

Family members typically play a major role in caregiving. Whether assuming full hands-on responsibility in the home setting or being an active participant within community-based facilities, families continue to provide caregiving to their loved ones. Even more than professional caregivers, families often require assistance and guidance in their caregiving journey. Community-based or facility caregiving staff may wish to share the following guidelines with family members as they embark on or continue with their caregiving activities.

Tips for Family Caregivers in Healthcare Facilities and Agencies: Caring for Persons With Advanced Dementia

Family caregivers can do several things to help ensure the best possible care for their family members who have advanced dementia and for themselves. The following section lists the interventions for best outcomes for you and your family member.

1. *Take care of yourself.* It is important to remember to take care of yourself, as you are caring for someone else. The care you are able to provide clearly depends on how well you are feeling. It can be stressful to provide care to someone who is ill. Stay current with your own physician visits, dental and vision care, and all other ways necessary to maintain health. Eat well, drink plenty of fluids, and rest as much as you are able. Do not neglect your own personal hygiene. Stay connected to your religious or faith community—they will be needed to support you as the illness progresses and after your family member dies. Each day, give yourself permission for yourself; whether that is a 5-minute break for meditation or a special coffee blend you buy yourself at the local store. It is easy to be consumed in caring for your loved one at your own personal expense. Ask for help when you need it, but above all, take care of yourself.

2. *Get plenty of rest.* When the person you are caring for rests, give yourself a break—either rest at the same time or do something just for you. Whether your loved one is still at home or is now in a facility, being a caregiver can be tiring. To continue to provide care, you must rest and take breaks. Take time for yourself to do something you enjoy. Instead of saying, "If I only had time," make the time to get a massage, get a manicure, golf, read a book without disturbance, take a nap, or go to church. Remember that you cannot be there for the person if you are not there for yourself.

3. *Recognize your limits—accept help when needed.* In order to care for someone, you need to stay well physically and emotionally. No one has superhero qualities, so know when to say when. Family, friends, and neighbors may *offer* help. Let them. Keep a list of all errands, food, chores, and appointments. When people ask how they can help, you will be able to suggest specific actions that may be beneficial. When you need help, *ask* for it. Asking early before you need it can help you avoid burnout later. Remember that all the people in your life can be players on your caregiving team—you can seek comfort from family, friends, support groups, religious affiliations, and more.

   At some point, caregiving for a loved one at home can become too demanding for one person to handle. Think about how many professional caregivers it takes to provide care for the residents in an assisted-living home, around the clock, in just 1 week's time! Consider additional help in the home. Recognize that placement in a facility is something that may need to happen at some point. Think about the need for respite care. Call your local Alzheimer's Association chapter for assistance, or connect with a geriatric care manager or social worker through the regional Area Agency on Aging or private service agency to help you and your family work through this process, as it can be very overwhelming.

If your loved one is already in a facility, you may still need some extra physical or emotional assistance. Traveling back and forth to a facility can be demanding. You may feel guilty if you do not see your loved one on some regular schedule. You may neglect your own needs so that you can be at the facility. Recognizing your limits and seeking out resources to help you with these caregiving demands are important in maintaining your own health and stamina.

4. *Maintain consistency.* Keep it simple. Maintain routines each day at home whenever possible to ease your caregiving stressors. Do things in the same way each day. Routine schedules are comforting for both the person receiving care and for the person providing the care. An idea that may be helpful is to write down exactly what you are doing to provide care in a 24-hour period. That way, if someone offers help or if you need to take a day off, the daily schedule is already outlined. Always have a "Plan B" in case situations change or a crisis develops.

If your loved one is in a facility, a daily or weekly routine is a good idea. Continuity and routines give some level of comfort and predictability to the person with advanced dementia. Be sure to budget in rest periods and time for yourself.

5. *Attend to meals.* Prepare a menu for a week in advance. If your meals are different from the person for whom you are providing care, have a separate menu planned for you. Having a menu will help you be more time efficient while preparing the meals and in keeping up with the grocery list. Do not forget to pay attention to your own nutritional needs. Even if the person for whom you are caring eats poorly, you need to eat healthy meals to keep your strength.

For those caregivers who have their family members in assisted-living or skilled nursing facilities, inquire if you can purchase a meal to eat during your visit. This allows opportunity to be with your family member and to have a prepared, well-balanced meal as well.

6. *Keep records and partner with your primary care provider.* Days are often alike and remembering everything can be difficult. Write down the things you need to remember such as medical appointments, prescription refills, or concerns such as decreased eating or a fall. Write down questions and ask the office nurse or the primary care provider to address them. You do not need to wait until the next scheduled appointment, home, or facility visit to ask your question. Get in contact with your primary care provider's office or answering service—the staff can ask the medical care provider your question for you. You should get an answer back usually within 24–48 hours. This will assist you with time management, as all concerns are addressed as they occur.

Creating a partnership with your medical provider and good communication with your doctor are very important and often take time and effort. Together with the family, the primary care provider should develop a reasonable plan for meeting the needs of the person with advanced dementia. Over time, these needs will change. Regular doctor visits at the office, your home, or facility setting (about every 6 months or right away if a sudden change occurs) will help you and your family get the best care. Care provided by everyone working together will best serve the needs of the person with advanced dementia.

If you have not completed advance directives for you or your family member with dementia, this is the time to do it. If these decisions have not been made already, it may be necessary to secure legal advice on how to ensure that an individual's wishes are protected. Be sure to include the appropriate family members or significant others in these discussions. If these decisions have been made already, make sure that your primary care provider and other healthcare providers, such as a long-term care facility, have a copy of the advance directives. Be sure that all family members and healthcare decision makers are aware of the advance directives for you and your loved one.

If your family member resides in an assisted-living or long-term care facility, make every effort to attend the quarterly care conferences. If you have noticed that your loved one is having increased problems, immediately bring it to the attention of the facility staff or your primary care provider. You are considered an integral part of the interdisciplinary team; your participation is vital in developing and executing a care plan that meets the needs of your loved one.

7. *Know the medications.* Keep a current list of medications available, whether the person is at home or in a facility. If possible, secure information on the dose, schedule, and purpose of each medication. When there is a new primary care provider, a new pharmacy, or a hospital admission, the list will be extremely helpful. Do this for both the person you are caring for and for yourself. If you are at home, check all prescription containers weekly, making sure prescriptions are filled before the medication runs out. Think ahead and plan accordingly, taking into account weekends and holiday schedules.

8. *Access resources in the community.* Use respite or in-home care services for extra help. You or the person you are caring for may be eligible for additional assistance from various community resources. Some resources include home delivered meals and home health aid workers who can assist with bathing and other care. Ask the physician's office if home health care or if hospice care can be considered, as each service provides in-home care and is covered by insurance. Your family member may receive registered nurse visits in the home, a certified nursing assistant to assist with bathing and dressing, and a social worker to contact community resources to see what is available to provide extra help, often at no additional cost, for your loved one and for yourself.

Know your community resources and ask yourself these important questions: What is available in the area? Does the facility you are considering have any complaints on file with the local Department of Health Services? Financial issues and resources for assistance also need to be explored during the caregiving journey. Contact your local Alzheimer's Association chapter, Area Agency on Aging, or health department for help—they can be of assistance providing guidance related to caregiving issues, finding long-term care placement, or for seeking out additional resources.

If your family member is in a facility, identify and access resources that are available within the facility, such as a social worker, to help with any of your caregiving needs. Counseling and support or help with financial matters may be needed. Depending on the type of facility and your family member's needs, you may be able to benefit from additional professional assistance in the facility, such as from a hospice. Explore these options with your primary care provider or facility professional resources.

9. *Enhance the connections.* As your family member has more difficulty in verbally expressing himself or herself, it is important that you focus on the development of new communication skills. You will need to learn to anticipate problems or difficult behaviors before they happen. Establish meaningful connections through activities. Accommodate the environment so that it is safe yet provides a sense of comfort and security. Whether you are at home or in a facility, adaptations and new approaches to the increasing care needs of the person with advanced dementia will be necessary.

   These approaches may help in making visits to the facility less disturbing and more meaningful for both of you:
   - Think of the visit as a shared experience—how both of you can achieve improved sensory awareness and connections during this time.
   - Think of four or five simple ways to establish a connection, such as themed visits or through the use of music, photos, or by holding hands and the sense of touch. Bring items to the visit that will awaken the senses.
   - Come to the visit free of expectations of how your loved one will respond.

   It also can be helpful for you to have meaningful connections with your loved one through spiritual experiences and activities. This includes prayer (a chance to say familiar words), scripture reading (a chance to hear encouraging and hopeful words), hymns and spiritual songs (a chance to sing and/or hear familiar songs), and pastoral presence (a chance to sit with the chaplain, clergy, or faith representative).

   Use the expertise of healthcare professionals in the community or the facility to give you new or modified activities and approaches to care that can enhance meaningful connections with your loved one.

10. *Secure additional education and support.* Attend a support group and an educational program. Support groups are valuable venues that provide a forum to help you identify your strengths as a caregiver, to share feelings, concerns, and information, and in supporting and encouraging each other. Knowing there are other individuals out there experiencing some of the same things you are experiencing can be a comfort and a relief. Support groups also afford the opportunity to learn about creative caregiving strategies and tools for making your caregiving experience less stressful. For those who cannot attend a support group, find a friend or confidant who can listen. There are other opportunities for sharing and support. Using Internet chat rooms and the variety of materials on authoritative Web sites, caregivers can improve their understanding while coping with the effects of dementia on their lives.

   Your own spiritual support should not be neglected. Individual prayer, prayer groups, meditation, and individual pastoral counseling may be supportive, comforting, and life affirming for both of you. Many healthcare facilities can assist families and their own staff in the caregiving journey to meet the comfort and quality of life needs for persons with advanced dementia. The opportunity exists to give meaningful and positive experiences for all caregivers providing palliative care to persons with advanced dementia.

Tips for Family Caregivers in the Hospital: Caring for Persons With Advanced Dementia

Family members can do several things to help ensure the best possible care for their family member who has advanced dementia and is hospitalized. The following section lists the interventions for best outcomes if hospitalization occurs.

1. *Do not expect dementia-capable care.* Most hospital staffs are not trained in dementia care. Encourage the nurses or other healthcare personnel at the bedside to get help from their supervisors if they are unfamiliar with advanced dementia. Bring in the person's life story from home or the facility and share it with hospital staff. Also post it at the bedside.

2. *Stay with the person as much as possible.* In the ED, the person with advanced dementia must have family or staff from the residential facility present in the examination with them at all times. Generally, the ED staff does not stay with any persons continuously. The potential for falls, wandering away, and other accidents is great without family present. The ED staff will not have information regarding the person's level of function, confusion, and potential for injury. Moreover, the caregiver must be able to provide the history of the emergency, other medical conditions, and the person's usual baseline function.

3. *Once admitted, the family should visit during critical times,* including during diagnostic tests, therapies, during meals, and in the evening throughout the hospitalization. Rotate visitation responsibilities so the burden is not on one person. If possible, have someone spend the night in the room, again rotating this responsibility. Discuss with the nursing staff as to when tests are being done so someone can accompany the person to these tests. The family provides an extra layer of supervision and interpretation for the person with advanced dementia. The caregiver provides familiarity, continuity, and reassurance during times when the person with advanced dementia is most likely to be confused.

4. *Do not hesitate to ask for help.* As family, you are your loved one's main advocate. Decide who will be the main spokesperson for your loved one. Write down the comments from the different physicians treating your loved one so you can keep them straight and report to other family members. Ask the nursing staff to try to keep the same staff taking care of your loved one as much as possible to avoid continuous new people.

5. *Strive for quiet, calm, and continuity in the person's room.* Bring the person's robe and pillow from home to assure continuity. The television should be off whenever the person is in the room. Limit visitors to only those who visit the person

at home on a regular basis. If family members are coming from a distance, have them make multiple small visits instead of staying in the room for hours.

6. *Report any changes in behavior* to the nursing staff, especially if you think your loved one might be in pain.

7. *Discuss with the physician what tests are necessary based on your loved one's advance directives.*

8. *Be aware of safety.* Persons with advanced dementia are unable to consider safety for themselves and are unable to inhibit behavior, thus they are at high risk for falls, elopement, injury on equipment and side rails, and removal of IVs and tubes. These mandate constant supervision. Family should be in the room of their loved one because he or she may be unable to ask for help.

9. *Make sure copies of all advance directives are brought to the hospital,* including the Medical Health Care Power of Attorney, living will, and guardianship papers. Discuss these documents with the primary attending physician.

10. *Discharge planning will start soon after your loved one is admitted.* Nursing staff will coordinate with the social worker, therapists, case managers, physicians, and family to determine where and when your loved one will be discharged. Family may need to visit long-term care facilities to determine which location will be best for the person. Ask questions regarding the ability to care for people with advanced dementia, what kind of provider support they have, and how family plays a part in the person's care. It is always best for facilities to collaborate with the family for optimum care and outcomes.

11. *Above all, continue to advocate for your loved one based on his or her wishes for care.* Continue to ask questions if you are confused or unclear regarding treatment or care issues. You and your loved one are the customers. You have a right to understand and to be understood.

CONCLUSION

Caregiving is a 24 hours a day, 7 days a week commitment. The caregiving journey for persons with advanced dementia may start at home or in a facility that provides supportive assistance. It is often difficult to navigate the complex healthcare system to determine the best setting, arrangements, and financial support for getting care in the advanced stages of the disease. Professional and family caregivers require education, support, and intervention strategies to help through this maze and ease the burden and stress of caregiving.

Although caregiving experiences vary from person to person and situation to situation, there are general issues that apply to almost everyone across the board. In this chapter, we outlined practical strategies for professional caregivers who work in healthcare facilities and agencies, as well as for those who work in hospitals, to use in providing care for persons with advanced dementia. We also listed strategies for families to use when their loved ones are residents of those facilities. Our goal was to help make life easier for professional and family caregivers alike and to help improve the quality of care and the quality of life for the individuals with advanced dementia for whom they care.

EXHIBIT 3.1

Standards of Care for Caregiving

A. The healthcare facility shall:
1. Develop policies and procedures to help family caregivers understand the trajectory of the dementia, common healthcare decisions, and common caregiving strategies for persons with advanced dementia.
2. Offer caregiving resources for families, such as the accompanying tip sheets, that enhance family caregiving for persons with advanced dementia.
3. Develop programming and resources for professional caregivers, such as the accompanying tip sheets, that will assist staff in providing dementia-specific supportive care for persons with advanced dementia and the family caregivers.
4. Develop and solidify interdisciplinary teams within healthcare facilities and agencies that support advanced dementia care practices.
5. Provide opportunities for additional education and support for families and professional caregivers of persons with advanced dementia.

B. Healthcare staff shall:
1. Actively incorporate family caregiving strategies into the care plans of persons with advanced dementia. This may include:
   a. Regular face-to-face meetings with family members;
   b. Ongoing education for family members, such as on helpful caregiving strategies; and
   c. An initial and ongoing assessment of the family's grief and loss with specific targeted interventions.
2. Attend orientation and continuing education activities that identify caregiving strategies and best practices of care for persons with advanced dementia.
3. Identify and make referrals to professional and supportive healthcare personnel and resources to assist the person with advanced dementia.
   a. Spiritual or religious supportive care
   b. Social services and financial counseling
   c. Access to other community resources

C. Persons with advanced dementia shall expect:
1. Supportive caregiving that affirms quality of life in all aspects, including physiological, psychological, social, and spiritual quality of life.
2. Their previously stipulated healthcare decisions are respected and honored.

▓ REFERENCES

AARP Public Policy Institute. (2007). *Valuing the invaluable: A new look at the economic value of family caregiving.* Retrieved January 23, 2010, from http://www.thefamilycaregiver.org/pdfs/NewLookattheEconomicValueofFamilyCaregivingIssueBrief.pdf

Ahronheim, J. C., Morrison, R. S., Morris, J., Baskin, S., & Meier, D. E. (2000). Palliative care in advanced dementia: A randomized controlled trial and descriptive analysis. *Journal of Palliative Medicine, 3*(3), 265–273.

Albert, S. M., Costa, R., Merchant, C., Small, S., Jenders, R. A., & Stern Y. (1999). Hospitalization and Alzheimer's disease: Results from a community-based study. *Journals of Gerontology Series A-Biological Sciences and Medical Sciences, 54*(5), M267–M271.

Alzheimer's Association. (2003). *Partnering with your doctor: A guide for persons with memory problems and their partners.* Retrieved January 23, 2010, from http://www.alz.org/national/documents/brochure_partneringwithyourdoctor.pdf

Alzheimer's Association. (2007). *Respite care guide.* Retrieved January 23, 2010, from http://www.alz.org/national/documents/brochure_respitecareguide.pdf

Alzheimer's Association. (2009). *Alzheimer's facts and figures (full report).* Retrieved January 23, 2010, from http://www.alz.org/alzheimers_disease_facts_figures.asp

Alzheimer's Association. (2009, March). *2009 Alzheimer's disease facts and figures (topic sheet).* Retrieved January 23, 2010, from http://www.alz.org/national/documents/ topicsheet_2009_facts_figures.pdf

Alzheimer's Association & National Alliance for Caregiving. (2004). *Families care. Alzheimer's caregiving in the US 2004.* Retrieved January 23, 2010, from http://www.alz.org/national/documents/report_familiescare.pdf

Andrieu, S., Reynish, E., Nourhashemi, F., Shakespeare, A., Moulias, S., Ousset, P. J., et al. (2002). Predictive factors of acute hospitalization in 134 patients with Alzheimer's disease: A one year prospective study. *International Journal of Geriatric Psychiatry, 17*(5), 422–426.

Balardy, L., Voisin, T., Cantet, C., Vellas, B., & REAL.FR Group. (2005). Predictive factors of emergency hospitalization in Alzheimer's patients: Results of one-year follow-up in the REAL.FR Cohort. *Journal of Nutrition, Health & Aging, 9*(2), 112–116.

Berg, L. (1988). Clinical dementia rating. *Psychopharmacology Bulletin, 24,* 637–639.

Bonsignore, M., & Heun R. (2003). Mortality in Alzheimer's disease. *Dementia & Geriatric Cognitive Disorders, 15*(4), 231–236.

Boss, P., Caron, W., Horbal, J., & Mortimer, J. (1990). Predictors of depression in caregivers of dementia patients: Boundary ambiguity and mastery. *Family Process, 29*(3), 245–254.

Cangelosi, P. R. (2009). Caregiver burden or caregiver gain? Respite for family caregivers. *Journal of Psychosocial Nursing, 47*(9), 19–22.

Cortes, F., Gillette-Guyonnet, S., Nourhashemi, F., Andrieu, S., Cantet, C., Vellas, B., et al. (2005). Recent data on the natural history of Alzheimer's disease: Results from the REAL.FR Study. *Journal of Nutrition, Health & Aging, 9*(2), 86–93.

Day, N., Musallam, K., & Wells, M. (1999). Observed behaviors of patients with probable Alzheimer's disease who are hospitalized for diagnostic tests. *Journal of Gerontological Nursing, 25*(11), 35–39.

Fillenbaum, G., Heyman, A., Peterson, B., Pieper, C. F., & Weiman, A. L. (2000). Frequency and duration of hospitalization of patients with AD based on Medicare data: CERAD XX. *Neurology, 54*(3), 740–743.

Fillenbaum, G., Heyman, A., Peterson, B. L., Pieper, C. F., & Weiman, A. L. (2001). Use and cost of hospitalization of patients with AD by stage and living arrangement: CERAD XXI. *Neurology, 56*(2), 201–206.

Freyne, A., Kidd, N., Coen, R., & Lawlor, B. A. (1999). Burden in carers of dementia patients: Higher levels in carers of younger sufferers. *International Journal of Geriatric Psychiatry, 14*(9), 784–788.

Kovach, C. R., Wilson, S. A., & Noonan, P. E. (1996). The effects of hospice interventions on behaviors, discomfort, and physical complications of end-stage dementia nursing home residents. *American Journal of Alzheimer's Disease, 11*(4), 7–10.

Leibson, C., Owens, T., O'Brien, P., Waring, S., Tangalos, E., Hanson, V., et al. (1999). Use of physician and acute care services by persons with and without Alzheimer's disease: A population-based comparison. *Journal of the American Geriatrics Society, 47*(7), 864–869.

Long, C. O. (2004). Community-based nursing and home care. In S. M. Lewis, M. M. Heitkemper, & S. R. Dirksen (Eds.), *Medical-surgical nursing. Assessment and management of clinical problems* (6th ed.). St. Louis, MO: Mosby.

Lucero, M. (2004). Enhancing the visits of loved ones of people in late-stage dementia. *Alzheimer's Care Quarterly, 5*(2), 173–177.

Luscombe, G., Brodaty, H., & Freeth, S. (1998). Younger people with dementia: Diagnostic issues, effects on carers and use of services. *International Journal of Geriatric Psychiatry, 13*(5), 323–330.

Mack, K., & Thompson, L. (2004). *A decade of informal caregiving: Are today's informal caregivers different than informal caregivers a decade ago?* Caregivers of Older Persons Data Profile. Washington, DC: Center on an Aging Society. Retrieved January 23, 2010, from http://ihcrp. georgetown.edu/agingsociety/ pubhtml/ caregiver1/ caregiver1.html

National Family Caregiver Association. (2005). *Common bonds of caregiving.* Retrieved January 23, 2010, from http://www.thefamilycaregiver.org/who_are_family_caregivers/common_bonds_of_caregiving.cfm

Phillips, L., Brusac, K., & Guo, G. (2005). Prevalence of Alzheimer's disease in Arizona: Future projections and implications. *Arizona Geriatrics Society Journal, 10*(2), 19–24.

Rabow, M. W., Hauser, J. M., & Adams, J. (2004). Supporting family caregivers at the end of life. "They don't know what they don't know." *The Journal of the American Medical Association, 291*(4), 483–491.

Schulz, R., & Beach, S. (1999). Caregiving as a risk factor for mortality. *Journal of the American Medical Association, 282*(23), 2215–2219.

Schulz, R., Belle, S. H., Czaja, S. J., McGinnis, K. A., Stevens, A., & Zhang, S. (2004). Long-term care placement of dementia patients and caregiver health and well-being. *The Journal of the American Medical Association, 292*(8), 961–967.

Schulz, R., & Sherwood, P. R. (2008). Physical and mental health effects of family caregiving. *American Journal of Nursing, 108*(9), 23–27.

Smith, G. E., Kokmen, E., O'Brien, P. C. (2000). Risk factors for nursing home placement in a population-based dementia cohort. *Journal of the American Geriatric Society, 48*(5), 519–525.

Wasow, M., & Coons, D. (1987). Widows and widowers of Alzheimer's victims: Their survival after spouses' death. *Journal of Independent Social Work, 2*(2), 21–23.

PROTECTING DIGNITY FOR THE PATIENT WITH DEMENTIA: ESTABLISHING AN ENVIRONMENT AND CAREGIVING STANDARDS

4

PERSONHOOD

Gary A. Martin, Judith Sgrillo, and Antonia Horton

▦ INTRODUCTION

In the broad and diverse field of dementia care, the 1990s hallmarked the introduction of the notion of "personhood" into the field. Led by Tom Kitwood, a social psychologist and gerontology professor at the University of Bradford in England, the concept of personhood and its tenets was applied to persons with dementia in an aggressive and eye-opening reconsideration of how dementia care should be conceptualized and practiced. This new direction emphasized a more humane and deeply empathic approach to dementia care by recognizing the person with dementia as an intrinsically valuable individual who deserves the full respect and dignity that all human beings share. Whereas in the past, persons with dementia were often defined by their disease or disabilities, Kitwood championed a new approach to dementia care called *person-centered care* that emphasized the uniqueness of individuals by listening to what they had to say and honoring their feelings. Before the 1990s, there was a one-size-fits-all mentality when it came to dementia and dementia care; in person-centered care, the focus changed so that each person was viewed as an individual, and the concept of personhood was the embodiment of this philosophy.

Even so, the notion of personhood is difficult to define, mostly because it is such a broad, holistic, and intangible construct. In simple terms, it means to be human—that we are all unique individuals with inestimable and irreplaceable worth, each having his or her own sets of needs, rights, values, and responsibilities. Every person is considered important and to have a singular status among others. No one is dispensable or interchangeable. Moreover, personhood carries with it an inviolable dignity that merits unconditional respect and, on the deepest level, all members of the human species share this dignity. Personhood is considered the essence of being human and is inextricably tied to the individual's sense of dignity and self-worth, as well as his or her place and standing within a social world.

In considering the concept of personhood, philosophers might emphasize the notions of free will and self-determination. Each individual has a conscious self-presence and a unique sense of efficacy, and is freely creative in his or her perceptions, attributions, and actions. There is an inherent value of the person as someone, rather than as something. In this regard, personhood constitutes the fundamental notion of that which gives meaning to all reality and constitutes its supreme value.

On the other hand, psychologists might look at personhood from a different perspective. They would say that personhood relates to the status and integrity of a person's sense of self-esteem, self-worth, and self-identity, and that maintaining an integrated sense of self requires that the individual receives recognition, respect, and trust from others within a social environment. From this perspective, personhood is viewed as a social phenomenon whereby an individual's sense of self is intimately linked to his or her social relationships—our perceptions of the feelings and actions of others toward us greatly influence, if not define, our sense of self and personhood.

Without digging any deeper into the philosophical and psychological underpinnings of personhood (where we all could most certainly drown in intellectual quicksand), Kitwood's conceptualization contained two critical points that relate to the personhood of persons with dementia. First, personhood is based in each individual's unique sense of self and the dignity and integrity that emanates from the self; and second, that personhood is defined and maintained only within a social context and is dependent on one's interactions with others.

▌ DEMENTIA AND PERSONHOOD

Dementia is a condition that is characterized by personal losses. Over time, people with chronic progressive dementias such as Alzheimer's disease will gradually lose the intellectual and functional skills that make them who they are. Their personalities will change, their memories will fade, their communication and social skills will break down, and they will become increasingly dependent on others.

The losses are enormous by the time they move to a long-term care setting, which, according to national statistics, will happen at some point in 9 out of 10 cases. As with most long-term care residents, they will lose their homes and most of their possessions, as well as their jobs, cars, mobility, independence, and sense of purpose. Close friends will be lost and family members may grow distant. Even when moving into the best of long-term care facilities, and under the best of circumstances, the losses that are incurred and the adjustments that must be made are huge.

However, it is the dementia that will cause the most devastation. By the time people reach the middle or moderate stages of their dementia, they are no longer able to engage in most lifelong hobbies and favorite activities (e.g., poets will no longer be able to write poems, tennis players will no longer be able to play tennis, gardeners will no longer be able to garden). Memory decline will be disorienting, eventually to the point where every place feels unfamiliar and every person is a stranger. Spouses and children may no longer be recognized, and they may come to the point of not knowing their own names. Skills will be lost, histories will be erased, and identities will disappear.

Moreover, throughout this slow-motion onslaught to one's sense of self, what happens to our personhood? What happens to our dignity, free will, and values? If we do not know where we are, how we got here, or even who we are, how are we to maintain our self-esteem, our sense of identity, or our self-worth? Does memory not presuppose identity? Does personhood not require some sense of who we are and how we fit into this world?

Moreover, what about our relations with others? Personhood requires a social context within which our sense of self is dependent on our perceptions of how people feel about us, including and especially our sense of respect for each other. If that is true, what happens to personhood when a person's communication and social skills deteriorate while friends and family disappear? And how does the notion of social dependence translate into a caregiving relationship where virtually all human contact is based on some stranger (after all, everyone is a stranger when you have no memory) assisting us with basic care needs.

The point here is that dementia is an assault on personhood. It not only robs individuals of their memories, it also robs them of their sense of who they are and how they fit into this world—their sense of self. Moreover, as the dementia progresses, the threats to one's personhood become even greater. By the time individuals reach the advanced stages of their dementia, there is little left of who they once were. They are severely confused, cannot control their own bodily functions, can no longer walk independently, have lost their language skills, and have become totally dependent on caregivers for all their needs.

In this light, it could be argued that the most important challenge for caregivers of persons with dementia is to help maintain and enhance their personhood despite all the losses and changes that they are and will be experiencing. This is no easy challenge given the broadscale ravages of dementia on the person, and the challenge grows greater and greater as the person descends further into the depths of the more advanced stages of his or her dementia.

There is a silver lining to the assault that dementia makes on personhood. Caregivers do have considerable impact and, with proper training and focus, can help maintain or strengthen an individual's sense of self and personhood. After all, one of the main tenets of personhood is that it is defined and maintained within a social context and is dependent on one's interactions with others. For persons with advanced dementia, the caregiving relationship *is* their most relevant social context, and the interactions they have with caregivers are one of the defining factors in maintaining their personhood. The personal and social identity of persons with dementia arises out of what is said and done by their caregivers depending, of course, on the sense of respect, dignity, compassion, and humanity that caregivers bring to the caregiving situation. Caregivers have the power to make a difference, and the quality of their interactions can determine whether the individual's personhood is enhanced or destroyed.

PERSON-CENTERED CARE AND ADVANCED DEMENTIA

Person-Centered Care

Kitwood's model of person-centered care was originally conceptualized as a philosophy and practice of care specifically for people with dementia but, over the years, has gained widespread international acceptance as a standard of care for all populations that are in care situations. The central premise of person-centered care is that the person being cared for is the center of all actions and decisions—this is in sharp contrast to more medically based models of care in which the facilities and/or the caregivers are the focal point of all decisions and actions.

In the person-centered care model, dementia care is focused on the whole person, not just on his or her diagnosis or symptoms, with emphasis on strengths and abilities rather than weaknesses and disabilities. This model of care strives to take into account each individual's life experiences, unique personality, and network of relationships within the context of his or her gender, ethnicity, family, and culture. As much as possible, efforts are made to identify and accommodate each individual's emotional needs and personal preferences. The care setting itself is designed to continually maintain a positive and supportive social environment, and caregiving assignments are based on building meaningful relationships rather than for staff convenience or speed and efficiency.

Although there is an impressive body of literature and research on person-centered care, very little has been written on applying it to the population with advanced dementia. This may be because it is assumed that the philosophy and practice of person-centered care is the same from one population to another or, more specifically, from one stage of dementia to the next. Moreover, there certainly is some truth to that assumption—after all, according to the model, every person has a right to dignity and deserves respect regardless of age, gender, race, culture, or diagnosis. On the other hand, the application of the person-centered model to the population with advanced dementia requires special consideration because of the unique challenges posed by persons with advanced dementia:

- Language deficits are so severe that persons with advanced dementia are severely impaired in the ability to verbalize their feelings, needs, or preferences.
- Cognition is severely impaired, including several areas of cognition that are highly relevant to the person-centered care model, including judgment, reasoning, insight, and orientation.
- Loss of social skills and social awareness, as well as major changes in the social environment (i.e., living in a care setting with other severely impaired persons with advanced dementia).
- Functional abilities are impaired to the point of not being able to participate in many traditional activities, including basic caregiving, to the extent where there is a massive loss of independence, control, and free will.

For a dementia program to be truly person-centered, these challenges must be recognized, addressed, and overcome. In particular, management and staff must have policies and practices in place that seek to better recognize and understand persons with advanced dementia. They must gather historical information, talk to family and friends, use trial-and-error strategies, and document and share what they learn so that others can use and continue to expand this knowledge base to better serve the resident. Most importantly, caregivers need to learn how the person with advanced dementia uniquely communicates in nonverbal ways, including through behaviors (see chapter 6 on behaviors). Caregivers must know well the individuals for whom they care to successfully implement the tenets of the person-centered care model.

It is worth noting that, more recently, we have seen the advent of an even more aggressive person-focused approach to person-centered care called *person-directed care*. This updated version of Kitwood's model gives long-term care residents active control over their care, allowing them to individually direct the way their care is given and how their needs are met. Residents living in this model determine what, where, and when they eat, have a custom-tailored menu of preferred activities available to them 24 hours a day, and have virtually any sort of assistance available to them on demand. The goal is to completely deinstitutionalize institutional living by allowing residents to have as much free will and control as they did when they were healthy and independent. Although this model sounds highly attractive to persons who do not have dementia, applying it to the population with advanced dementia requires a deep and intimate knowledge of the individual, including his or her personality characteristic, communication patterns, values, and preferences— an enormous challenge that may not be entirely possible.

Caregiving

Person-centered care is a comprehensive, holistic, and multifaceted model of care where all aspects of care are examined and translated into a context that strives to maintain the personhood of those who live and work within that model. No single element or discipline within that model is more important or potent than the hands-on caregivers—it is the caregivers who have the power to make or break the personhood of those persons for whom they provide care. Their approaches, skills, values, demeanor, and priorities greatly affect the quality of their care as well as the sense of respect, dignity, and self-identity experienced by persons with advanced dementia.

For persons with dementia, the focus is always comfort. We teach a "soft" approach that emphasizes a warm, friendly, and respectful approach to care. Equally important are the caregiving skills and techniques caregivers bring to the caregiving situation. Caregiving for persons with advanced dementia is *not* intuitive. It does not come naturally and requires caregivers to have special training for them to do it correctly and humanely. Throughout the chapters of this book, we describe highly effective caregiving techniques available to caregivers that are specifically designed for persons with advanced dementia, including in areas of intake and nutrition (see chapter 9), bathing (see chapter 13), and pain management (see chapter 7), among others. These techniques universally focus on comfort (i.e., helping the person stay comfortable while getting the job done), and without these skills caregivers are much more likely to violate an individual's sense of trust, dignity, respect, and well-being. For it to be effective, the person-centered care model demands that caregivers be trained and skilled in delivering comfort-based care specifically geared to persons with advanced dementia.

To maintain a person-centered model of care for a population with advanced dementia, caregivers must really know the person for whom they care (see chapters 3 and 6). This requires spending significant amounts of quality time with persons with advanced dementia—getting to know their personalities, their emotional responses to various stimuli, the nonverbal nuances of their communication patterns, their likes and dislikes, and their comfort levels. This cannot be overstated—only through knowing and understanding their residents can caregivers effectively maintain their residents' personhoods and meet the goals of the person-centered care model for persons with advanced dementia.

When training caregivers in advanced-dementia care, we emphasize a very basic principle that is virtually universal in its application: figure out what the person with advanced dementia likes then do it over and over again. This principle applies to meals and snacks, activities, bathing, and other activities of daily living (ADL)-specific approaches, pain management, and virtually all other aspects of caregiving. This requires that caregivers institute a trial-and-error mentality to caregiving, determining what the person likes and does not like, then discarding what they do not like and aggressively repeating what they do like. For example, if a person with advanced dementia likes ice cream, we offer it many times a day, or if he or she is comfortable and cooperative with towel baths, we discontinue showers and bathe them using the towel bath technique. The trick, of course, is reading their expressions, gestures, and behaviors well enough to uncover what they like.

Finally, the person-centered care model emphasizes the importance of honoring and maintaining the personhood of caregivers, too. Kitwood (1997) wrote that there is "a close parallel between the way employees are treated by their seniors, and the way clients themselves are treated. If employees are supported and encouraged, they will take their own sense of well-being into their day-to-day work" (p. 103). Personhood is a construct that applies to every human being—in the person-centered model of care, all people have an inherent dignity and deserve unconditional respect, including the caregivers.

The Milieu

The person-centered care literature puts great emphasis on the environment in which people live. *Home* is a central theme and the adjective *homelike* is a commonly used descriptor. As with other aspects of care within the model, facility residents are given great authority and discretion in the design and content of the environment, making it as homelike as they require. Who could argue? We all would rather live in our own homes than in institutions, and most would agree that being homelike is an important, if not critical, attribute for all long-term care and other institutional settings.

In the context of advanced-dementia care, we prefer the label and concept of milieu to that of environment because milieu suggests not only the physical aspects of the setting, but also the subjective impact (or ambience) that setting has on the individual. In addition, the concept of milieu connotes the therapeutic qualities of the environment that impact the residents' well-being.

For persons with advanced dementia, we also emphasize the person's *surroundings*—a subset of the milieu that refers to those elements of the environment that immediately touch the senses of the individual. To translate the concept of environment into an advanced-dementia care setting, the person-centered care model needs to emphasize the immediate sensory aspects of the milieu and personal surroundings—the closer the stimulus, the more important and impactful it is to the person with advanced dementia. With this in mind, the pictures on the wall and the color of the paint are not as relevant to the person with advanced dementia as the softness of the bed linen or the warmth of a sweater. In this context, caregivers must determine what feels good to the individual and what does not, taking into account everything the person sees, hears, touches, tastes, and smells. Moreover, because every person with advanced dementia is unique and different, each requires custom-tailored surroundings designed to maximize comfort and enhance his or her quality of life (see chapter 5 for a more in-depth discussion of milieu, environment, and surroundings).

Activities

Activity programming for persons with advanced dementia should be designed to promote personal comfort, personhood, quality of life, and human dignity. Unlike traditional and institutional-based activity programming, which relies on an inflexible and restricted schedule (e.g., exercises at 9:00 A.M., bingo at 1:00 P.M., etc.), activity programming for persons with advanced dementia must be individualized and flexible. It must take into account the individual difference of the participants, including their unique abilities, interests, and attention spans, and it must be fluid in allowing participants to start and stop according to what works best for them.

Individualized activities are preferred, although very small and intimate group activities can be effective as long as the caregiver can engage the person with dementia and they are doing something that draws on a warm and meaningful connection between them. Such connections are important in helping persons with advanced dementia reaffirm their sense of self and maintain their sense of personhood.

As with other aspects of advanced dementia care, when considering activities it is important to follow the axiom of "figure out what they like to do and do it often." There should be no fixed schedule for following this approach, so activity programming should be a round-the-clock phenomenon in which all caregivers, family, and friends participate. In this light, every activity should be made meaningful, including and especially caregiving activities (i.e., ADLs), because all acts of caregiving include elements of sensory stimulation and social interaction that can be reframed into positive meaningful activities. For example, many grooming activities such as brushing hair or manicuring nails can become pleasant and comforting personal contacts when done right.

Many of the more traditional activities may no longer be relevant. Most persons with advanced dementia can no longer do arts and crafts, read books, cook, or even play bingo. Movies and television shows are often impossible to follow and may, in fact, be overly stimulating or distressing. Activities that are well suited for the population with advanced dementia include various types of music activities, food-related activities, walks outside, light massages, and personal grooming, although the list must be individualized and account for personal tastes (not everyone with advanced dementia likes Frank Sinatra or chocolate ice cream). It is especially important to know the individual's activity history, including such diverse areas as occupation and avocations, family history, interests and hobbies, and religious background—once again, knowing and understanding the individual well becomes a critical factor in engaging and connecting with persons with advanced dementia.

This flexible, highly individualized, and personal approach to activity programming fits well within the philosophy and practices of the person-centered care model. In that model, activities are a cornerstone for helping individuals maintain their sense of self and personhood, especially given that people's self-esteem and self-identities tend to emanate from the activities that they do and the self-attributions they make when doing them. However, for the person-centered care model to be truly effective with the population with advanced dementia, it must once again make necessary adjustments to account for the more severe limitations and deficits found in that population, with every effort made to understand and accommodate each individual's activity needs in spite of those deficits (see chapter 14 for a more detailed discussion on activity programming).

Residential Care Programs for Persons With Advanced Dementia

There are roughly one million people with advanced dementia in the United States, with 90% of them residing in long-term care facilities. Those facilities include nursing homes, assisted-living centers, group homes, and adult foster care homes. Many serve mixed populations, and some specialize in dementia care. The majority of the advanced dementia population resides in programs designed for persons with chronic health problems who do not have dementia (e.g., persons diagnosed with hip fractures, strokes, lung disease, heart failure, diabetes, AIDS, kidney failure, liver disease, etc., along with a growing number of persons with psychiatric disorders and developmental disabilities). In fact, more than one quarter of all persons residing in mixed-population long-term care facilities have advanced dementia.

A much smaller percentage of the population with advanced dementia resides in secured wandering dementia programs that are specifically designed for persons with moderate-stage dementia who wander. Some of these dementia-specific programs allow for residents who do not wander (i.e., most persons with advanced dementia do not ambulate or wander), but many have policies requiring that residents with nonwandering dementia be transferred to the unlocked mixed-population programs mentioned previously. Ironically, only a relatively small number of persons with advanced dementia reside in programs designed specifically for advanced dementia, because there are only a handful of such programs in existence around the country.

People with advanced dementia tend to reside in long-term care programs that are not designed for them, with the vast majority being in nonspecialized programs where they are side by side with persons who do not have dementia. Even in the best of such facilities, persons with advanced dementia are prone to get only the most basic care and very little else. Yes, they will be cleaned and changed when incontinent, fed at mealtimes, bathed on shower days, and put to bed at bedtime, but very little more is done for them. Meals and snacks are not geared for them and they tend to become malnourished and lose weight (which is usually blamed on the dementia rather than on caregiving practices). Social and recreational activities in these programs are not appropriate for them and completely miss the mark. Caregivers in these programs are rarely trained in dementia care and hardly ever receive advanced-dementia training, which means they do not know or understand their residents with advanced dementia, do not anticipate their needs, do not alleviate their discomforts, and do not know how to manage their behaviors; plus, the prescribing of psychoactive medications is not just common, it is rampant. In addition, the truly sad thing about all this is that administrators, doctors, and caregivers do not seem to realize that this sort of care is negligent and abusive, and that there are much better alternatives.

Person-centered care is a wonderful care model for persons with dementia that translates well into an advanced-dementia care context. The model's holistic focus on the individual and his or her personhood is a highly effective antidote to the terrible toll dementia takes on a person's dignity and sense of self. But to overcome the harsh realities experienced by persons with advanced dementia in today's long-term care settings, including the relentless degradation and loss of their personhood, tenets of the person-centered care model need to again be reconsidered, this time relative to the population with advanced dementia. Administrators and doctors need to be reoriented, caregivers need to be retrained, and programs need to be retooled. This book provides a foundation for such a reconceptualization, offering professionals information on many critical issues pertaining to advanced-dementia care, and providing fodder for program changes that, among other things, help to maintain the personhood of the individuals residing in those programs.

EXHIBIT 4.1

Standards of Care to Honor the Integrity of the Individual

A. The healthcare facility shall:
 1. Adopt a care philosophy and programwide core values that recognize and honor the intrinsic worth and personhood of each individual within the program setting, including persons with advanced dementia and their caregivers.
 2. Institute and maintain program policies and procedures that support and honor the personhood of each individual within the program setting, including persons with advanced dementia and their caregivers.
 3. Incorporate the fundamental principles and practices of personhood into all aspects of the program, including the milieu, activities, and caregiving practices.

Continued

Exhibit 4.1 *Continued*

4. Provide ongoing education and training on issues of personhood to all caregiving staff.
5. Develop staffing and scheduling practices that ensure that the persons with advanced dementia are cared for by caregivers who know them well, ensuring good continuity of care and enhancing a sense of familiarity and understanding between caregivers and the persons for whom they care.

B. Healthcare staff shall:
1. Receive specialty training in advanced dementia in a caring and non-threatening manner while promoting the key concepts related to personhood.
2. Interact with persons with advanced dementia in a caring and non-threatening manner while promoting the key concepts of personhood, including:
   a. Understanding the individuality and uniqueness of each individual;
   b. Recognizing and honoring the inherent dignity of the individual;
   c. Unbridled respect for the individual;
   d. Helping the individual maintain a sense of self; and
   e. The importance and impact of social relations.
3. Ensure that the care plan reflects the physiological, psychological, social, cultural, and spiritual aspects of each resident who has advanced dementia.

C. Persons with advanced dementia shall expect:
1. Individualized activity programming.
2. A milieu that is safe, comfortable, and attends to personal needs.
3. That his or her personhood is maintained and enhanced as much as possible, and is honored by all persons within the caregiving setting.
4. The caregiving situation to be safe and comfortable, and that they will be treated in a dignified, humane, respectful, and nonthreatening manner.

▨ REFERENCES

Bell, V., & Troxel, D. (2001). *The best friends staff: Building a culture of care in Alzheimer's programs.* Baltimore, MD: Health Professions Press.

Bell, V., & Troxel, D. (2003). *The best friends approach to Alzheimer's care* (Rev. ed.). Baltimore, MD: Health Professions Press.

Brooker, D. (2007). *Person-centered dementia care: Making services better.* Philadelphia, PA: Jessica Kingsley Publishers.

Buron, B. (2008). Levels of personhood: A model for dementia care. *Geriatric Nursing, 29*(5), 324–332.

Chaudhury, H. (2002). Place-biosketch as a tool in caring for residents with dementia. *Alzheimer's Care Quarterly, 3*(1), 42–45.

Cohen, D., & Eisdorfer, C. (1986). *The loss of self: A family resource for the care of Alzheimer's disease and related disorders.* New York: W. W. Norton.

Downs, M., Small, N., & Froggatt, K. (2006). Person-centered care for people with severe dementia. In A. Burns & B. Winblad (Eds.), *Severe dementia* (pp. 193–204). Hoboken, NJ: John Wiley & Sons, Inc.

Edvardsson, D., Winblad, B., & Sandman, P. O. (2008). Person-centred care of people with severe Alzheimer's disease: Current status and ways forward. *Lancet Neurology, 7*(4), 362–367.

Fazio, S. (2008a). *The enduring self in people with Alzheimer's: Getting to the heart of individualized care.* Baltimore, MD: Health Professions Press.

Fazio, S. (2008b). Person-centered care in residential settings: Taking a look back while continuing to move forward. *Alzheimer's Care Today, 9*(2), 155–161.

Hughes, J., Lloyd-Williams, M., & Sachs, G. (2010). *Supportive care for the person with dementia.* Oxford, UK: Oxford University Press.

Jones, M. (1999). *Gentle care: Changing the experience of Alzheimer's disease in a positive way.* Point Roberts, WA: Hartley & Marks.

Kitwood, T. (1997). *Dementia reconsidered: The person comes first.* London: Open University Press.

Kovach, C. R. (1997). Maintaining personhood: Philosophy, goals, program development and staff education. In C. R. Kovach (Ed.), *Late-stage dementia care: A basic guide* (pp. 25–43). Washington, DC: Taylor & Francis.

Long, C. O. (2009). Palliative care for advanced dementia. *Journal of Gerontological Nursing, 35*(11), 19–24.

Martin, G. A. (2004). Personhood. In C. O. Long (Ed.), *Palliative care for advanced dementia: Train-the-trainer manual* (pp. P2-Suppl.-8). Phoenix, AZ: Alzheimer's Association, Desert Southwest Chapter.

Post, S. G. (2006). Respectare: Moral respect for the lives of the deeply forgetful. In J. C. Hughes, S. J. Louw, & S. R. Sabat. (Eds.), *Dementia: mind, meaning, and the person* (pp. 223–234). New York: Oxford University Press.

Touhy, T. A. (2004). Dementia, personhood, and nursing: Learning from a nursing situation. *Nursing Science Quarterly, 17*(1), 43–49.

CREATING THE OPTIMAL MILIEU FOR CARE

Gary A. Martin, Judith Sgrillo, and Antonia Horton

■ INTRODUCTION

All healthcare professionals know that palliative care means comfort care. What many do not know is that dementia care also means comfort care. Persons with dementia who feel physically and emotionally comfortable tend to be at their best and do their best. They are less confused, exhibit fewer behavior problems, and function at a higher level. Pain will cause a person with dementia to become more confused and to potentially act out; so will virtually all other forms of physical discomfort, like being hungry or thirsty, hot or cold, sitting in uncomfortable positions, or wearing ill-fitted clothing (to name just a few). Because dementia care is comfort care, one of the most critical goals in dementia care at every level is to maximize comfort, and it is the caregiver's job to do everything possible to help persons with dementia to be as comfortable as possible.

However, achieving the goal of comfort with persons who have advanced dementia can be challenging. First, comfort can be compromised from a thousand different directions and it is difficult to control all the physical and emotional variables that influence a person's subjective sense of comfort. Second, persons with advanced dementia are severely limited in their ability to deal with their own discomforts and must rely on others to do so. Third, persons with advanced dementia are not well attuned to identifying, discriminating, and mentally processing their perceptions and feelings. Although they feel and react to discomfort and emotional distress, they cannot readily organize and process their thinking enough to understand those feelings. Finally, and perhaps the most important, persons with advanced dementia cannot verbalize and articulate their discomforts and the reasons why they are uncomfortable so that others can understand and help them with the problem.

This issue of trying to maximize comfort is a perfect storm for persons with advanced dementia: they are more likely to suffer physical and emotional discomforts, do not have the skills to alleviate their discomforts, and cannot tell others about it. As a result, their discomforts often go unresolved and they become increasingly helpless, distressed, and confused as the unresolved discomfort worsens. This results in an all-too-common vicious cycle of discomfort and decline that, left unchecked, leaves the person with a tragically diminished quality of life that is avoidable and unnecessary (see chapter 6 for further discussions about the importance of comfort in late-stage dementia care).

Although many care-related issues affect a person's level of comfort, none is as immediate and influential as the environment in which the person lives. For persons with advanced dementia, that environment is usually a care facility of one type or another. In the past years, persons with advanced dementia mostly resided in nursing homes. More recently, there has been a shift of sorts to other care settings like group homes, assisted-living centers, and adult foster care homes. Interestingly, that shift started in the 1990s when consumer-oriented families went looking for more comfortable and homelike settings in which to place their loved ones. At first, these residential alternatives to nursing homes catered to persons who were frail but cognitively intact. As time passed, they opened their doors to persons with more substantial problems, including those with mild and moderate dementia. Most recently, we have seen a significant influx of persons with advanced dementia residing in those alternative care settings.

Regardless of the setting, the environment is a critical concern when caring for persons with advanced dementia. An uncomfortable environment means that those persons living (and working) there will be uncomfortable. It is the responsibility of the owners, managers, and caregivers from those settings to not only make the environment safe and therapeutic, but to also make sure that it is as comfortable as possible and, in the case of persons with advanced dementia, to do so in a manner that shows understanding and sensitivity to each individual resident's special needs. As a general rule, this means that the environment must be as warm, homelike, personable, and noninstitutional as possible by considering and controlling such key aspects as temperature, lighting, furnishings, floorings, windows, decorations, colors, fabrics, room sizes, and outside areas.

There is a relatively large body of literature in the field of dementia care that addresses the issues of environmental design, some of which are listed in the bibliography section of this chapter. That literature tends to focus on general design principles for persons with dementia without specifying any particular stage of dementia, suggesting that those principles apply to all stages of dementia. Recommendations tend to cover issues like the use of space, furniture placement, seating arrangements, personalizing space, accessibility of activity props, and dining arrangements. They also include discussions about decorations, colors, floor materials, and window treatments. Unfortunately, there has been very little research and few articles that specifically focus on environmental design for persons with advanced dementia. Therefore, by default, these writings lead the reader to assume that their principles and recommendations apply equally to all persons with dementia, including those with advanced dementia. For the most part, this is not the case.

▦ THE MILIEU AND ADVANCED DEMENTIA

Definitions

Environmental design literature tends to refer to people's living space as the environment. However, when considering the living space of persons with dementia, we find the word *environment* somewhat limited because it tends to connote only the physical elements of a setting (e.g., furniture, floorings, window treatments, pictures, plants, etc.). In developing these guidelines and standards for persons with advanced dementia, we believe it is important to broaden the context of a person's living space to include the intangible aspects of the environment, including the mood, atmosphere, and feel of the setting to those people who live there.

With that in mind, we prefer the broader and deeper meaning of the word *milieu* in describing the individual's environment and how the environment affects the individual. This is an especially important notion when considering that persons with advanced dementia may not be aware of their general surroundings or the details of their environment, and are more likely to respond to their environment on a more visceral and emotional level. Their subjective experience with the environment has little to do with aesthetics and everything to do with personal comfort. Milieu better captures the importance of this effect.

The word *milieu* also adds a therapeutic context to the environment. In the sociology and social psychology fields, milieu is commonly used as an important aspect of many therapies (also referred to as *milieu therapy*). This includes the practice of immersing individuals in living and social settings that require participation in activities and social interactions designed to address emotional and interpersonal needs. The therapeutic value of the milieu cannot be overstated, including and especially for persons with advanced dementia.

The concept of milieu also includes the notion of how all the elements of the environment, including people, add up to an overall effect that influences a person's sense of comfort and well-being. In effect, the milieu has a gestaltlike quality that suggests it has a nature and bearing that is far greater than the sum of its parts.

Guiding Principles

Care facilities can be unpleasant places that have bright lights, hard surfaces, cold hallways, loud noises, and unpleasant odors. Starting before dawn and going until well after dusk there is often a constant commotion as caregivers do their jobs, residents engage in activities, visitors come and go, housekeepers clean, and maintenance workers make repairs. The sounds of televisions, call bells, overhead intercoms, telephones, alarms, and cleaning equipment combine with the often loud voices emanating from activity programs, staff conversations, and residents moaning or yelling from subjective distress. The cacophony of sound found in care facilities easily rivals what is heard in shopping malls and on busy street corners. Added to this are the onerous smells of disinfectants, detergents, and urine that fill the air. Moreover, at mealtimes, dining rooms virtually explode into chaos, whereas at shift-change times, nurses' stations often turn into bedlam.

With all this in mind, for persons with advanced dementia, the milieu should be designed for comfort. For that to happen, the loud, busy, and noxious care home qualities must be neutralized. Telephone ringtones, call bells, and alarms should be eliminated or converted to more pleasant sounds, such as musical tones or nature sounds. Overhead intercoms should be disconnected, perhaps replaced by individually-carried pagers or other portable electronic devices.

Floor plans should be redesigned to include smaller activity areas that are self-contained, soundproofed, and do not spill over into other parts of the living space. Staff should be trained to keep their voices down and to respect the integrity of the residents and their environment. Lighting should be modified to emphasize ambient light, eliminating direct exposure to bright lamps and fluorescent lights. Cleaning fluids should be odorless or pleasantly scented. The overall milieu should be made as warm as possible by using homelike fabrics and decorations. Items that are cold and hard to the touch should be replaced by items that are warm, soft, and pleasing. Overall, the milieu should focus on sensory stimuli that are calming and soothing, but should also include stimuli that are interesting and engaging. It should be as stress free as possible, and should be aggressively sensitive to the less-tangible aspects of the residents' subjective experience, such as ambience, culture, spirituality, and social contact.

In this spirit, we suggest the following guiding principles when designing a milieu for persons with advanced dementia:

- Comfort comes first. All elements of the milieu must be geared toward maximizing the residents' comfort level.
- Each resident is a unique individual who may respond differently to aspects of the milieu than other residents.
- Those elements of the milieu that are closest to the individual have the greatest impact; this is especially true for persons with advanced dementia who are affected most by what they can touch and what touches them.
- People have an effect on the milieu, just as the milieu has an effect on people.
- Milieus have a ripple effect. When the milieu affects one person (e.g., his or her moods and behaviors), he or she, in turn, affects others. In this way, aspects of the milieu that might not directly impact persons with advanced dementia can still affect them via the milieu's impact on their caregivers.
- Administrators and caregivers have considerable control over most aspects of the milieu—it is usually within their power to change the milieu (for better or worse).
- Making changes in the milieu will result in associated changes in the people within that milieu.

SURROUNDINGS AND ADVANCED DEMENTIA

Definition

When considering the living environment for persons with advanced dementia, we also prefer the narrower and more specific meaning of the word *surroundings* in describing those aspects of the setting that envelop and touch the individual and are part of his or her immediate primary sensory experience. These are the most salient aspects of the milieu for persons with advanced dementia that have the greatest impact on the individual's comfort. The surroundings include any part of the environment that has immediate sensory contact with the individual through touch, hearing, vision, smell, and taste.

Surroundings can be divided into two categories: shared and individual. Shared surroundings are those aspects of the milieu that have immediate sensory contact with the individual but that are also in contact with, or available to, other individuals in that setting. This mainly involves public areas like dining rooms, day rooms, lounges, patios, and hallways, and may include shared bathrooms, shared bedrooms, and other semiprivate living areas. The primary goal in designing a milieu's public areas is to make the shared surroundings as comfortable and therapeutic as possible for all individuals who live there.

Personal surroundings refer to those elements of the milieu that have immediate sensory contact with the individual but not with other persons who reside in that setting. In public areas, personal surroundings are mainly those things that physically touch the individual—sights, sounds, and smells are more likely sensory events that are shared with others. Moreover, in personal areas such as private bedrooms and bathrooms, all sensory stimuli should be considered as part of an individual's personal surroundings. The primary goal in designing these private areas is to customize and personalize the stimuli to best fit the comfort zone of the one unique individual who lives there.

Guiding Principles

Shared surroundings must try to strike a common chord for everyone, rather than cater to one individual. For example, the music played in public areas needs to appeal to the broader audience. For persons with advanced dementia, this might include smooth jazz, traditional 1950s and 1960s popular music (e.g., Frank Sinatra, Dean Martin, Barbara Streisand), or perhaps big band era jazz or even 1950s rock and roll, but could also include country or classical music (depending on the makeup and histories of the resident population). In a similar vein, thermostats in public areas need to be set at temperatures that best suit all the individuals in the room, not just the one or two exceptions who prefer it extremely warm or extremely cool. It should be noted that older adults generally prefer warmer temperatures, so for persons with advanced dementia it is usually best to keep common-area thermostats at moderately warm settings.

The most important pieces of furniture in shared surroundings are the chairs in which residents sit. Persons with advanced dementia generally do not ambulate so they spend almost all of their time in beds or chairs. When getting them out of bed, caregivers usually place persons with advanced dementia in wheelchairs where they might sit for hours at a time. Although wheelchairs may be convenient for caregivers, they are not especially comfortable for the persons who sit in them, especially for frail elders with advanced dementia who cannot easily reposition themselves. Other and more comfortable seating options should be used. Consequently, the chairs located in public areas must be as comfortable as possible, providing adequate support, a soft feel, and fabrics that are pleasing to the touch. This suggests upholstered chairs, rather than wood, metal, or plastic, and that these chairs have the ability to recline.

To be truly resident friendly and comforting to persons with advanced dementia, all aspects of the shared surroundings must be considered and controlled to evoke the maximum comfort possible for everyone. Examples of the more significant aspects of the shared surroundings that should be considered include the following:

- Entertainment-oriented sounds (e.g., music, television, DVDs, radios, etc.)
- Acoustic qualities of the room
- Other noises from the workplace (e.g., telephones, call bells, alarms, intercoms, cleaning equipment, furnaces and air conditioners, squeaky wheelchairs, shuffling walkers, etc.)
- Voices of others in the milieu (e.g., caregivers, activity programs, other residents, visitors, medical providers, etc.)
- Room temperature
- Furniture for seating
- Lighting (e.g., lamps, fixtures, windows, etc.)
- Public-area odors (e.g., cleaning solutions, urine, deodorizers, aromatherapies, food odors, etc.)
- Perfumes and colognes worn by other people in the immediate area

Personal surroundings are an entirely different matter. Although comfort continues to be the driving force behind the design of personal surroundings, it is only the individual's comfort that is considered. Every person with advanced dementia is unique, and his or her personal surroundings must be tailored to his or her unique tastes and comfort levels. Whereas the masses may be most comfortable with middle-of-the-road soothing music selections, an individual may be most comfortable listening to the Beatles or Beethoven, depending on his or her taste. Most persons with advanced dementia become distressed with the loud soundtracks to action adventure movies or to news reports, game shows, and reality shows on television, but a given individual might be the exception to the rule and actually derive comfort from those types of shows. Moreover, although most older adults, including those with advanced dementia, prefer warmer room temperatures, there certainly are individuals who are more comfortable when it is cooler or even cold.

Any individual with advanced dementia can be the exception to almost any general rule we apply to persons with advanced dementia. Our goal in designing the individual's living space to take into account the individual's unique comfort preferences and infuse those preferences into his or her personal space. There are two main ways of accomplishing this. First, caregivers must obtain a detailed personal history that includes information on specific lifelong preferences for such things as music, television shows, foods, bedding, perfumes or colognes, fabric softeners, and anything else that pertains to the individual's current personal surroundings. Once collected, that information can be used in the initial design of the individual's personal living space. Then second, caregivers should use a trial-and-error approach to virtually all sensory aspects of the individual's personal surroundings, trying various stimuli with an eye toward emphasizing and repeating those stimuli that enhance comfort and discarding those stimuli that appear to be uncomfortable. Using these approaches over time, astute caregivers can put together a uniquely-designed mosaic of personal surroundings that maximizes personal comfort and greatly improves the individual's quality of life.

For personal surroundings, caregivers should consider the following:

- *Bedding:* Mattresses, pillows, sheets, pillowcases, blankets, comforters
- *Clothing:* Nightclothes and day clothes; fabric and fit (e.g., loose, warm, nothing rough, stiff, or scratchy); color is not as important as feel and fit
- *Seating:* Upholstered with soft, comfortable fabrics; adjustable positions (e.g., recliners); adequate support; use of comforters, blankets, lap robes, and so forth, to enhance comfort; minimize time in wheelchairs
- *Bathing:* Type of bathing experience (e.g., shower, tub bath, towel bath); water and room temperature; soap and shampoo; wash cloths and towels (see chapter 13, on bathing)
- *Temperature:* Thermostat set to preference (usually warmer rather than cooler); may change from one moment to the next; clothing can help to modulate; look for signs of discomfort (e.g., sweating, disrobing, shivering, cold skin)
- *Lighting:* Ambient light; not too bright or too dim; keep in mind the person will often be lying down or have their head back, looking into ceiling fixtures—adjust lighting accordingly
- *Entertainment:* Music, depending on preference, played over high-quality speakers that give a true, rich tone (not tinny or distorted); spare use of television focusing on shows that are tried-and-true; greater use of recorded shows (DVD, VHS) played on television, also depending on preference and are tried-and-true; keep volume down; do not turn on television just because it is there—only use it strategically and therapeutically
- *Smells:* Focus on personal history, also use trial and error; watch for pleasing responses to smells; use lifelong and tried-and-true products (e.g., perfumes, scented oils and lotions, and scented grooming and hygiene products); familiar fabric softener smell in bedding and clothing; consider aroma therapy and use of essential oils, but only on a trial-and-error basis; foods with pleasing smells (e.g., bread, coffee, cinnamon toast, popcorn)
- *Sounds:* Eliminate or control excessive and undesirable noises that inevitably come from the care home environment; give the room a soundproof quality through the use of noise-deadening carpeting, fabrics (e.g., curtains, framed fabrics on the wall, decorative quilts, etc.); mask problem noises with pleasant music or nature sounds; use headphones, if tolerated
- *Food and drink:* Offer frequent preferred drinks and snacks (see chapter 9)

CONCLUSION

Like with palliative care, comfort is the key to good dementia care. For persons with advanced dementia, optimizing comfort can be extremely challenging. This is especially the case because their disabilities make them susceptible to discomforts and they cannot do anything to alleviate or communicate their discomforts on their own. The environment is a critical factor in the individual's physical and emotional comfort, so much so that we believe the terminology needs to be fine-tuned to better reflect this causal affect. For broad issues relating to the environment and its impact on residents living there, we prefer the term *milieu*, which suggests a more holistic definition that includes the individual's feelings associated with the environment as well as the therapeutic value of the environment. In addition, we use the term *surroundings* to describe any aspects of the milieu that directly touch the person's senses. For persons with advanced dementia, immediate sensory experiences are more important to subjective comfort than any other aspects of the milieu. Therefore, the main focus in considering and designing a milieu for persons with advanced dementia should be on comfort-based and sensory-oriented aspects of the individual's shared and personal surroundings (see Exhibit 5.1).

EXHIBIT 5.1

Standards of Care for Milieu Environment

A. The healthcare facility shall:
1. Develop and implement policies and procedures that address the milieu as a means of promoting comfort and dignity for persons with advanced dementia.
2. Design an environment and shared surroundings that are therapeutic, safe, and homelike.
3. Provide assistance and guidance to families and caregivers in promoting a milieu that supports palliative care for persons with advanced dementia.
4. Create a positive and supportive milieu for the persons with dementia and their caregivers.
5. Provide unit enhancements (e.g., beanbag chairs, Merry Walker, special dining room seating arrangements, Snoezelen cart/room) to promote comfort.
6. Identify aspects of the milieu that provide comfort or discomfort. Draft policies and procedures that identify the need for caregivers to note and address these items in the person's plan of care.

B. Healthcare staff shall:
1. Complete the life story or biosketch and conduct interviews with family members to determine which aspects of the milieu work best in providing a comfortable and person-centered setting in which to live.
2. Work with family members to create personal surroundings within the milieu that are comfortable, warm, and pleasing for person with advanced dementia.
3. Be attentive to those aspects of the milieu that provide comfort or discomfort to persons with advanced dementia. Document and address such issues in respective care plans.

4. Be attentive to the milieu, including the environment and shared or personal surroundings, by adjusting and adapting it to meet the person's changing needs.

C. Persons with advanced dementia shall expect:

1. A milieu that is comfortable, homelike, warm, personable, supportive, and safe, which includes attention to the environment, including shared and personal surroundings.

2. Whenever possible, customized personal surroundings that are designed with detailed input from family and friends who know the person best.

3. The milieu, including the environment and shared or personal surroundings, to be continually adjusted and adapted to meet their changing needs.

▨ REFERENCES

Brawley, E. C. (2001). Environmental design for Alzheimer's disease: A quality of life issue. *Aging & Mental Health, 5*(Suppl. 1), S79–S83.

Calkins, M. P. (1997). A supportive environment for people with late-stage dementia. In C. R. Kovach (Ed.), *Late-stage dementia care: A basic guide* (pp. 101–112). Washington, DC: Taylor & Francis.

Calkins, M. P. (2001). The physical and social environment of the person with Alzheimer's disease. *Aging & Mental Health, 5*(Suppl. 1), S74–S78.

Calkins, M. P. (2005). Environments for late-stage dementia. *Alzheimer's Care Quarterly, 6*(1), 71–75.

Chalfont, G. (2007). *Design for Nature in Dementia Care*. Philadelphia: Jessica Kingsley Publishers.

Cutler, L. J. (2007). Physical environments of assisted living: Research needs and challenges. *The Gerontologist, 47*(SI2), 68–82.

Day, K., Carreon, D., & Stump, C. (2000). The therapeutic design of environments for people with dementia: A review of the empirical research. *The Gerontologist, 40*(4), 397–416.

Dewing, J. (2009, June). Caring for people with dementia: Noise and light. *Nursing Older People, 21*(5), 34–39.

Fazio, S., Seman, D., & Stansell, J. (1999a). Redesigning care programs. In S. Fazio, D. Seman, & Stansell, J. (Eds.), *Rethinking Alzheimer's care* (pp. 113–135). Baltimore: Health Professions Press.

Fazio, S., Seman, D., & Stansell, J. (1999b). Reshaping the environment. In S. Fazio, D. Seman, & J. Stansell (Eds.), *Rethinking Alzheimer's care* (pp. 91–112). Baltimore: Health Professions Press.

Fazio, S. (2008). Physical and social environments that recognize the self. In S. Fazio (Ed.),*The enduring self in people with Alzheimer's: Getting to the heart of individual care* (pp. 75–97). Baltimore, MD: Health Professions Press.

Geboy, L. (2009). Linking person-centered care and the physical environment: 10 design principles for elder and dementia care staff. *Alzheimer's Care Today, 10*(4), 228–231.

Kovach, C. R. (1997). Behaviors associated with late-stage dementia. In C. R. Kovach (Ed.), *Late-stage dementia care: A basic guide* (pp. 127–141). Washington, DC: Taylor & Francis.

Perritt, M. R., McCune, E. D., & McCune, S. L. (2005). Research informs design: Empirical findings suggest recommendations for carpet pattern and texture. *Alzheimer's Care Quarterly, 6*(4), 300–305.

Rabig, J., Thomas, W., Kane, R. A., Cutler, L. J., & McAlilly, S. (2007). Radical redesign of nursing homes: Applying the green house concept in Tupelo, Mississippi. *The Gerontologist, 46*(4), 533–539.

Samus, Q. M., Rosenblatt, A., Steele, C., Baker, A., Harper, M., Brandt, J., et al. (2005). The association of neuropsychiatric symptoms and environment with quality of life in assisted living resident with dementia. *The Gerontologist, 45*(SI1), 19–26.

Sloane, P. D., Noell-Waggoner, E., Hickman, S., Mitchell, M., Williams, C. S., Preisser, J. S., et al. (2005). Implementing lighting intervention in public areas of long-term care facilities: Lessons learned. *Alzheimer's Care Quarterly, 6*(40), 280–293.

Troxel, D. (2005). The last great frontier in long-term care: Let's get our elders outside. *Alzheimer's Care Quarterly, 6*(4), 332–334.

Werezak, L. J., & Morgan, D. G. (2003). Creating a therapeutic psychosocial environment in dementia care: A preliminary framework. *Journal of Gerontological Nursing, 29*(12), 18–25.

Zeisel, J., Hyde, J., & Shi, L. (1999). Environmental design as a treatment for Alzheimer's disease. In L. Volicer & L. Bloom-Charette (Eds.), *Enhancing the quality of life in advanced dementia* (pp. 206–222). Philadelphia: Brunner/Mazel.

6

MANAGING BEHAVIOR PROBLEMS ASSOCIATED WITH ADVANCED DEMENTIA

Gary A. Martin and Marianne McCarthy

■ INTRODUCTION

Much has been written about the behaviors associated with Alzheimer's disease and related dementias, and how to conceptualize and address problems associated with those behaviors. In virtually all cases, the emphasis of those write-ups has been on the sometimes severe behaviors exhibited by persons with middle- or moderate-stage dementia—those persons with dementia who are still verbal and ambulatory and, although significantly impaired, have maintained partially intact cognitive, functional, and communication skills. Although that population has been well considered and researched relative to their often very challenging behavior problems, the population with advanced dementia has, for the most part, been ignored or, more commonly, lumped together with their less-impaired brethren with the assumption that their behavioral issues are the same. They are not.

Unlike the statistics available on persons with early- and moderate-stage dementia, incidence rates on behavior problems exhibited by persons with advanced dementia are sparse and not well documented. Reports suggest that roughly two-thirds of all persons with advanced dementia exhibit some sort of significantly agitated behavior (e.g., physical restlessness, disruptive vocalizations, resisting care).

The behavior problems exhibited by persons with advanced dementia can be described as less severe and more limited than those exhibited by persons with early- or moderate-stage dementia. Persons with advanced dementia are more likely to exhibit behaviors that are considered a nuisance, but not considered dangerous. They are rarely hospitalized in psychiatric settings for their behaviors, are not prone to injure caregivers or others, and do not need the more aggressive psychoactive medications such as antipsychotics or tranquilizers. When they do have behavior problems, their behaviors are often described as disruptive or agitated, but rarely as dangerous or unmanageable. The only truly dangerous behaviors that are commonly exhibited by persons with advanced dementia are those behaviors that might result in the person harming himself or herself, such as with falls or poor intake.

The list of common behavior problems for persons with advanced dementia is short, as compared to that of persons in the earlier stages of dementia and includes such things as resisting or fighting care, physical agitation and physical restlessness, distressed vocalizations (e.g., yelling, moaning, crying), poor oral intake, and falling. Because of their loss of mobility, strength, and communication skills over time, persons with advanced dementia do not have the wherewithal to wander, rummage, or elope. They are generally not in a position to assault peers, act out sexually, strip off their clothes, or intrude on others. Their resistance to care is usually more a matter of thrashing and flailing their arms or pulling away from their caregivers than of closed-fisted combativeness, and their diminished strength means that caregivers, more often than not, can get care done safely without incident, even when the person is actively resisting and fighting. Yelling or crying out is a common problem—after all, persons with advanced dementia are generally nonambulatory and only those who are unable to walk or get around on their own are prone to yell out. However, this is viewed more as a nuisance rather than a danger by most caregivers (although loud, constant screamers can be quite disruptive and are not well tolerated in many long-term care settings).

Interestingly, the more truly dangerous behaviors exhibited by persons with advanced dementia are falls and poor intake, yet these problems are often not considered behavior problems at all. Experts view falls as somewhat unique and distinct from behavior problems. This area has its own rapidly expanding body of research, literature, and intervention protocols that are well-known and almost universally followed (see chapter 12 on ambulation and mobility), including the use of unique safety options and passive restraints that are found in virtually no other setting (e.g., low beds, Merry Walkers, geriatric chairs) and are readily available and widely used within the long-term care industry. Moreover, although eating is certainly a behavior, suggesting that diminished intake is indeed a behavior problem, poor intake and associated weight loss seem to be accepted as an expected and unavoidable result of the progressive decline caused by the dementia. We take exception to this assumption and believe that poor intake is, in fact, a behavior problem that can be effectively addressed (see chapter 9 on eating and nutrition, for further discussion).

All in all, the behavior problems exhibited by persons with advanced dementia are well tolerated by most caregivers and most long-term care facilities, and we do not hear a lot of serious complaints about these behaviors. In fact, it is often taken for granted that these behaviors will occur and that they can be easily managed by virtually any professional caregiver (trained or untrained) without much effort or difficulty in a long-term care setting.

However, let us be clear. The most critical issues are not the magnitude, severity, and manageability of the behaviors exhibited by persons with advanced dementia. The most critical issues here are those relating to maintaining the personhood of the individual. Behavior problems exhibited by persons with advanced dementia should be viewed as red flags or alarms. Behavior problems are the alarms that signal the violation in some way of an individual's personhood; that his or her dignity has been diminished; that he or she is not receiving the respect they deserve; that his or her quality of life has been compromised; or that his or her comfort has been breeched. Although it may be our job as caregivers to get the job done by doing our best to make sure that our dementia residents are dry, bathed, clothed, and fed, it is also our responsibility to make sure we accomplish these goals in such a fashion as to maximize comfort, maintain dignity, give unwavering respect, and maximize the quality of their lives. The behavior problems exhibited by persons with advanced dementia usually suggest that we are not doing our best to realize these goals—that the person with advanced dementia is in some way uncomfortable or distressed, and that we are not adequately understanding or addressing the situation. It is their right to get better care, and it is our responsibility to give it.

That said, most caregivers are really trying their hardest and doing their best. They truly care for, if not love, the people for whom they provide care. However, when it comes to caring for persons with advanced dementia, especially when considering behavior problems, most caregivers are quite naïve and poorly trained in how to best do their job. Behavior problems are often ignored. Disruptive and agitated behaviors are generally accepted as being part of the dementia and, as such, untreatable. Psychotropic medications are prescribed when behaviors are more severe (and sometimes when they are not so severe). Environmental and behavioral interventions are either unknown or dismissed as not appropriate for this population.

The remainder of this chapter addresses these issues directly. First, we review the etiology of behaviors—why most persons with advanced dementia exhibit behavior problems. Second, we discuss ways to prevent behavior problems in the first place by maximizing comfort, anticipating needs, and considering and controlling antecedents to those behaviors. Finally, we outline interventions that are effective in diminishing or resolving behavior problems that do arise, including a brief discussion on psychopharmacologic interventions.

ETIOLOGY OR CAUSES OF BEHAVIOR PROBLEMS

Confusion

Perhaps the most basic and obvious hallmark of Alzheimer's disease and related dementias is the profound sense of confusion that the person with dementia experiences—the more advanced the dementia, the more severe the confusion. At the heart of virtually all dementia-related behavior problems at any stage is this sense of confusion. People with early-stage dementia become confused with handling money, driving their cars, and managing their lives, resulting in misunderstandings, missteps, accidents, and increased frustration and depression. People with moderate-stage dementia have difficulty understanding their surroundings and others' actions, including and especially caregivers, to the point of acting on their confusion in highly problematic ways (e.g., wandering, intrusions, defensive aggression, elopement, paranoid actions, etc.).

For persons with advanced dementia, the extent of their confusion makes it nearly impossible for them to understand their surroundings and what is going on around them. Caregivers' well-meaning but highly invasive actions are often physically and emotionally discomforting and distressing to persons with advanced dementia. Sights and sounds can be startling and overwhelming. They have problems identifying, understanding, and controlling basic feelings such as pain, discomfort, and distress—the expression of subjective discomfort and distress is often reduced to basic and reflexive emotional and behavioral responses (e.g., fight or flight reactions, physical restlessness, distressed vocalizations).

Brain Changes

The direct and deleterious effects of dementia, such as Alzheimer's disease, on the brain play a major role in why persons with advanced dementia experience behavior problems. Along with the confusion caused by the decline of cognitive abilities like memory, executive functions, visuospatial skills, and language abilities, many dementias also directly affect areas of the brain that are involved with emotional control, such as the amygdala, cingulate gyrus, insula, inferior frontal cortex, the temporal cortex, and the parietal cortex. As a result, there is a much greater chance of individuals exhibiting increased volatility, emotional liability, impulsivity, restlessness, and other affective and behavioral problems that greatly influence overall behavior.

Caregiving

Persons with advanced dementia have a greater need for hands-on care than with virtually any other care population. Most are completely dependent on others for the majority of their daily living activities. They cannot dress or groom themselves, bathe themselves, or attend to their own basic hygiene issues. They are incontinent and require others to clean them and change their clothes. They cannot ambulate independently and rely on others to assist them in walking or to push their wheelchairs. A few can feed themselves, but only with extensive setup and cuing, but most must be fed by caregivers if they are to eat or drink at all.

Because of their need for total care with all care tasks, caregiving for persons with advanced dementia involves highly personal, intimate, and intrusive actions on the caregiver's part. These actions can be, and often are, physically and emotionally uncomfortable and distressing to persons with advanced dementia, especially because they are so profoundly confused and do not understand their own need for care or the actions of their caregivers. The extreme intrusiveness and physicality of caregiving, combined with the severe level of confusion on the part of persons with advanced dementia, triggers reflexive emotional and behavioral responses, including resisting and fighting, yelling and crying, and other symptoms of emotional distress. In other words, caregiving itself is a frequent and repeated trigger for behavior problems (see chapters 8–11 for a more in-depth discussion of caregiving issues for persons with advanced dementia).

Pain

Persons with advanced dementia have a high incidence rate of untreated pain, yet they cannot identify, describe, locate, or otherwise verbalize their pain. Instead, they tend to express their pain indirectly through their emotions and behaviors.

Many common behavior problems exhibited by persons with advanced dementia (e.g., resisting care, not eating, yelling, crying, restlessness, disturbed sleep) are actually very basic and reflexive responses to pain (see chapter 7 for a more in-depth discussion of pain issues for persons with advanced dementia).

Acute Medical Problems

Persons with advanced dementia are at increased risk of developing acute medical conditions, such as infection, electrolyte imbalances, dehydration, and metabolic disturbances. In addition, because of their physical fragility, persons with advanced dementia exhibit an increasing vulnerability to adverse reactions from many medications. Persons with advanced dementia have an increased likelihood of delirium and of suffering adverse reactions to medications. It is significant to note that the superimposition of delirium on dementia has been estimated to be high, ranging from 66%–88%. Delirium is an acute, fluctuating disorder of attention and cognition that is often associated with significant morbidity, mortality, and resource use. Because of their poor cognition and limited functional abilities, it can be difficult to distinguish delirium from dementia in persons with advanced dementia, or to recognize delirium superimposed on dementia. As a result, delirium is often not recognized and underlying acute medical disorders such as infection, adverse drug reactions, electrolyte imbalance, dehydration, and metabolic disturbances go undiagnosed and untreated.

In persons with advanced dementia, sudden changes in behavior are often indicative of a delirium. These changes simultaneously accompany changes in consciousness and attention levels. In nearly all persons with advanced dementia, delirium will cause a significant decline in cognitive, behavioral, and functional abilities. Associated behaviors may include agitation, restlessness, extreme lethargy, crying or moaning, repetitive vocalizations (including yelling), changes in appetite, and/or changes in sleep pattern. Moreover, persons who develop delirium may also experience psychotic features such as hallucinations, paranoia, and delusions.

Many researchers have demonstrated the association between delirium and the increased risk of death. Because delirium is such a grave prognostic sign, caregivers must be suspicious of its occurrence whenever they observe behavioral changes in persons with advanced dementia. Moreover, caregivers must report these changes immediately and refer persons demonstrating these changes to healthcare providers.

Environmental Stressors

The behaviors of persons with advanced dementia often reflect obvious or subtle characteristics of their surroundings, environment, and milieu. If the setting is either overstimulating or understimulating, or if it has a noxious, disturbing, or sterile (i.e., institutional) quality to it, the person with advanced dementia will often behave in a distressed or agitated fashion. Environmental stressors can take many forms: uncomfortable bedding, darkness or bright lights, high volumes on televisions or stereos, heavy foot traffic and intrusions by peers and caregivers, loud and busy meals, high-energy activity programs, loud talking and laughing from nursing stations—the list of possible culprits goes on and on. Add to this list all the very idiosyncratic sensory stimuli that uniquely affect each individual, and there is an unlimited potential for environmental stressors to adversely affect virtually anyone with advanced dementia. However, the person affected is probably unable to tell anyone what it is that is bothering him or her. The behaviors could go on indefinitely with unsuspecting caregivers never identifying or figuring out that the environment is the cause of the problem, with the behaviors being either ignored and/or medicated (see chapter 5 for a more in-depth discussion on the effects of milieu on caring for persons with advanced dementia).

■ GUIDING PRINCIPLES I: PREVENTION OF BEHAVIOR PROBLEMS

Comfort

Dementia care is comfort care. Making the person with dementia comfortable, both physically and emotionally, should be a primary consideration in the care of all persons with dementia. Persons with dementia who are truly comfortable will generally be less confused, more functional, and exhibit fewer behavior problems than those who are in some way uncomfortable. Persons with dementia who are comfortable rarely hit, scream, moan, or cry, and are much less likely to be agitated or act restless.

When working with persons with dementia and their caregivers, we often reference a simple equation to explain behavior problems:

$$CONFUSION + DISCOMFORT = BEHAVIOR\ PROBLEMS$$

The severity of the behavior problems often depends on either the severity of the confusion or the severity of the discomfort—higher levels of confusion, and/or higher levels of discomfort, will result in more severe behavior problems. Although realizing that this relationship is not absolute, we have found it to be true much of the time and to be an excellent guideline in helping others understand the importance of comfort in working with persons with dementia.

Comfort becomes an even more critical issue when it comes to persons with advanced dementia. These are the people at the far end of the dementia spectrum who are often helpless and are dependent on others for everything. Their sense of comfort is totally in the hands of their caregivers. To complicate this issue even further, persons with advanced dementia generally suffer from severe language and communication deficits. They generally cannot say what they need, ask for assistance, or explain their discomforts, nor can they describe their pain, request a drink of water, or ask to lie down. Additionally, they are unable to verbalize their likes and dislikes, or even complain about the care they are getting (ironically, nursing home staffs often list these total care residents as being among the easiest to care for, mostly because they make no demands and voice no complaints).

Comfort care is synonymous with good dementia care and should be the common denominator for all actions taken by caregivers. Keeping persons with advanced dementia truly comfortable is the key to minimizing, if not completely preventing, many of the behavior problems that persons with advanced dementia commonly exhibit. Skilled and conscientious caregivers who focus on comfort issues will see far fewer behavior problems than those caregivers who do not have such skills or focus.

A Soft Caregiving Approach

The manner in which caregivers approach persons with advanced dementia has an enormous impact on what behaviors will occur during caregiving, especially whether the individual will become resistive or combative during care (one of the most commonly reported behavior problems). Many of the behavior problems reported by caregivers are actually caused by those same caregivers because of their acting abrupt, rushed, cold, or sterile while giving care.

It is incumbent on caregivers to make every effort to keep the caregiving situation comfortable for the person with advanced dementia, even though the act of caregiving is highly intimate and intrusive. In our work, we advocate a soft caregiving approach that requires the caregiver to use a soft touch, soft voice, and soft expressions, gestures, and actions. There are other well-published names for this type of caregiving (e.g., Best Friends approach, Gentlecare), and they all stress the importance of caregivers making a warm and personal connection with the individual by maintaining a gentle, friendly, and respectful demeanor throughout caregiving. This includes smiling, making eye contact, using calm and soothing voice tones, applying a gentle touch, and going slow. The process should never be rushed or abrupt and should always focus on creating a safe, comfortable, and comforting situation in which care is given. The goal is to get the caregiving job done as comfortably and enjoyably as possible—if a feeling of comfort is maintained, it is likely that the person with advanced dementia will not resist or fight the caregiver. The concept is a universal one: A friendly approach elicits a friendly response; respect will be returned with respect; and a smile begets a smile. Preventing behavior problems is often just that easy.

Anticipating Needs

There has been much discussion in the dementia literature about the relationship between unmet needs and behavior. Persons with advanced dementia communicate via nonnormative behaviors when primary and secondary needs are not met (e.g., hungry or thirsty, hot or cold, incontinent, sick, in pain, tired, lonely, etc.). Need-driven behaviors are caused by unmet needs. These behaviors may be caused by unintentional physical or psychological discomfort imposed by well-meaning but inadequately trained caregivers who may not be recognizing and consequently not meeting the needs of the persons for whom they are providing care. In this regard, behaviors exhibited by persons with advanced dementia should be viewed as a direct expression of their discomfort and should alert caregivers that they have unmet needs that must be addressed.

More to the point, caregivers should make every effort to anticipate the needs of persons with advanced dementia instead of simply responding to them after they arise. Preventing pain in the first place is much preferable to treating it once it is there ("an ounce of prevention is worth a pound of cure"). Similarly, it is best to offer food and drink before individuals become hungry or thirsty, to reposition them before they become stiff and sore, to dress them warmly before they get cold, and to put them to bed before they are exhausted. Anticipating problems, rather than reacting to them, is one of the keys to preventing behavior problems in the first place.

Anticipating needs is not easy and requires caregivers to have a deep, comprehensive, and intimate knowledge of the persons for whom they provide care. This is especially true because, even in the advanced stages, persons with dementia have widely different needs, preferences, experiences, and perceptions. We often hear highly skilled and experienced nursing home certified nursing assistants say that, by far, the single most important element in good caregiving is to *know your resident*. They go on to explain that only in knowing your resident can caregivers truly understand and anticipate their residents' needs and make them comfortable on all levels. Moreover, of course, this challenge is made all the more difficult because persons with advanced dementia cannot describe their histories, talk about their families and friends, and express their preferences. Given those limitations, it is not always easy to know your resident well enough to anticipate his or her needs and truly make him or her comfortable.

Knowing the person with advanced dementia well enough to anticipate needs and maximize comfort requires effort. Facilities and individual caregivers should strive to gather relevant personal and historical information on persons for whom they provide care. Families should be asked to help in providing information, past and present, that could help in better knowing and understanding the person with advanced dementia. Caregivers should have consistent caregiving assignments (e.g., unchanging or monthly assignment rotations). Trial-and-error efforts should be made to learn about individual differences, subtle nuances, and personal preferences, including and especially learning about how an individual nonverbally communicates needs and comfort levels. Moreover, all of this should be clearly documented and communicated from one caregiver to the next so that everyone has the benefit of the accumulated knowledge being gathered.

■ GUIDING PRINCIPLES II: NONPHARMACOLOGIC INTERVENTIONS

Problem-Solving Strategies

Behavior management techniques are closely linked to sound caregiving techniques and ultimately rely on the knowledge, skills, and understanding caregivers bring to the caregiving situation. However, even when the soundest prevention measures are used with persons with advanced dementia, behavior problems will still occur—although in most cases they should be less frequent and less intense than when preventative measures are not used. Caregivers and other healthcare professionals should not assume that behavior problems are a direct symptom of the dementia and therefore cannot be resolved. There is always a reason why a person with advanced dementia acts the way he or she does. It is essential that caregivers make efforts to assess and treat these behaviors systematically and effectively.

It is recommended that caregivers and other healthcare professionals take a problem-solving approach to assessing and addressing behavior problems. Try to treat such problems empirically through a trial-and-error process:

- First, look for and treat all possible sources of physical discomfort. Persons with advanced dementia who are in pain will often express their pain by acting out behaviorally (e.g., resisting or fighting care, yelling, moaning, crying, etc.). Similarly, other causes of physical discomfort can be the source of the problem, such as being hot or cold, hungry or thirsty, wet or constipated, or simply tired.
- Second, consider the environment and the person's sensory needs and resolve any problematic issues. The environment may be overly stimulating with sound, light, or activity. Conversely, the setting may be too dark or too quiet, or in some other way understimulating, or the person may simply be bored. There may also be a new problem with vision or hearing that needs to be addressed.
- Third, assess the people who are nearby and may be adversely affecting the individual. Loud or intrusive peers could be triggering an upset. Caregivers may be using uncomfortable techniques or approaches when giving care, upsetting and distressing the person. Persons with advanced dementia may respond more negatively to certain caregivers than others—attempt to match them up with more compatible caregivers to facilitate a more positive care relationship.
- Fourth, assess for acute medical problems that could be causing an undiagnosed delirium that might trigger or exacerbate behaviors. Presently, healthcare professionals recognize that urinary tract infections can cause behavioral changes and are quick to test for them; however, they often stop there without looking for other acute medical causes. Further investigation, including possible laboratory tests, may be warranted to discover other possible medical causes. It is also important to assess for possible medication reactions as a reason for the change in behavior.

Antecedent Control

The use of antecedent control techniques is extremely effective in managing dementia-related behaviors for persons with late-stage dementia. Unlike learning-based techniques (e.g., cognitive retraining, operant conditioning, modeling, classical conditioning) often used in dealing with other challenging populations, antecedent control does not require the individual to remember or learn anything in order for behaviors to change and be managed.

The principles behind antecedent control are simple and intuitive:

- First, clearly define and describe the behavior at issue, including the frequency, duration, and intensity of the behavior.
- Second, assess the circumstances under which the behavior occurs, including locations, times of day, people involved, elements of the environmental (e.g., lighting, noise, etc.) activities that were going on when the behavior occurred, the

surrounding people's actions, and any other salient antecedents that may affect or influence the behavior.

■ Third, look for obvious cause-and-effect relationships between the identified antecedents and the behavior. If there are no obvious antecedents, begin a process of systematically altering all identified antecedents until the behavior problem improves or resolves.

■ Finally, identify alternative antecedents that do not trigger the behavior problem, or, better still, identify antecedents that actually elicit a positive behavior. Once identified, antecedents can be used to help manage behaviors. Eliminate those antecedents that trigger problems while simultaneously introducing or enhancing those antecedents that elicit more positive behaviors.

Examples:

■ Loud news or game shows played on television might elicit an agitated or disruptive response from some persons with advanced dementia. On the other hand, playing golden oldies or soothing classical music might trigger a more calm and comfortable response. In the future, caregivers should make sure that the calming music is played and the news and game shows are not.

■ A male caregiver experiences resistive combative behaviors from certain women with advanced dementia, whereas female caregivers have no such problems. It would be appropriate for only female caregivers to provide care to those individuals.

■ Most all advanced dementia residents of a nursing home unit become agitated and combative with a specific caregiver, but other caregivers have no such problems. Closer inspection finds that the caregiver's rushed and abrupt approach is upsetting the residents. Training the caregiver in using a soft approach resolves the problem, with her new caregiving skills eliciting more cooperative behaviors from the residents.

Although the principles behind antecedent control are simple, in practice, the process can be complicated given the myriad of possible antecedents to a specific behavior problem. Sometimes the situation is obvious and can be resolved instantly, such as with these examples. At other times, the situation can be complicated and may require several systematic interventions before the relevant antecedents can be identified, changed, and controlled.

Back Off, Distract, and Engage

Untrained caregivers often make the mistake of handling upsets head-on, either by pushing their way through the task (e.g., aggressively giving care even though the individual is resisting or fighting) or by trying to explain what they are doing, reasoning with the individual, or admonishing them for their behavior. This confrontational approach is usually ineffective and only serves to increase the discomfort, upset things even more, and worsen the problem.

A better response is to back off, slow down, and try to distract and engage the person with advanced dementia with something soothing and pleasant. For example, if an individual is resisting and fighting during incontinence care, caregivers might briefly stop what they are doing, smile and emphasize the soft approach described previously, and maybe offer the individual a favorite snack or treat. Once the upset has subsided, the caregiver can offer more treats, establish a better rapport, and begin the process of reapproaching the caregiving situation. If signs of the upset return, the caregiver can repeat the process by slowly and comfortably getting the job done bit by bit over time without ever triggering a major upset. This technique of backing off, distracting, pleasantly engaging, then reapproaching the caregiving task, can be highly effective in managing many difficult hands-on caregiving situations.

Distraction and engagement can also be effective in dealing with disruptive behavior such as yelling, crying, or moaning. Directly addressing the behavior will, more often than not, worsen the problem. Instead, caregivers should identify those activities (e.g., preferred snacks, favorite songs, going outside, brushing hair, gentle massage) that positively engage the person with advanced dementia, and use those activities as an effective intervention to quickly calm the person and help them to feel comfortable again. Remember, comfortable people do not hit, do not yell, and do not cry.

GUIDING PRINCIPLES III: PSYCHOPHARMACOLOGIC INTERVENTIONS

According to most published guidelines, the use of *psychotropic medication* to manage behavioral symptoms in dementia should be considered as a last resort, especially in older persons. Their use should be limited to the treatment of psychosis or severe and persistent agitation when these symptoms cause suffering, pose a danger, or interfere with needed care. Foundation for this precautionary stance is predicated on evidence regarding increased risk of significant adverse effects in older adults that range from sedation to an increased incidence of cerebrovascular events and death.

Despite a lack of evidence, the off-label use of antipsychotic agents is becoming routine in treating agitation and psychosis in persons with dementia. Although some clinicians believe that the risks for adverse effects may be lower with atypical antipsychotic agents such as quetiapine and risperidone as compared to a conventional agent such as haloperidol, the limited available evidence does not convincingly support this claim. In fact, because of the paucity of data and limitations of existing studies, there is currently no consensus as to which antipsychotic agent is preferred when treating persons with dementia who are exhibiting problematic behaviors. Other medications (e.g., benzodiazepines, antidepressants, mood stabilizers, cholinesterase inhibitors) have also been used to treat problematic behaviors demonstrated by persons with dementia, but clinical trials that support these approaches are also lacking.

Therefore, regardless of agent, the potential benefit of using psychoactive and antipsychotic agents in the management of problematic behavior in persons with advanced dementia must be weighed against potential risks, including increased falls, confusion, weight gain, slowing of movement and thinking, accelerating heart disease, and, in rare instances, death. Clinicians are cautioned to use a very conservative and cautious approach when prescribing and administering psychotropic medications in treating behavior problems. A general rule of thumb is to start low and go slow. Persons with advanced dementia are very frail. The recommended dosages for most psychoactive medications are considerably lower for this population than for persons with earlier stages of dementia. Additionally, polypharmacy with psychoactive and other medications must be avoided whenever possible.

Another important consideration is treatment duration. Psychoactive agents should be used for the briefest time necessary to address and manage the targeted behaviors. Clinicians and caregivers are directed to conduct monthly medication reviews to evaluate the continued indication, efficacy, dose, and existence of adverse side effects related to prescribed psychoactive agents. The necessity of continuing medication management of behaviors must be routinely considered and medications shown to be either ineffective or associated with adverse effects should be discontinued (see Exhibit 6.1).

EXHIBIT 6.1

Standards of Care for Managing Behaviors

A. The healthcare facility shall:
   1. Develop and implement policies and procedures for behavior management strategies that are consistent with established dementia care standards. This shall include:
      a. Criteria for admission and discharge;
      b. Proper documentation of behavior problems, especially when the safety and well-being of the person or other people are jeopardized;
      c. Proper reporting of significant behavior-related problems to primary care providers, consulting behavioral health specialists, oversight agencies, and responsible parties, especially when the safety and well-being of the person or other people are jeopardized;
      d. Policy and procedures for pain treatment that are sensitive to the possibility that disruptive behaviors may be an indicator of pain;
      e. Policy and procedures for the recognition of delirium that are sensitive to the possibility that disruptive behaviors may indicate acute confusion caused by an underlying physical illness or adverse drug reaction;
      f. Policy and procedures for the nonpharmacologic treatment of behavior problems;

    g. Policy and procedures for determining the appropriateness of making referrals to qualified professionals for assistance in assessing and treating behavior problems; and

    h. Policy and procedures for the routine and timely review of psychoactive medications.

2. Provide initial and ongoing training to care staff in the principles of:

    a. Understanding and using good caregiving techniques and approaches in caring for persons with advanced dementia, including emphases on comfort and on addressing unmet needs;

    b. Systematically assessing unmet needs by addressing the following areas: basic comfort, emotional needs, pain, and/or other illnesses;

    c. Recognizing and reporting changes in condition that could be indicative of pain, acute medical conditions, or other unmet needs;

    d. Properly assessing and addressing problematic behaviors; and

    e. The use of nonpharmacologic interventions in effectively treating problematic behaviors.

3. Provide a milieu that is dementia friendly and is neither overstimulating nor understimulating to people with advanced dementia.

4. Have available healthcare professionals and behavioral specialists who are qualified to assess and treat significant behavior problems.

5. Establish a policy and procedure for drafting life stories on all persons with advanced dementia:

    a. Life stories are to be included in persons' care plan to assist in improving comfort levels of persons.

    b. Life stories are to be made available to all caregivers so that they can better know and understand the individuals for whom they are caring.

B. Healthcare staff shall:

1. Make every effort to know the persons for whom they provide care by:

    a. Drafting schedules that emphasize consistent assignments to allow caregivers to get to know their patients;

    b. Matching caregivers with patients to increase positive interactions;

    c. Reading and learning the life stories of their patients; and

    d. Being observant of their patients' behavior patterns so that aberrant behavior can be promptly detected and reported.

2. Attend educational sessions designed to increase their skills in working with persons with advanced dementia, including training specific to the understanding and management of behavior problems. Specific training topics should include:

    a. Sound caregiving techniques (e.g., addressing behavior trigger, redirection strategies, etc.);

    b. Sound caregiving approaches (e.g., soft approaches, comfort care, etc.);

    c. Recognition, assessment, treatment of pain;

    d. Understanding behaviors and what they are communicating;

Continued

Exhibit 6.1 *Continued*

  e. Recognizing and anticipating needs;
  f. Techniques for meaningful engagement; and
  g. Nonpharmacologic approaches to behavior problems.
3. Anticipate and meet the broad range of comfort needs exhibited by persons who suffer from advanced dementia.
4. Provide flexibility in care and scheduling (e.g., individualized bathing schedules, offering snacks that are appealing to the patient).

C. Persons with advanced dementia shall expect:
  1. Caregivers who are trained in advanced dementia care and who demonstrate at least a rudimentary expertise in providing it.
  2. Caregivers who strive to make them comfortable physically and emotionally.
  3. To have access to adequate pain management and to be as free from physical and emotional pain as possible.
  4. To have their behaviors assessed in a systematic fashion that strives to determine causes of discomfort. These causes might include:
      a. Unmet basic comfort needs (e.g., hunger or thirst, hot or cold, positioning problems, bowel or bladder requirements, etc.);
      b. Unmet emotional needs (e.g., discomforts associated with environmental stressors, sensory stimulation, lack of meaningful human contact, poor caregiving approaches);
      c. Pain of any type; and
      d. Illness that is acute or chronic.
  5. Use of the least amount of medications possible to control behaviors on those occasions when pharmacological treatment is necessary.
  6. Referrals to qualified healthcare and behavioral healthcare specialists if discomfort, pain, suspected delirium, or behavior needs warrant.

▦ REFERENCES

Alexopoulos, G. S., Streim, J., Carpenter, D., & Docherty, J. P. (2004). Using antipsychotic agents in older patients. *Journal of Clinical Psychiatry, 65*(Suppl. 2:5–99), 100–104.

Algase, D. L., Beck, C., Kolanowski, A., Whall, A., Berent, S., Richards, K., et al. (1996). Need-driven dementia-compromised behavior: An alternative view of disruptive behavior. *American Journal of Alzheimer's Disease, 11*(6), 10–19.

Alzheimer's Association. (2009). *Alzheimer's disease facts and figures 2009.* Retrieved January 5, 2010, from http://alz.org/national/documents/report_alzfactsfigures2009.pdf

Alzheimer's Disease International. (2009). *World Alzheimer report executive summary 2009.* Retrieved January 5, 2010, from www.alz.co.uk/research/files/WorldAlzheimerReport-ExecutiveSummary.pdf

American Geriatrics Society and the American Association for Geriatric Psychiatry. Consensus statement on improving the quality of mental health care in U.S. nursing homes: Management of depression and behavioral symptoms associated with dementia. *Journal of the American Geriatrics Society, 51,* 1287–1298.

Ancoli-Israel, S., Martin J. L., Gehrman, P., Shochat, T., Corey-Bloom, J., Marler, M., et al. (2003). Effect of light on agitation in institutionalized patients with severe Alzheimer Disease. *American Journal of Geriatric Psychiatry, 11*(2), 194–203.

Arlt, S., & Jahn, H. (2006). Pharmacological treatment of non-Alzheimer dementias. *Current Opinion in Psychiatry, 19*(6), 642–648.

Ballard, C. (2008). Antipsychotics: No quick fix for people with dementia. *British Journal of Neuroscience Nursing, 4*(6), 261–262.

Ballard, C., Hanney, M. L., Theodoulou, M., Douglas, S., McShane, R., Kossakowski, K., et al. (2009). The dementia antipsychotic withdrawal trial (DART-AD): Long-term follow-up of a randomized placebo-controlled trial. *The Lancet Neurology, 8*(2), 151–157.

Beck C. K., Vogelpohl, T. S., Rasin, J. H., Uriri, J. T., O'Sullivan, P., Walls, R., et al. (2002). Effects of behavioral interventions on disruptive behavior and affect in demented nursing home persons. *Nursing Research, 51*(4), 219–228.

Boettger, S., & Breitbart, W. (2005). Atypical antipsychotics in the management of delirium. A review of the empirical literature. *Palliative & Supportive Care, 3*(3), 227–237.

Buffum, M. D., Hutt, E., Chang, V. T., Craine, M. H., & Snow, A. L. (2007). Cognitive impairment and pain management: Review of issues and challenges. *Journal of Rehabilitation Research & Development, 44*(2), 315–330.

Cohen-Mansfield, J. (2001). Nonpharmacologic interventions for inappropriate behaviors in dementia: A review, summary, and critique. *American Journal of Geriatric Psychiatry, 9*(4), 361–381.

Cohen-Mansfield, J., & Jensen, B. (2008). Assessment and treatment approaches for behavioral disturbances associated with dementia in the nursing home: Self-reports of physicians' practices. *Journal of the American Medical Directors Association, 9*(6), 406–413.

Cohen-Mansfield, J., & Mintzer, J. (2005). Time for change: The role of nonpharmacological interventions in treating behavior problems in nursing home residents with dementia. *Alzheimer Disease and Associated Disorders, 19*(1), 37–40.

Cohen-Mansfield, J., & Werner, P. (1997). Management of verbally disruptive behaviors in nursing home residents. *Journal of Gerontology Series A, Biological Sciences and Medical Sciences, 52* (6), M369–M377.

Colombo, M., Vitali, M., Cairati, R., Vaccaro, G., Andreoni, A., & Guaita, L. (2007). Behavioral and psychotic symptoms of dementia (BPSD) improvements in a special care unit: A factor analysis. *Archives of Gerontology and Geriatrics, 44*(Suppl. 1), 113–120.

Cummings, J. L., Schneider, E., Tariot, P. N., Graham, S. M., & Memantine MEM-MD-02 Study Group. (2006). Behavioral effects of memantine in Alzheimer disease patients receiving donepezil treatment. *Neurology, 67*(1), 57–63.

Davis, G. C. (1997). Chronic pain management of older adults in residential settings. *Journal of Gerontological Nursing, 23*(6), 16–22.

De Deyn, P. P. (2006). Drug treatment: Treatment of behavioral and psychological symptoms of dementia with neuroleptics. In A. Burns & B. Winblad (Eds.), *Severe dementia* (pp. 193–204). Hoboken, NJ: John Wiley & Sons, Inc.

Dewing, J. (2009, June). Caring for people with dementia: Noise and light. *Nursing Older People, 21* (5), 34–38.

Dolan, M. M., Hawkes, W. G., & Zimmerman, S. I., Morrison, R. S., Gruber-Baldini, A. L., Hebel, J. R., et al. (2000). Delirium on hospital admission in aged hip fracture patients: Prediction of mortality and 2-year functional outcomes. *Journal of Gerontology Series A Biological Science and Medical Sciences, 55*(9), M527–M534.

Edlund, A., Lundström, M., Brännström, B., Bucht, G., & Gustafson, Y. (2001). Delirium before and after operation for femoral neck fracture. *Journal of the American Geriatrics Society, 49*(10), 1335–1340.

Fick, D. M., Agostini, J. V., & Inouye, S. K. (2002). Delirium superimposed on dementia: A systematic review. *Journal of the American Geriatrics Society, 50*(10), 1723–1732.

Fick, D. M., Cooper, J. W., Wade, W. E., Waller, J. L., Maclean, J. R., & Beers, M. H. (2003). Updating the Beers criteria for potentially inappropriate medication use in older adults: Results of a U.S. consensus panel of experts. *Archives of Internal Medicine, 163*(22), 2716–2724.

Fick, D. M., & Foreman, M. D. (2000). Consequences of not recognizing delirium superimposed on dementia in hospitalized elderly individuals. *Journal of Gerontological Nursing, 26*(1), 30–40.

Fick, D. M., & Mion, L. (2007). Assessing and managing delirium in older adults with dementia. *Annals of Long-term Care,* D8. Retrieved November 15, 2009, from http://www.annalsoflong-termcare.com/article/7861

Fick, D. M., & Mion, L. C. (2008). Delirium superimposed on dementia: An algorithm for detecting and managing this underrecognized confluence of conditions. *American Journal of Nursing, 108*(1), 52–60.

Foreman, M. D. (1996). Nursing strategies for acute confusional states. *American Journal of Nursing, 96*(4), 44–51.

Franco, K. N., & Messinger-Rapport, B. (2006). Pharmacological treatment of neuropsychiatric symptoms of dementia: A review of the evidence. *Journal of the American Medical Directors Association, 7*(3), 201–202.

Gauthier, S., Wirth, Y., & Möbius, H. J. (2005). Effects of memantine on behavioural symptoms in Alzheimer's disease patients: An analysis of the Neuropsychiatric Inventory (NPI) data of two randomised, controlled studies. *International Journal of Geriatric Psychiatry, 20*(5), 459–464.

Gerdner, L., Buckwalter, K., & Hall, G. (2005). Temporal patterning of agitation and stressors associated with agitation: Case profiles to illustrate the progressively lowered stress threshold model. *Journal of the American Psychiatric Nurses Association, 11,* 215–222.

Holmes, C., Wilkinson, D., Dean, C., Vethanayagam, S., Olivieri, S., Langley, A., et al. (2004). The efficacy of donepezil in the treatment of neuropsychiatric symptoms in Alzheimer's disease. *Neurology, 63*(2), 214–219.

Holmes, C., Hopkins, V., Hensford, C., MacLaughlin, V., Wilkinson, D., & Rosenvinge, H. (2002). Lavender oil as a treatment for agitated behaviour in severe dementia: a placebo controlled study. *International Journal of Geriatric Psychiatry, 17*(4), 305–308.

Hooker, K., Bowman, S. R., Coehlo, D. P., Lim, S. R., Kaye, J., Guariglia, R., et al. (2002). Behavioral change in persons with dementia: Relationships with mental and physical health of caregivers. *The Journals of Gerontology Series B, Psychological Sciences and Social Sciences, 57*(5), P453–P460.

Jacobson, S. A., Pies, R. W., & Katz, I. R. (2007). *Clinical manual of geriatric psychopharmacology* (1st ed.). Arlington, VA: American Psychiatric Publishing, Inc.

Jeste, D. V., Meeks, T. W., Kim, D. S., & Zubenko, G. S. (2006). Research agenda for DSM-IV: Diagnostic categories and criteria for neuropsychiatric syndromes in dementia. *Journal of Geriatric Psychiatry and Neurology, 19*(3), 160–171.

Kelly, K. G., Zisselman, M., Cutillo-Schmitter, T., Reichard, R., Payne, D., & Denman, S. (2001). Severity and course of delirium in medically hospitalized nursing facility persons. *American Journal of Geriatric Psychiatry, 9*(1), 72–77.

Kerssens, C. J., & Pijnenburg, Y. A. (2008). Vulnerability to neuroleptic side effects in frontotemporal dementia. *European Journal of Neurology: The Official Journal of the European Federation of Neurological Societies, 15*(2), 111–112.

Keys, M. A., & DeWald, C. (2005). Clinical perspective on choice of atypical antipsychotics in elderly patients with dementia, part I. *Annals of Long-Term Care: Clinical Care and Aging, 13*(2), 26.

Kirshner, H. S. (2008). Controversies in behavioral neurology: The use of atypical antipsychotic drugs to treat neurobehavioral symptoms in dementia. *Current Neurology and Neuroscience Reports, 8*(6), 471–474.

Kovach, C. R., Noonan, P. E., Schlidt, A. M., & Wells, T. (2005). A model of consequences of need-driven, dementia-compromised behavior. *Journal of Nursing Scholarship, 37*(2), 134–140.

Lachs, M. S., Williams, C. S., O'Brien, S., & Pillemer, K. A. (2002). Adult protective service use and nursing home placement. *The Gerontologist, 42*(6), 734–739.

Leslie, D. L., Zhang, Y., Bogardus, S. T., Holford, T. R., Leo-Summers, L. S., & Inouye, S. K. (2005). Consequences of preventing delirium in hospitalized older adults on nursing home costs. *Journal of the American Geriatrics Society, 53*(3), 405–409.

Lenzer, J. (2005). FDA warns about using antipsychotic drugs for dementia. *British Medical Journal, 330*(7497), 922.

Lindsey, P., & Buckwalter, K. (2009). Psychotic events in Alzheimer's disease: Applications of the PLST model. *Journal of Gerontological Nursing, 35*(8), 20–37.

Long, C. (2009). Palliative care for advanced dementia. *Journal of Gerontological Nursing, 35*(11), 19–24.

Markowitz, J. D., & Narasimhan, M. (2008). Delirium and antipsychotics: A systematic review of epidemiology and somatic treatment options. *Psychiatry, 5*(10), 29–36.

McCarthy, M. (2003). Situated clinical reasoning: Distinguishing acute confusion from dementia in hospitalized older adults. *Research in Nursing & Health, 26*(2), 90–101.

Merrilees, J. (2007). A model for management of behavioral symptoms in frontotemporal lobar degeneration. *Alzheimer Disease and Associated Disorders, 21*(4), S64–S69.

Passant, U., Elfgren, C., Englund, E., & Gustafson, L. (2005). Psychiatric symptoms and their psychosocial consequences in frontotemporal dementia. *Alzheimer Disease and Associated Disorders, 19*(Suppl. 1), S15–S18.

Pelland, C., & Trudel, J. F. (2009). Atypical antipsychotic efficacy and safety in managing delirium: A systematic review and critical analysis. *Psychology and Neuropsychiatry, 7*(2), 109–119.

Richardson, S. (2003). Delirium: Assessment and treatment of the elderly patient. *American Journal for Nurse Practitioners*, 9–15.

Seitz, D. P., Gill, S. S., & van Zyl, L. T., (2007). Antipsychotics in the treatment of delirium: A systematic review. *Journal of Clinical Psychiatry, 68*(1), 11–21.

Semla, T. P., Belzer, J. L., & Higbee, M. D. (2009). *Geriatric dosage handbook* (14th ed.). Hudson, OH: Lexi-Comp.

Sink, K. M., Holden, K. F., & Yaffe, K. (2005). Pharmacological treatment of neuropsychiatric symptoms of dementia: A review of the evidence. *The Journal of the American Medical Association, 293*(5), 596–608.

Souder, E., & O'Sullivan, P. (2003). Disruptive behaviors of older adults in an institutional setting: Staff time required to manage disruptions. *Journal of Gerontological Nursing, 29*(8), 31–36.

Srikanth, S., Nagaraja, A.V., & Ratnavalli, E. (2005). Neuropsychiatric symptoms in dementia-frequency, relationship to dementia severity and comparison in Alzheimer's disease, vascular dementia and frontotemporal dementia. *Journal of the Neurological Sciences, 236*(1–2), 43–48.

Swanberg, M. M. (2007). Memantine for behavioral disturbances in frontotemporal dementia: A case series. *Alzheimer Disease and Associated Disorders, 21*(2), 164–166.

Tariot, P. N. (2003). Medical management of advanced dementia. *Journal of the American Geriatrics Society, 51*(Suppl. 5), S305–S313.

Volicer, L. (2008). End-of-life care for people with dementia in long-term care settings. *Alzheimer's Care Today, 9*(2), 84–102.

Vossel, K. A., & Miller, B. L. (2008). New approaches to the treatment of frontotemporal lobar degeneration. *Current Opinion in Neurology, 21*(6), 708–716.

Wittenberg, D., Possin, K. L., Rascovsky, K., Rankin, K. P., Miller, B. L., & Kramer, J. H. (2008). The early neuropsychological and behavioral characteristics of frontotemporal dementia. *Neuropsychology Review, 18*(1), 91–102.

7

ASSESSING AND ADDRESSING PAIN

Jan Dougherty, Judith Sgrillo, and A. Elizabeth Swan

INTRODUCTION

Pain is prevalent in care homes to a far greater degree than many people might expect. Of the more than two million elders living in nursing homes today, reports suggest that as many as 65% suffer from some form of persistent pain. However, even though persistent pain is common in nursing homes, less than half of the residents who experience pain are prescribed routine pain medications. Worse still, although persons with cognitive impairment experience pain at a higher rate than those who are cognitively clear, they are even less likely to receive routine pain medications. This is the case even though most individuals in the mild and moderate stages of dementia can still talk, and at least to some extent, can still express their needs and verbalize their pains.

Pain negatively affects quality of life and must be addressed vigorously. However, what happens to the people suffering from advanced dementia who are in pain but are unable to say so? How do we know when such patients are in pain? How would they express their pain? Moreover, what can we do to help them? Unnoticed pain leads to unnecessary suffering, and persons with advanced dementia are the most likely to have their pain go unnoticed. These individuals cannot use call lights, cannot voice needs, cannot make complaints, and cannot tell anyone about their pains.

However, persons with advanced dementia do communicate their pain in nonverbal ways through their behaviors. In the past, it was believed that escalating behaviors were directly caused by cognitive impairment. Now it is recognized that persons with advanced dementia often express pain through their emotions and behaviors, and that many common behavior problems exhibited by persons with advanced dementia are actually very basic reflexive reactions to pain. However, it is still common practice to give tranquilizers or other psychoactive drugs for these behaviors instead of first considering pain as a possibility. In a surprisingly high percentage of cases, it makes more sense and is more effective to give pain medications for behavior problems than it is to give tranquilizers.

This chapter outlines the recommended pain assessment process, pain tools, pharmacologic and nonpharmacologic interventions, and outcomes to treating pain and promoting comfort in persons with advanced dementia.

GUIDELINES FOR ASSESSING PAIN IN PERSONS WITH ADVANCED DEMENTIA

Pain assessment is more challenging for persons with advanced dementia than with most other populations. When older persons who do not have dementia experience pain, they can tell their medical providers and receive appropriate treatment. However, persons with advanced dementia do not have the verbal skills to voice their pain and, instead, exhibit behavioral changes that are easy to misinterpret. As a result, pain in these individuals is more difficult to assess and more difficult to treat.

Physicians who treat persons with dementia demonstrate good reliability and validity for detecting and diagnosing when working with persons who are in the mild-to-moderate stages of dementia. However, their reliability and validity for detecting pain drops significantly when assessing persons in the later stages, with pain often being underestimated or missed altogether. One reason for this is the communication problem—persons with advanced dementia cannot answer simple questions like, "Do you have pain?" Another reason is that symptom presentation is confounded by other possible discomforts, including emotional distress, constipation, cold, hunger, fatigue, or positioning issues. Psychotropic medications can also be a problem because they tend to mask symptoms of pain.

Caregivers' attitudes and actions may also hinder the detection of pain in persons with advanced dementia. Caregivers may be sensitized to pain and attribute pain-related behaviors to cognitive or psychiatric problems. Nurses may avoid giving pain medications in fear of inducing delirium or drug dependencies, or they may be reluctant to use opioids without a clear diagnosis. It is also common for frequent caregiver rotations to result in caregivers not knowing their residents well enough to recognize their highly individual and subtle indicators of pain.

When considering pain management issues for persons with advanced dementia, facilities should strive to keep abreast of the research and literature. Keeping current with up-to-date evidence-based pain management protocols and guidelines can ensure that best practices are being used with this extremely challenging population.

PAIN ASSESSMENT STRATEGIES

Research has demonstrated that those persons with Mini-Mental State Exam (MMSE) scores of less than 15 cannot reliably use any of the traditional pain scales that require verbal responses from patients. There are several such pain assessment tools that are commonly used in pain assessment. These includes the following:

■ *Wong-Baker Pain Scale.* The Wong-Baker Pain scale, also known as the "Faces Scale," asks individuals to look at the picture and pick the face that represents how he or she feels. This tool is too abstract for persons with dementia and relies on the caregiver to fit the picture to the person, making the instrument an unreliable predictor of pain. This scale is for persons who are cognitively intact and should not be used with persons who have dementia at any level.

▨ *Visual Analog Scale (VAS)*. The VAS asks individuals to mark where on the line he or she would rate his or her pain. This tool is too complex for persons with moderate or severe dementia, but is acceptable for persons who are cognitively intact or who exhibit mild cognitive impairment.

▨ *Verbal Rating Scale (VRS)*. The VRS uses a rating scale of 1 to 10 to rate pain by asking the question, "On a scale of 0 to 10, with 0 meaning *no pain* and 10 meaning the *worst pain* you can imagine, how much pain are you having now?" This requires patients to then rate their pain by ascribing it a number in response to the question. Some long-term care facilities have simplified the scale to 0 to 5, but even these ratings are too abstract for persons with moderate or severe dementia. This scale is for persons who are cognitively intact and perhaps persons with mild dementia, but should not be used with persons beyond the early stages of dementia.

▨ *McGill Pain Scale*. This scale uses verbal descriptors and, interestingly, does best with persons who have mild and moderate dementia. The scale requires patients to pick words that best describe their pain: *no pain* (0), *mild* (1), *discomforting* (2), *distressing* (3), *horrible* (4), or *excruciating* (5). This is an acceptable tool for persons who are cognitively intact, a reasonable tool for those who are somewhat cognitively impaired, but not appropriate for persons with advanced dementia because they cannot understand the directions and do not have the necessary language skills to process and say the descriptor words.

▨ *Pain Assessment in Advanced Dementia (PAINAD)*. The PAINAD (Table 7.1) uses nonverbal cues as indicators of pain and is therefore recommended for use with those persons who have advanced dementia. A score greater than 4 indicates the need to provide pain intervention.

Assessing pain for those with dementia is necessary but difficult. Another, more comprehensive approach to pain assessment that is recommended for persons with advanced dementia, is the Assessment of Discomfort in Dementia (ADD) used by the Palliative Care Center at Medical College of Wisconsin. The ADD protocol was developed as a way to identify sources of physical and affective discomfort, which it does through a five-step process.

Step 1: Look for physical causes of discomfort. If the source of discomfort is identified, meet the person's needs. For example, determine if the person is hungry or thirsty, hot or old, wet or soiled, or has other sensory-related issues (e.g., bored, lonely, sad, missing glasses, hearing aids out of place). The person is asked to point to himself or herself to assist the caregiver in determining if pain is present, with an objective being to identify the physical cause of the individual's discomfort.

Step 2: Obtain a current history and physical (H&P). Review the H&P and assess current clinical findings, looking for comorbidities that could be sources of pain. Reexamine old problems identified on the H&P and look for new problems that might have arisen. Note behavioral symptoms such as facial expressions (e.g., grimacing, frowning, worried), changes in mood (e.g., irritable, withdrawn, agitated), verbal expressions and voice (e.g., yelling, whining, moaning), body language (e.g., tense, restless, hypoactive, abusive), and behavior (change in appetite, sleep, gait). Also, note nonverbal measures of pain such as crying, yelling, moaning, grimacing, restlessness, tense muscles, agitation, combativeness, pulling away when touched,

TABLE 7.1

Pain Assessment in Advanced Dementia

	0	1	2	Score
Breathing independent of vocalization	Normal	Occasional labored breathing, short period of hyperventilation	Noisy labored breathing, long period of hyperventilation, Cheyne-Stokes respirations (see "PAINAD Item Definitions")	
Negative vocalization	None	Occasional moan or groan, low level of speech with a negative or disapproving quality	Repeated troubled calling out, loud moaning or groaning, crying	
Facial expression	Smiling or inexpressive	Sad, frightened, frowning	Grimacing	
Body language	Relaxed	Tense, distressed pacing, fidgeting	Rigid, fists clenched, knees pulled up, pulling or pushing away, striking out	
Consolability	No need to console	Distracted or reassured by voice or touch	Unable to console, distract, or reassure	

Note: Total scores greater than 4 require intervention for pain.   Total: _____

Note. "Development and Psychometric Evaluation of the Pain Assessment in Advanced Dementia (PAINAD) Scale" by V. Warden, A. C. Hurley, and L. Volicer, 2003, *Journal of the American Medical Directors Association*, *4*, 9–15. Copyright 2003 by Elsevier. Reprinted with permission from Victoria Warden, May 25, 2004.

PAINAD Item Definitions

Breathing

1. *Normal breathing.* DESCRIPTION: Characterized by effortless, quiet, rhythmic (smooth) respirations.
2. *Occasional labored breathing.* DESCRIPTION: Characterized by episodic bursts of harsh, difficult, or wearing respirations.
3. *Short period of hyperventilation.* DESCRIPTION: Characterized by intervals of rapid, deep breaths lasting a short period of time.
4. *Noisy labored breathing.* DESCRIPTION: Characterized by negative sounding respirations on inspiration or expiration. They may be loud, gurgling, wheezing. They appear strained or worn down.
5. *Long period of hyperventilation.* DESCRIPTION: Characterized by an excessive rate and depth of respirations lasting a considerable time.
6. *Cheyne-Stokes respirations.* DESCRIPTION: Characterized by rhythmic waxing and waning of breathing from very deep to shallow respirations with periods of apnea (cessation of breathing).

Negative Vocalization

1. *None.* DESCRIPTION: Characterized by speech or vocalization that has a neutral or pleasant quality.
2. *Occasional moan or groan.* DESCRIPTION: Characterized by mournful or murmuring sounds, wails, or lamentation. Groaning is characterized by louder-than-usual inarticulate involuntary sounds, often abruptly beginning and ending.
3. *Low-level speech with a negative or disapproving quality.* DESCRIPTION: Characterized by muttering, mumbling, whining, grumbling, or swearing in a low volume with a complaining, sarcastic or caustic tone.
4. *Repeated troubled calling out.* DESCRIPTION: Characterized by phrases or words being used over and over in a tone that suggests anxiety, uneasiness, or distress.
5. *Loud moaning or groaning.* DESCRIPTION: Characterized by mournful or murmuring sounds, wails, or laments in much louder-than-usual volume. Loud groaning is characterized by louder-than-usual inarticulate involuntary sounds, often abruptly beginning and ending.
6. *Crying.* DESCRIPTION: Characterized by an utterance of emotion accompanied by tears. There may be sobbing or quiet weeping.

Facial Expression

1. *Smiling or inexpressive.* DESCRIPTION: Characterized by upturned mouth, brightening of the eyes, and a look of pleasure or contentment. Inexpressive refers to a neutral, at ease, relaxed, or blank look.
2. *Sad.* DESCRIPTION: Characterized by an unhappy, lonesome, sorrowful, or dejected look. There may be tears in the eyes.
3. *Frightened.* DESCRIPTION: Characterized by a look of fear, alarm, or heightened anxiety. Eyes appear wide open.
4. *Frown.* DESCRIPTION: Characterized by a downward turn of the corners of the mouth. Increased facial wrinkling in the forehead and around the mouth may appear.
5. *Facial grimacing.* DESCRIPTION: Characterized by a distorted or distressed look. The brow is more wrinkled, as is the area around the mouth. Eyes may be squeezed shut.

Body Language

1. *Relaxed.* DESCRIPTION: Characterized by calm, restful, or mellow appearance. The person seems to be taking it easy.
2. *Tense.* DESCRIPTION: Characterized by a strained, apprehensive, or worried appearance. The jaw may be clenched. (Exclude contractures of any extremities.)
3. *Distressed pacing.* DESCRIPTION: Characterized by activity that seems unsettled. There may be a fearful, worried, or disturbed element present. The rate may be faster or slower.
4. *Fidgeting.* DESCRIPTION: Characterized by restless movement, such as squirming about or wiggling in the chair. Repetitive touching, tugging, or rubbing body parts can also be observed.
5. *Rigid.* DESCRIPTION: Characterized by stiffening of the body. The arms and/or legs are tight and inflexible. The trunk may appear straight and unyielding. (Exclude any contractures.)
6. *Fists clenched.* DESCRIPTION: Characterized by tightly closed hands, which may be opened and closed repeatedly or held tightly shut.
7. *Knees pulled up.* DESCRIPTION: Characterized by flexing the legs and drawing the knees up toward the chest. The person may have an overall troubled appearance. (Exclude any contractures.)

Continued

Table 7.1 *Continued*

8. *Pulling or pushing away.* DESCRIPTION: Characterized by resistiveness on approach or to care. The person may try to escape by yanking or wrenching free or by shoving you away.
9. *Striking out.* DESCRIPTION: Characterized by hitting, kicking, grabbing, punching, biting, or other form of personal assault.

Consolability

1. *No need to console.* DESCRIPTION: Characterized by a sense of well-being. The person appears content.
2. *Distracted or reassured by voice or touch.* DESCRIPTION: Characterized by a disruption in the behavior when the person is spoken to or touched. The behavior stops during the period of interaction with no indication that the person is at all distressed.
3. *Unable to console, distract, or reassure.* DESCRIPTION: Characterized by the inability to soothe the person or stop a behavior with words or actions. No amount of comforting, either verbal or physical, will alleviate the behavior.

and rubbing or holding body parts. This is also the point where the PAINAD scale might be used.

Step 3: If the assessment is negative for clear indicators of pain, caregivers should try nonpharmacologic interventions to deal with the behaviors at hand. Interventions would include comfort measures that address the individual's comfort needs, antecedents and distracters that help the person engage in activities that are interesting and comforting, and therapeutic changes in the milieu and social setting.

Step 4: If nonpharmacologic interventions are unsuccessful, medical providers and caregivers should then try pharmacologic interventions designed to directly treat pain. This should be done by following the World Health Organization's (WHO) 3-Step Pain Relief Ladder, which was originally designed for cancer pain relief, but is highly applicable for pain control with persons who have advanced dementia. In this case, start with nonopioids (e.g., Tylenol, aspirin) and see if they work. If necessary, move up to mild opioids (e.g., codeine). If that proves ineffective, try stronger opioids (e.g., morphine) until the person is free of pain. Additional drugs, "adjuvants," can be used at any level of the ladder to deal with ancillary symptoms, and drugs should be given routinely rather than on demand for maximum affect.

Step 5: If pain medications and other nonpharmacologic interventions fail to resolve the behavior, then psychotropic medications may be considered (refer to chapter 6, on behaviors, and chapter 8, on medications, for more information).

▦ PAIN INTERVENTIONS REQUIRE ONGOING EVALUATION

Caregivers should complete a pain assessment using the PAINAD and the ADD guidelines on a daily basis whenever behaviors first appear, escalate, or change. They should continue to use these tools until the person's PAINAD score is less than 4. Regularly scheduled pain interventions, such as the use of pain medications, should be put into place. Also, caregivers should always be sure to evaluate the outcomes that result from the pain intervention relative to the intended result.

Caregivers should consider using the analgesic trial to address pain, documenting all pain outcomes by noting changes in behaviors as they correspond to treatments. Similarly, caregivers should document changes in the use of psychotropic drugs and corresponding behavior changes, and they should note the use and effects of nonpharmacologic interventions. The goal is to take a systematic approach to assess the effects of all iatrogenic elements to the individual's treatment regimen in order to learn what works and what does not work in the treatment of the individual's pain.

The implications of this approach to assessing and treating pain in persons with advanced dementia are significant. First, behavioral observations are a key to discerning if persons with advanced dementia have pain, especially because they cannot be reliably assessed using traditional pain measurement tools. Second, caregivers are a critical link in the pain assessment chain—they are the ones who are most likely to notice and report behavioral indicators of pain. As such, it is important that caregivers have staffing assignments that allow them to truly get to know their residents over time. Third, pain medications should be used in dealing with behavior problems before using psychotropic medications. Fourth, pain medications should be prescribed on a routine basis rather than as needed in order to be effective. Finally, the interdisciplinary team, including the clinical pharmacist, should evaluate the appropriate use of pain medications and psychotropic medications on a regular basis.

Facilities should consider quality indicators that address pain management that can be adopted for long-term care and are applicable to those with advanced dementia. Staff and families need to be adequately informed about pain management. Pain intensity measures should be coupled with appropriate pain rating scales, and those measures should be documented at frequent intervals. A multimodal approach should be used when assessing and addressing pain, such as the one found in the ADD guidelines. The goal in treating persons with advanced dementia is to prevent and control pain to a degree that maximizes function and quality of life and to do so as accurately and effectively as is seen with persons who do not have advanced dementia.

EXHIBIT 7.1

Standards of Care Related to Assessing and Managing Pain

A. The healthcare facility shall:
1. Adopt a care philosophy that respects the person's right to effective pain management.
2. Have two separate policies and procedures to address the assessment, interventions, and evaluation of pain for:
    a. Persons with advanced dementia or those who are cognitively impaired, and
    b. Persons who are not cognitively impaired.

Continued

Exhibit 7.1 *Continued*

3. Institute a policy and procedure that supports regular consultation by a clinical pharmacist of the person's medication profile to ensure that the person with advanced dementia:
   a. Is free of inappropriate psychotropic medications when psychosis and severe agitation are no longer present, and
   b. Receives adequate and appropriate pain medications.
4. Adopt a standardized and relevant process (ADD) and pain assessment tool (PAINAD) that measures pain for those who have advanced dementia or those who are cognitively impaired.
5. Adopt the WHO's 3-Step Pain Relief Ladder as the means for determining pharmacologic interventions for pain.
6. Ensure that accurate and timely documentation occurs on the medical record as it relates to pain assessment, planning, interventions, and evaluation.
7. Execute regular quality improvement audits to determine if staff is regularly assessing, intervening, and evaluating pain.
8. Provide orientation and regular training programs for the interdisciplinary team related to current pain management strategies.
9. Provide assurances that ongoing training programs are current and contain up-to-date clinical information.

B. Healthcare staff shall:
1. Receive initial and ongoing annual training in pain management strategies that includes assessment, intervention, and evaluation strategies for individuals who have advanced dementia, who are cognitively impaired, or for others who are cognitively intact.
2. Implement the healthcare facility pain policies and procedures.
3. Anticipate and meet the basic needs for individuals who have discomfort and pain through the following measures:
   a. Conduct regular pain assessments and provide the requisite intervention whenever a person verbalizes pain or discomfort or displays new or exacerbated behaviors. Communicate findings to the primary care provider.
      ▪ A pain assessment will be completed on each new admission to a facility.
      ▪ A pain assessment will be completed on any change in a person's behavior or if a new behavior is exhibited.
      ▪ Pain assessments will be conducted during the most uncomfortable time of the day or most discomforting event for that person.
   b. Complete a comprehensive pain assessment when the person with dementia scores greater than 4 on the PAINAD scale. Communicate these findings to the primary care provider.
   c. Provide effective pain management using routine pharmacologic and routine nonpharmacologic interventions. Offer pain medications on a regular schedule and not on an as needed basis. The WHO's 3-Step Pain

Relief Ladder will be used when providing pharmacologic management for those persons in pain. Nonpharmacologic management includes, but is not limited to, massage, heat or cold applications, and other modalities that meet pain needs and provide meaningful connections.

    d. Continue to evaluate the person's pain daily, and more frequently as needed, until the scores drop below a score of 4.

C. Persons with advanced dementia shall expect:
1. The appropriate assessment and plan for successful pain management.
2. Implementation of pain protocols that use the WHO's 3-Step Pain Relief Ladder.
3. The evaluation of the pain intervention to determine the effectiveness and corresponding relief.
4. To be free of inappropriate psychotropic medications when psychosis and severe agitation is no longer present.
5. That behaviors will be regarded as manifestations of pain first before progressing to psychotropic medications.

▓ REFERENCES

American Geriatrics Society Panel on Pharmacological Management of Persistent Pain in Older Persons. (2009). Pharmacological management of persistent pain in older persons. *Journal of the American Geriatrics Society, 57*(8), 1331–1346.

Brown, R. C. (2001). Persistent pain in nursing home residents. *Journal of the American Medical Association, 286*(7), 788.

Buffum, M. D., Hutt, E., Chang, V. T., Craine, M. H., & Snow, A. L. (2007). Cognitive impairment and pain management: Review of issues and challenges. *Journal of Rehabilitation Research & Development, 44*(2), 315–330.

Center for Gerontology and Health Care Research. (2004). *Persistent severe pain: Arizona.* Retrieved September 16, 2004, from http://www.chcr.brown.edu/dying/azpspdata.htm

Chibnall, J. T., Tait, R. C., Harman, B., & Luebbert, R. A. (2005). Effect of acetaminophen on behavior, well-being, and psychotropic medication use in nursing home residents with moderate-to-severe dementia. *Journal of the American Geriatrics Society, 53*(11), 1921–1929.

Cohen-Mansfield, J., & Lipson, S. (2002). Pain in cognitively impaired nursing home residents: How well are physicians diagnosing it? *Journal of the American Geriatrics Society, 50*(6), 1039–1044.

Cohen-Mansfield, J., & Mintzer, J. E. (2005). Time for change: The role of non-pharmacological interventions in treating behavior problems in nursing home residents with dementia. *Alzheimer Disease & Associated Disorders, 19*, 37–40.

Epps, C. D. (2001). Recognizing pain in the institutionalized elder with dementia. *Geriatric Nursing, 022*(2), 71–77.

Feldt, K. S. (2000). Improving assessment and treatment of pain in cognitively impaired nursing home residents. *Annals of Long-Term Care, 8*(9), 36–42.

Fries, B. E., Simon, S. E., Morris, J. N, Flodstrom, C., & Bookstein, F. L. (2001). Pain in U.S. nursing homes: Validating a pain scale for the minimum data set. *The Gerontologist, 41*(2), 173–179.

Gordon, D. B., Pellino, T. A., Miaskowski, C., McNeill, J. A., Paice, J. A., Laferriere, D., et al. (2002). A 10-year review of quality improvement in pain management: Recommendations for standardized outcome measures. *Pain Management in Nursing, 3*(4), 116–130.

Hutt, E., Pepper, G. A., Vojir, C., Fink, R., & Jones, K. R. (2006). Assessing the appropriateness of pain medication prescribing practices in nursing homes. *Journal of the American Geriatrics Society, 54*(2), 213–239.

Kovach, C. R., Griffie, J., Muchka, S., Noonan, P. E., & Weissman, D. E. (2000). Nurses' perceptions of pain assessment and treatment in the cognitively impaired elderly. It's not a guessing game. *Clinical Nurse Specialist, 14*(5), 215–220.

Kovach, C. R., Weissman, D. E., Griffie, J., Matson, S., & Muchka, S. (1999). Assessment and treatment of discomfort for people with late-stage dementia. *Journal of Pain and Symptom Management, 18*(6), 412–419.

Last Acts. (2002). *Means to a better end: A report on dying in America today.* Washington, DC: Author.

Marquette University, & the Palliative Care Program at the Medical College of Wisconsin. (1997). *Improving management of physical pain and affective discomfort for people with dementia in long-term care.* Milwaukee, WI: Authors.

Mitchell, S. L., Morris, J. N., Park, P. S., & Fries, B. E. (2004). Terminal care for persons with advanced dementia in the nursing home and home care settings. *Journal of Palliative Medicine, 7*(6), 808–816.

Teno, J. M., Weitzen, S., Wetle, T., & Mor, V. (2001). Persistent pain in nursing home residents. *Journal of the American Medical Association, 285*(16), 2081.

Warden, V., Hurley, A. C., & Volicer, L. (2003). Development and psychometric evaluation of the Pain Assessment in Advanced Dementia (PAINAD) scale. *Journal of the American Medical Directors Association, 4,* 9–15.

World Health Organization. (1990). *Cancer pain relief and palliative care.* Geneva, Switzerland: Author.

Wynne, C. F., Ling, S. M., & Remsburg, R. (2000). Comparison of pain assessment instruments in cognitively intact and cognitively impaired nursing home residents. *Geriatric Nursing, 21,* 20–23.

8

ENSURING THE APPROPRIATE USE OF MEDICATIONS IN ADVANCED DEMENTIA

Marianne McCarthy, Maribeth Gallagher, and Marwan Sabbagh

▨ INTRODUCTION

Healthcare professionals are generally faced with challenges when it comes to the appropriate use of medications in the elderly. Many physiological changes occur with aging and these changes can affect the pharmacokinetics (the action of a drug in the body over a period of time, including the processes of absorption, distribution, metabolism, and excretion) and/or pharmacodynamics (the duration and magnitude of response to a drug observed relative to the concentration of the drug) of medications.[1] Most drugs on the market do not have clear dosing recommendations for the elderly. Polypharmacy (prescribing multiple drugs to a patient), another common problem among the elderly people, can heighten the potential for adverse drug reactions. In the United States, residents in long-term care settings take an average of 6.67 medications each day, 27% of them take nine or more.

Persons with dementia present particular challenges, and those in the terminal stages of dementia present the greatest of all. For instance, drugs presently prescribed for the treatment of agitation are considered *off label*. A medication is off label when it is prescribed for a purpose other than its approved use. To date, the Food and Drug Administration (FDA) has not approved medication for the treatment of dementia-related psychosis or agitation. Complicating matters, the FDA has required black box warnings regarding moderate but statistically significant cardiac and cerebrovascular risks and risks of death associated with the use of antipsychotic agents that are generally prescribed to treat psychosis and agitation in people with dementia. (The FDA has required manufacturers of atypical antipsychotics to put the labeling of moderate but statistically significant cardiac and cerebrovascular risks and risks of death associated with the use of antipsychotic agents that are generally prescribed to treat psychosis and agitation in people with dementia [commonly known as a black box warning]).

---

[1] The shorthand forms are PK, what the body does to the drug, and PD, what the drug does to the body.

93

With both older adults in general and Alzheimer's patients in particular, it is advisable to start low and go slow when it comes to medications. With Alzheimer's patients, however, special considerations apply in treating dementia-related symptoms such as cognitive and functional decline, psychosis, and behavioral disturbances.

PHARMACOLOGIC MANAGEMENT: PHILOSOPHY AND GENERAL TREATMENT STRATEGIES

Medications are used to manage various medical, psychiatric, and behavioral symptoms manifested by people with advanced dementia. This section describes general treatment strategies.

With behavioral problems, before initiating pharmacologic intervention, caregivers and healthcare providers are urged to consider a nine-step approach that includes:

1. Giving attention to meet the patient's basic needs;
2. Completing a history and physical;
3. Using of nonpharmacologic interventions first;
4. Using of pharmacologic approaches with psychotropic medications (see chapters 6 and 7 for more specifics);
5. Making efforts to decrease polypharmacy by discontinuing all unessential drugs, especially those with anticholinergic properties (e.g., diphenydramine and oxybutinin; discussed at greater length later in this chapter);
6. Introducing new drugs one at a time and titrate to therapeutic effect;
7. Performing a comprehensive review of all medications monthly, per the Omnibus Reconciliation Act (OBRA), or with every medication change;
8. Considering ethnopharmacological issues when treating diverse populations. Ethnopharmacology examines the relationship between ethnicity and drug response including drug absorption, distribution, metabolism, and excretion (see chapter 15 for additional information);
9. Considering coexistent diseases, for example, it would be important to consider when or if it is necessary to withdraw medication management in a coexisting condition. Ideally, these issues will have been predetermined and documented in a person's advanced directives.

MEDICAL MANAGEMENT STRATEGIES

This section provides guidelines for selecting and managing medications that modify dementing illnesses and disease progression.

Primary Dementia Pharmacotherapy

Treatment recommendations given here are primarily related to the pharmacologic management of Alzheimer's disease (AD). Other dementias will be addressed later on.

Cholinesterase Inhibitors

Cholinesterase inhibitors enhance acetylcholine activity and thereby improve memory and cognition. Examples of these drugs include donepezil hydrochloride (Aricept, the only donepezil hydrochloride that is used for both severe and mild-to-moderate AD), galantamine, rivastigmine tartrate (approved to treat mild-to-moderate AD and Parkinson's disease dementia), and tacrine hydrochloride. Tacrine is no longer used commonly in the United States. They can produce a modest decrease in disease progression; slow cognitive and functional decline; modestly decrease psychotic symptoms such as delusions, paranoia, and hallucinations; and have a modest effect on apathy, agitation, and possibly anxiety.

The major side effects are gastrointestinal in nature (e.g., nausea, vomiting, diarrhea). Cholinesterase inhibitors are approved by the FDA for the treatment of mild-to-moderate dementia. When used at this stage, they may delay the need for nursing home placement by up to 6–12 months.

Memantine HCl

The FDA has also approved memantine HCl for moderate-to-severe dementia. The drug works through a different mechanism of action. Specifically, it partially blocks the NMDA receptor (N-Methyl D-Aspartate) thereby reducing a cellular event called excitotoxicity. This agent is commonly prescribed in conjunction with cholinesterase inhibitors in the later stages of the disease. However, use as a monotherapy may also be considered. A 3-month trial of memantine HCl is recommended for evaluating efficacy. Preassessments and postassessments of the patient's cognitive and functional status should be conducted to determine whether therapy is effective.

Ongoing Assessment and Management

Although significant results can be obtained with different cholinesterase inhibitors and memantine HCl, the disease will eventually progress to an advanced stage despite treatment, at which point, the discontinuation of this treatment should be considered. Indicators that a patient has reached this stage include inability to ambulate or to recognize family members. A standardized rating scale such as the Functional Assessment Staging Tool (FAST), the Global Deterioration Scale (GDS), or the Clinician's Interview-Based Impression (CIBI) can be used in determining decline in functional status. With the FAST scale, for example, advancement to level 7b or 7c might be an indicator for discontinuation.

Discussion with family members is essential when making decisions to terminate treatment. Additionally, consideration must be given to clinical evidence that suggests that withdrawal of these medications likely accelerates cognitive and functional decline. Some families elect to continue treatment even when it may be that the medications are no longer efficacious in the advanced stage.

Behavioral and Psychological Symptoms Manifested by Persons Receiving Dementia Pharmacotherapy

As many as 90% of people with dementia develop significant behavioral problems during the course of their disease. Common behavioral and psychological symptoms of dementia (BPSD) include agitation, aggression, paranoia, sleep disturbances, and mood disorders. These behaviors, as previously mentioned, are often the result of unmet needs and management can be accomplished by addressing these needs. Persons with dementia frequently experience psychotic features. As many as 70% of agitated persons with dementia will manifest hallucinations, delusions, illusions, and paranoia; however, not all psychotic features are disturbing to the persons experiencing them, and behaviors associated with them might be modified with nonpharmacologic interventions alone.

Caution in Prescribing

If nonpharmacologic approaches are ineffective and the features are disturbing to the patient, pharmacologic treatment may be considered. Several factors should be kept in mind, however. Elderly persons are generally vulnerable to untoward effects of antipsychotic agents, such as extrapyramidal symptoms (EPS) that cause gait disturbances, imbalance, tremor, muscle rigidity, diminished postural reflexes, an increased risk of falls, and sedation. Persons with dementia are even more vulnerable, so extreme caution must be used when prescribing these drugs. Appropriate indications for the use of antipsychotic medications are outlined in the OBRA of 1987. These guidelines require that antipsychotics be used to treat specific conditions and not solely for behavior control. It is important to discriminate between psychotic agitation (accompanied by delusions, hallucinations, paranoia) and nonpsychotic agitation, realizing that most agitation in these individuals is nonpsychotic. There is no clear evidence that most typical antipsychotic drugs are useful for treating neuropsychiatric or nonpsychotic symptoms. There might be a slight benefit for haloperidol with aggression, but it is unclear if this benefit outweighs the possible serious adverse effects, including tardive dyskinesia, falls, or EPS. It is generally agreed that the use of these agents should be discouraged in persons with dementia.

Managing Psychosis and Agitation

Recent expert opinion guidelines concluded that atypical antipsychotics are the first line in treating psychosis and agitation associated with dementia. Although there is no clear consensus on treatment of agitation without psychosis, atypical antipsychotics are the most agreed-upon choice. For psychosis and BPSD, consider judicious (meaning a very low dose) use of atypical antipsychotic agents such as risperidone, olanzapine, and quetiapine fumarate. Keep in mind the warnings, side effects, and complications, including EPS, diabetes, and weight gain.

However, as practitioners, be mindful of black box warnings for all antipsychotic medications for the treatment of behavioral complications in dementia. This class of medications may be associated with an increase of morbidity and mortality in dementia patients.

Managing Nonpsychotic Agitation

For nonpsychotic agitation that has not responded to nonpharmacologic interventions, clinicians may consider mood-stabilizing agents such as valproic acid and derivatives (divalproex sodium). However, it must be noted that this behavior is among the most challenging to manage and medications may be of limited benefit. Studies have demonstrated small but statistically significant benefit from cholinesterase inhibitors when used to treat BPSD. Memantine HCl may be of benefit in cognitive and functional domains but there does not appear to be a clinically significant benefit in the treatment of neuropsychiatric symptoms for persons with moderate-to-severe dementia. Although neither agent should be considered as first-line therapy for the treatment of BPSD, clinicians should assess their effect on these symptoms in persons already receiving these drugs for disease management. Consider, too, using drug combinations such as cholinesterase inhibitors and atypical antipsychotic agents or mood stabilizers for their synergistic effects.

Managing Anxiety and Depression

Persons with dementia are at risk for anxiety and depression, both of which have been shown to respond to pharmacotherapy. Apathy, another frequently manifested feature of dementia, will not generally respond to drug treatment, however, so attempts should be made to differentiate between apathy and depression. With depression, consider treatment early in the course of the dementing illness and then throughout its progression if drug therapy continues to be effective. Selected tricyclics, MAO-B inhibitors, and selective serotonin reuptake inhibitors (SSRIs) or combination drugs that address both serotonin and norepinephrine are advised; however, caution must be taken when combining MAO inhibitors with cholinesterase inhibitors.

Of the five clinical trials that have investigated the use of serotonergic antidepressants (sertraline, fluoxetine, citalopram, and trazodone) for the treatment of BPSD, only the trial of citalopram found benefit. Therefore, although well-tolerated, serotonergic agents do not appear to be very effective in the treatment of neuropsychiatric symptoms of dementia other than depression and their use should be limited to that condition. SSRIs may offer some benefit with better tolerability than other antidepressants in persons with dementia.

Medications to Avoid

There are medications that should be avoided too. Avoid bupropion hydrochloride when treating depression with anxiety features because this drug might be more negatively activating (i.e., prone to increase agitation) than other agents.

The anticholinergic effects of paroxetine hydrochloride make this agent less attractive as a first choice for treatment of depression in older persons with dementia. Fluoxetine hydrochloride, with its long half-life and potential for drug–drug interactions, is usually not recommended in the geriatric populations. Beers Criteria and OBRA Regulations strongly urge the avoidance of benzodiazepines (BDZs), such as diazepam or alprazolam, for the management of anxiety in older people, in general, and patients with dementia, specifically, as they carry a risk of increased cognitive impairment and falls.

Managing Sleep Disturbance

Treatment of poor sleep is a high priority for persons with AD. Insomnia adds an extra burden to their already compromised functioning and impaired quality of life. Sleep disturbances are extremely common in this group, affecting an estimated 44%. Before doing anything else, attempt to assess first whether insomnia is caused by a medical or psychiatric condition, and, if that is a possibility, consult the healthcare provider.

In general, several strategies have proved useful, some involving medication, others not. Always try a nonpharmacologic approach first. Again, consider that the priority is to treat the patient and not the staff—medications should be used judiciously.

Recommended nonpharmacologic interventions include use of music, massage, lavender oil (many people find its scent calming), a consistent bedtime routine, and warm milk. Darkening the room or reducing noise may help. Rather than following an institutional schedule, people with dementia should be encouraged to maintain their usual sleep schedules to enhance restfulness. Avoid caffeinated beverages after midday.

Avoid over-the-counter drugs such as diphenhydramine (found in Benadryl or Tylenol PM), which can increase confusion, falls, urinary retention, and constipation in elderly persons, especially those with dementing illnesses. Melatonin, a sleep-promoting hormone, has not been shown to be effective and is not recommended for the treatment of sleep disturbance in dementia, but is generally considered safe.

If nonpharmacologic strategies are ineffective, treatment with hypnosedatives may be considered. Controversies regarding the use of these medications in persons with dementia revolve around issues of efficacy and potential toxicity. Currently, the short-acting BDZs and imidazopyridines (zolpidem, zaleplon) are used as effective hypnosedatives in the general population, but no controlled studies have evaluated their specific effects on people with dementia. A comprehensive review has determined that the imidazopyridines may have less adverse effects on psychomotor and cognitive function than BDZ and may be a better choice. Consider zolpidem 2.5–10 mg. Trazodone, a tetracyclic antidepressant, may also be relatively safe in small doses (25–50 mg) for sleep induction in older persons, including those with dementia. If people are being treated for certain co-occurring problems, consider using the following agents to facilitate sleep: mirtazapine in low doses (15 mg) or ramelteon at 8 mg. Mirtazapine can stimulate appetite, which is an added benefit in a population that often experiences weight loss. Quetiapine, although it is highly sedating and is commonly used as a sleep adjuvant, should be avoided because of the black box warnings mentioned earlier; however, in patients with paranoia and psychosis, particularly at night, and when other options have been tried without success, an appropriate choice may be at low doses (25–75 mg).

The use of tricyclic antidepressants, such as amitriptyline or doxepin, to promote sleep in institutionalized older adults is not recommended given their significant anticholinergic side effects.

Managing Pain

Persons with advanced dementia may experience pain for several reasons, including osteoarthritis, ischemic pain, postherpetic neuropathy (a health history should detail whether the patient has had chicken pox, to alert staff to the possibility that pain is being caused by shingles), and peripheral neuropathies. Because patients are unable to clearly express discomfort, healthcare professionals must anticipate and meet their needs. Nonpharmacologic and pharmacologic treatment are both options (see chapter 7 for more information).

Consider the following factors when prescribing pain relief medication for the individual with AD.

Start with a trial dose of routine acetaminophen (650–1,000 mg every 8 hours). Later on, in some cases, a topical anagelsic might be used to compound the pain-relieving effects. Do not exceed 3 g of acetaminophen per day. Avoid nonsteroidal anti-inflammatory drugs such as ibuprofen or naprosyn over prolonged periods of time because of the risk of gastrotoxicity and nephrotoxicity. Consider judicious use of adjuvant drugs based on the type and origin of pain. For example, in managing neuropathic pain, low-dose tricyclic antidepressant agents such as nortriptyline hydrochloride, desipramine hydrochloride, and anticonvulsant agents (e.g., pregabalin and gabapentin) are effective. However, it is important to evaluate the anticholinergic or sedating side effects against the benefits.

Remember to discontinue or decrease acetaminophen when administering opioid agents such as oxycodone and acetaminophen or hydrocodone and acetaminophen for pain management. Morphine sulfate, an immediate-release preparation, is useful. Additionally, morphine sulfate is efficacious when used at the end of life, as it often decreases restlessness and breathing difficulties.

▨ MEDICAL MANAGEMENT CONSIDERATIONS FOR NON-ALZHEIMER DEMENTIAS

The four most common types of dementia are dementia with Lewy bodies, frontotemporal dementia, vascular dementia, and Alzheimer's dementia. Although there are many common features shared by the four, there are specific features that must be considered when providing pharmacologic intervention for each one. The following is an overview of specific characteristics associated with non-Alzheimer dementias.

Frontotemporal Dementia

This is a relatively uncommon type of dementia, with an earlier age of onset (40–65) than Alzheimer's dementia. Many frontotemporal dementias (FTDs) are linked to genetic mutations on chromosome 17 called the *tauopathies*. Symptoms include prominent language changes like anomia (inability to name), aphasia (inability to generate language), echolalia (repetition of the examiner), and perseverative speech. Patients lose social skills. They display inappropriate behavior and judgment, disinhibition, and lack of insight. Treatment tends to be difficult and is mainly focused on management of behavioral complications, although approved medications do exist to treat this condition. Memantine HCl and cholinesterase inhibitors are considered ineffective with FTD but there is anecdotal evidence of benefit with memantine.

Dementia With Lewy Bodies

This dementia is characterized by progressive slowness of movements and Parkinson's-like features, well-formed hallucinations (particularly visual hallucinations), rapidly progressing dementia, fluctuations of clarity followed by confusion, and sensitivity to medication. Lewy bodies are abnormal inclusions that accumulate within neurons, most commonly associated with Parkinson's disease. What distinguishes dementia with Lewy bodies (DLB) from Parkinson's from a pathological standpoint is that Lewy bodies are concentrated in one part of the brain in Parkinson's (the substantia nigra), but are widely distributed in DLB.

Caution should be taken when treating patients with DLB as they can be sensitive to medications. For cognitive symptoms, rivastigmine is approved and an appropriate choice. Persons with DLB are particularly vulnerable to the extrapyramidal effects of antipsychotic agents and because of this, these agents should be used with great caution. If use of these drugs becomes necessary, quetiapine fumarate is the antipsychotic drug of choice when treating psychosis in persons with DLB. Among the atypical antipsychotics, risperidone has been associated with an increase in EPS and increased incidence of neuroleptic malignant syndrome. Olanzapine may also exacerbate EPS in people suffering from DLB. Parkinsonian motor features associated with DLB should not be pharmacologically treated unless necessary because of medication sensitivity (e.g., dopamine agonists such as pramipexole and ropinirole can trigger psychotic symptoms in DLB), in which case, levodopa is the safest choice.

Vascular Dementia

This dementia is caused by a stroke. After a stroke, memory loss, cognitive decline and other symptoms of dementia can begin fairly abruptly. A diagnosis of VD is supported by extensive cerebrovascular changes on a brain scan, an abnormal neurological examination, or a history of stroke. This type of dementia may not progress and can even improve with the right type of treatment. Especially in the early and moderate stages, it is important to control risk factors for vascular disease using lipid management, blood pressure management, or low-dose aspirin therapy as that might reduce risk of further strokes, which could exacerbate the dementia. Treatment can also include standard pharmacotherapy of AD.

EXHIBIT 8.1

Standards of Care for Medication Management

A. Healthcare facilities shall:
1. Adhere to the OBRA 1987 guidelines as they relate to medication administration in long-term care facilities to ensure the highest practical, physical, medical, and psychological well-being of every resident.
2. While addressing ongoing medical and emotional health problems, adopt an approach of care that avoids polypharmacy.
3. Institute a policy and procedure that supports regular consultation of the person's medication profile by a consulting pharmacist to ensure that the person with advanced dementia:
   a. Is not being prescribed psychotropic medications if psychosis is no longer present, and
   b. Receives adequate pharmacologic treatment of co-occurring medical and emotional health problems.
4. Ensure that accurate and timely documentation occurs in the medical record.
5. Provide orientation and regular training programs in medication administration geared to the interdisciplinary team.
6. Make assurances that ongoing training programs are up to date.

B. Healthcare staff shall:
1. Receive initial and ongoing annual training in medication administration and monitoring as related to cognitively intact older adults and those with advancing and advanced dementia, including information on:
   a. The efficacy of initiating, maintaining, and terminating pharmacologic interventions in persons with advanced dementia;
   b. Dosing and usage of agents commonly prescribed for persons with advanced dementia;
   c. Assessing the effect of medications on targeted symptoms and behaviors;
   d. Suggestions for selecting medications that modify dementing illnesses and their progression, treat depression and anxiety, manage sleeplessness, agitation, and pain; and
   e. Specific pharmacologic management strategies for common types of dementing illnesses.

Continued

Exhibit 8.1 *Continued*

2. Implement medication monitoring policies and procedures, whereby:
   a. A pharmacist reviews each person's drug regimen monthly;
   b. A consultant pharmacist reports the results to the attending physician and the director of nursing; and
   c. The reviews are acknowledged and acted on.
3. Complete a medication assessment on each new admission.
4. Complete a medication assessment on any change in a person's behavior.
5. Complete a medication assessment whenever a person progresses from one level of dementia to another.

C. The person with advanced dementia shall expect:
   1. To be free from polypharmacy while having co-occurring medical and emotional health problems adequately managed with medication as deemed necessary and appropriate.
   2. To be free of inappropriate psychotropic medications when psychosis and severe agitation are no longer present.

▨ REFERENCES

Agronin, M. (2004). The man with aggression and agitation. In P. Aupperle (Ed.), *Managing moods: Diagnosis and treatment of mood problems and behavioral issues in the elderly* (pp. 29–40). New York: McMahon Publishing Group.

Agronin, M. E., & Tangalos, E. G. (2003). *Cholinesterase inhibitors in the treatment of dementia: A continuing education monograph.* Temple, TX: Scott & White and the Center for Health Information.

Alexopoulas, G. S. (2005, March). *Antidepressants and anxiolytics in the elderly: A focus on safety. Depression in the elderly: Clinical Manifestations, Treatment, Safety, and Comorbidity.* Presented at the annual meeting of the American Association for Geriatric Psychiatry, San Diego, CA.

Alexopoulas, G. S., Streim, J., Carpenter, D., Docherty, J. P., & Expert Consensus Panel for Using Antipsychotic Drugs in Older Patients. (2004). Using antipsychotic agents in older patients. *Journal of Clinical Psychiatry, 65*(Suppl. 2), 5–99.

Baine, J., Birks, J., & Dening, T. (2009). Antidepressants for treatment depression in dementia. *Cochrane Database System Review, Issue 1*. Retrieved January 24, 2010, from www.thecochrane-library.com

Ballard, C. G., Waite, J., & Birks, J. (2008). Atypical antipsychotics for aggression and psychosis in Alzheimer's disease. *Cochrane Database System Review, Issue 4.* Retrieved January 24, 2010, from www.thecochranelibrary.com

Baskys, A., & Duke, L. (2004). Dementia of the Lewy body type. In G. T. Grossberg (Ed.), *Atypical antipsychotic medications in dementia.* New York: AKH, Inc. and McMahon Publishing Group.

Birks, J. (2009). Cholinesterase inhibitors for Alzheimer's disease. *Cochrane Database System Review, Issue 1.* Retrieved January 24, 2010, from www.thechocranelibrary.com

Chibnall, J., Tait, R., Harman, B., & Luebbert, R. (2005). Effect of Acetaminophen on behavior, well-being, and psychotropic medication use in nursing home residents with moderate-severe dementia. *Journal of the American Geriatrics Society, 53*(11), 1921–1929.

Cohen-Mansfield, J., & Mintzer, J. (2005). Time for change: The role of nonpharmacologic interventions in treating behavior problems in nursing home residents with dementia. *Alzheimer Disease Associated Disorders, 19*(1), 37–40.

De Deyn, P. P. (2006). Drug treatment: Treatment of behavioral and psychological symptoms of dementia with neuroleptics. In A. Burns & B. Winblad (Eds.), *Severe Dementia* (pp. 193–204). Hoboken, NJ: John Wiley & Sons, Inc.

Doody, R. S. (2003). Current treatments for Alzheimer's disease: Cholinesterase inhibitors. *Journal of Clinical Psychiatry, 64*(Suppl. 9), 11–17.

Doody, R. S., Stevens, J. C., Beck, C., Dubinsky, R. M., Kaye, J. A., Gwyther, L., et al. (2001). Practice parameter: Management of dementia (an evidenced-based review). Report of the Quality Standards Subcommittee of the American Academy of Neurology. *Neurology, 56*(9), 1154–1166.

Fick, D. M., Cooper, J. W., Wade, W. E., Waller, J. L., Maclean, J. R., & Beers, M. H. (2003). Updating the Beers criteria for potentially inappropriate medication use in older adults: Results of a U.S. consensus panel of experts. *Archives of Internal Medicine,163*(22), 2716–2724.

Grossberg, G. T. (2004). Treating depression and anxiety in long-term care. *Annals of Long-Term Care (Suppl.), 12*, 1–6.

Herrmann, N. (1998). Valproic acid treatment of agitation in dementia. *Canadian Journal of Psychiatry, 43*, 68–72.

Holmes, H. M., Sachs, G. A., Shega, J. W., Hougham, G. W., Cox Hayley D., & Dale, W. (2008). Integrating palliative medicine into the care of persons with advanced dementia: Identifying appropriate medication use. *Journal of the American Geriatric Society, 56*(7), 1306–1311.

Jeste, D. V., & Finkle, S. I. (2000). Psychosis of Alzheimer's disease and related dementias. Diagnostic criteria for a distinct syndrome. *American Journal of Geriatric Psychiatry, 8*, 29–34.

Kaufer, D. (2004). Dementia with Lewy bodies: The management of cognitive and behavioral symptoms. *Annals of Long-Term Care, 7*(Suppl.), 4–6.

Keys, M. A., & De Wald, C. (2005). Clinical perspectives on choice of atypical antipsychotics in elderly patients with dementia, part 1. *Annals of Long-Term Care, 2*(13), 26–32.

Knopman, D. S., Knapp, M. J., Gracon, S. I., & Davis, C. S. (1994). The clinician Interview-Based Impression (CIBI): A clinician's global change rating scale in Alzheimer's disease. *Neurology, 44*(12), 2315–2321.

Lykestos, C. G., & Lee, H. B. (2004). Diagnosis and treatment of depression in Alzheimer's disease: A practical approach for the clinician. *Dementia and Geriatric Cognitive Disorders, 17*, 55–64.

Marquette University & the Palliative Care Program at the Medical College of Wisconsin. (1997). *Improving management of physical pain and affective discomfort for people with dementia in long-term care.* Milwaukee, WI: Authors.

Montsinger, C. D. (2003). Use of atypical antipsychotic drugs in patients with dementia. *American Family Physician, 67*, 2335–2340.

Omnibus Budget Reconciliation Act (OBRA), Public Law No. 100-203 (22 December 1987).

Reisberg, B. (1988). Functional assessment staging (FAST). *Psychopharmacology Bulletin, 24*(4), 653–659.

Reisberg, B., Ferris, S. H., de Leon, M. J., & Crook, T. (1982). The Global Deterioration Scale for assessment of primary degenerative dementia. *American Journal of Psychiatry, 139*(9), 1136–1139.

Reynolds, B. (2004). Optimizing care for patients with Alzheimer's disease: Emerging treatment strategies. *Supplement to Journal of the American Academy of Nurse Practitioners, 16*(1), 3.

Rogers, J. C., Holm, M. B., Burgio, L. D., Hsu, C., Hardin, J. M., & McDowell, B. J. (2000). Excess disability during morning care in nursing home residents with dementia. *International Psychogeriatrics, 12*(2), 267–282.

Selma, T. P., Beizer, J. L., & Higbee, M. D. (2005). *Geriatric dosage handbook* (5th ed.). Cleveland, OH: Lexi-Comp, Inc.

Sink, K. M., Holden, K. F., & Yaffe, K. (2005). Pharmacological treatment of neuropsychiatric symptoms of dementia. *The Journal of the American Medical Association, 293*(5), 596–608.

State Operations Manual Certification, Transmittal 232 (1989, September) Washington, DC: Health Care Financing Administration, Department of Health and Human Resources.

Tariot, P. N., Farlow, M. R., Grossberg, G. T., Graham, S. M., McDonald, S., Gergel, I., et al. (2003). Memantine/donepezil dual-therapy is superior to placebo/donepezil therapy for the treatment of moderate to severe Alzheimer's disease (abstract). *Journal of the American Geriatrics Society, 51*(S4), S225–S226.

Tariot, P. N. (2003). Medical management of advanced dementia. *Journal of the American Geriatrics Society, 51*(5), S305–S313.

Tracktenberg, R. E., Weiner, M. F., Patterson, M. B. Teri, L. & Thal, L. J. (2003). Comorbidity of psychopathological domains in community-dwelling persons with Alzheimer's disease. *Journal of Geriatric Psychiatry Neurology, 16*(2), 94–99.

Tran, R. N. (2005). Sleep problems in Alzheimer's disease. *Journal of the Arizona Geriatrics Society, 10*(3), 20–23.

Wagner, J., & Wagner, M. L. (2000). Non-benzodiazepines for treatment of insomnia. *Review of Sleep Medicine, 4*(6),551–581.

Wild, R., Pettit, T., & Burns, A. (2003). Cholinesterase inhibitors for dementia with Lewy bodies. *Cochrane Database of Systematic Reviews,* (3), CD003672.

Wimo, A., Winblad, B., Stöffler, A., Wirth, Y., & Möbius, H. J. (2003). Resource utilization and cost analysis of memantine in patients with moderate to severe Alzheimer's disease. *Pharmacoeconomics, 21*(5), 327–340.

Winblad, B., & Poritis, N. (1999). Memantine in severe dementia: Results of the 9M-Best Study (benefit and efficacy in severely demented patients during treatment with memantine). *International Journal of Geriatric Psychiatry, 14*(2),135–146.

Zhong, K., Tariot, P., Mintzer, J., Minkwitz, M. C., & Devine, N. A. (2004). Quetiapine for the treatment of agitation in elderly institutionalized patients with dementia: A randomized, double-blind trial. Paper presented at 9th International Conference on Alzheimer's Disease and Related Disorders, Philadelphia, PA.

MANAGING ACTIVITIES OF DAILY LIVING

9

EATING AND NUTRITION

Lori Eddings, Tena Alonzo, Anna de Jesus, and Antonia Horton

■ INTRODUCTION

It is a commonly held belief among healthcare professionals that weight loss is inevitable in persons with advanced dementia. They are right; but they are also wrong. They are right because people with advanced dementia usually do lose weight and, more often than not, waste away as their dementia progresses into the later stages. But they are wrong in believing that weight loss is inextricably linked to dementia and that persons with dementia will inevitably lose weight as a result of the disease process alone. Weight loss in persons with advanced dementia is *not* inevitable, but it does happen and will continue to happen more often than it should as long as caregivers continue to hold on to outdated notions of what and how to feed persons with advanced dementia, and as long as practitioners hold on to the myth that weight loss *is* inevitable and that there is nothing they can do about it.

For persons with advanced dementia, weight loss may occur if caregivers forget the value of food as comfort, do not pay attention to food preferences, or misread the behaviors of the person they are taking care of. Individuals may appear not to be interested in food when, in fact, they simply are no longer able to express hunger or thirst. This makes persons with advanced dementia vulnerable to dehydration and inadequate nutrition. Caregivers need to assess individual preferences and anticipate nutritional and hydration needs, particularly as the person's dementia progresses.

Caregivers' decisions about food and the dining environment can serve to either limit or enhance eating pleasure. Done right, care facilities can experience almost no weight loss among their residents by, for instance, providing various snacks between meals. The following set of guidelines specifies a philosophy of nutrition and offers interventions designed to maintain intake, promote good nutrition, and minimize weight loss for persons with advanced dementia.

■ GENERAL PRINCIPLES TO SUPPORT EATING AND NUTRITION NEEDS IN PERSONS WITH ADVANCED DEMENTIA

Weight loss is a concern for persons with advanced dementia. As mentioned earlier, it is not always true that a person with advanced dementia is unwilling to eat. Weight loss can occur because of cognitive or behavioral problems, comorbidities, chewing and swallowing difficulties, and caregivers' failure to appropriately meet nutritional needs.

A person with dementia will face a progressive loss of skills. The following levels identify a typical progression with regard to eating. Assessment is necessary to determine the person's feeding needs.

- Level 1. Persons with dementia are independent in eating but may need to have food prepared for them.
- Level 2. Persons with dementia are independent in eating but may need to be reminded to finish the meal (i.e., they may need prompting and cueing).
- Level 3. Persons with dementia require cueing as well as additional staff assistance. They may play with their food or make a mess. They may be unable to use their utensils or bring food to their mouth. They may exhibit frustrations related to their difficulty with eating.
- Level 4. Persons with dementia require total assistance but cooperate with feeding efforts by the staff. There is little choking and they are generally able to eat most, if not all, of the food given to them.
- Level 5. Persons with dementia require total assistance and tend to resist the efforts of healthcare staff during dining. They tend to take the longest to eat. They tend to pocket their food and need lots of cueing to eat. They may forget to chew and swallow. It may be difficult for them to receive adequate nutrition even when given three large meals per day.

Providing Comfort Through Nutrition

People with advanced dementia need comfort food. Comfort food, as defined here, is any food that a person will accept, eat, and tolerate. Healthcare staff can provide comfort through nutrition by using the following approaches:

- Provide food no matter what the hour is.
- Offer food that is soft and sweet, particularly if the person rejects other types of food.
- Make available the foods that the person likes to eat.
- Consider feeding as an activity that reestablishes meaningful connections.
- Offer assistance, if needed, employ eye contact, light touch, and soothing or comforting conversation.
- Participate in dining with the individual—this will provide visual cues to encourage them to eat.
- Use the accept-and-swallow approach to feeding, meaning that the goal is for the person to readily accept food and fluid into their mouth and then continue to process and swallow it.

Other Important Considerations

It is important to focus on food texture, food consistency, and palatability with this population. Eliminate dietary or therapeutic restrictions. This honors dignity and respects the preferences and comfort of the person with advanced dementia. Take care to use terminology that maintains dignity. Examples include saying *clothing protector* instead of *bib* and avoiding the use of the word *feeder*. Remember that you are not offering the person a *feeding* program but a *dining* program.

General Approaches to Improving Eating and Nutrition

There are all sorts of reasons why someone with dementia may be having trouble eating. Their caregiver may not be able to recognize behaviors that indicate their preferences with food. Assess the environment for problems that can interfere with the individual's comfort level during their dining program. These problem areas can include:

- Noise and commotion in the dining area;
- Physical stressors, including untreated pain, discomfort, constipation, infection, acute illness, depression, and other maladies;
- Poor dentition (e.g., an abscessed tooth or ill-fitting dentures);
- Difficulty paying attention caused by environmental distractions or a change in the routine or caregiver;
- Poor attentiveness related to fatigue;
- Unappealing food; and
- Changes in food preferences.

Be alert to the nature of the disease progression or comorbidities that may result in apraxia, dysphagia, or other deficits that compromise the eating process. When attending to eating and nutrition in people with Alzheimer's disease, it is important for caregivers to be as flexible as possible while providing palliative care.

Making food a comfort can be accomplished using a four-step IDEA approach— identify, develop, evaluate, and act accordingly regarding the specific needs of the person with dementia.

1. *Identify* what the person likes to eat. Ask family members for both a baseline history of their likes and dislikes and an overview of their nutrition history. Recognize cultural and ethnic food preferences, as well as any food allergies. Elicit the support of the interdisciplinary team to identify preferences and approaches.
2. *Develop* a food plan that incorporates various foods and beverages the person enjoys. Assess the range of foods that will be served according to taste, textures, colors, variations in hot and cold dishes, and opportunities for attractive presentation of the food items. Gauge overall nutritional value of the food plan to be sure it meets the individual's estimated needs. Include interventions that address distractions in the dining environment and caregiver approaches to feeding. Accommodate individuals who will not eat various foods by offering foods they will accept. Initiate the food and fluid plan.
3. *Evaluate* the plan to determine whether it works for the person with dementia. Observe for signs of comfort and pleasure such as smiles and willingness to accept food and signs that the food and fluid plan is not working, such as a

grimace or unwillingness to accept anything by mouth. Monitor progress. Ensure adequate intake and determine if the food and fluid selections are meeting the person's needs for comfort, nourishment, weight maintenance, and hydration.

4. *Act* accordingly. If the plan is working continue with it if not keep trying with other types of food/fluid, changes in the environment, caregiver approaches to feeding and other factors that can contribute to a comfortable and supportive dining experience.

Strategies to Enhance the Dining Experience and Promote Nutrition

▨ Meal plans need to take into account daily habits. Modify breakfast schedules to be sure food is available when people wake up in the morning. If food is available when they rise, individuals may be more willing to eat. Start serving meals early for those persons who need more time to eat.

▨ Use special devices or adaptive eating utensils that allow individuals to feed themselves (e.g., curved plates, Sippy Cups, plates with lids, utensils with built-up handles). Ensure the safe and effective use of these devices. Occupational therapy staff may help with the proper use. Provide encouragement and support during mealtimes with appropriate cueing and attention to the person's field of vision. Tableware that is easy to see (bigger or brightly colored) may help draw the person's attention to their environment and assist them in eating and drinking. Avoid stimulation overload by moving meals to times that minimize or eliminate noise and other distractions. Consider small portions or offering one food item at a time; large amounts of food on a plate may be overwhelming for some people. Determine the temperature of food the person prefers. Again, be flexible. What works one day may not work the next day.

▨ Create a dining environment that is conducive to eating, because this can lead to improved food consumption. To achieve this, make the environment as stress free as possible. Ensure adequate staffing to adequately assist people. Ensure that meals are not rushed. Consider specialized dining experiences that will be appealing, such as small table arrangements or specific dining partners; for example, consider placing loud people with those who are hard of hearing, or place quiet tablemates with those who may be easily distracted or agitated. Play soft and soothing music. Use quiet tones of voice. Be sure the dining room temperature is set at a comfortable level. Investigate whether people might be allowed to eat in satellite dining areas—the dining room, hallway, by the nurse's station, in their own room, or wherever they are most likely to consume foods.

▨ Explore ways to make meals special, with celebrations or by having the aroma of warm bread or baking cookies in the dining area. Invite family members to share with you special connections between favorite smells, foods, and memories the person may have (a special meal or special event in their life associated with food). Encourage staff to interact or dine with people. Quiet mealtime interaction provides a sense of family and camaraderie.

▦ Identify snacks that people enjoy. Provide foods and snacks that are nutritionally dense. Good examples of these include sandwich halves, various fruits, oatmeal, pudding, and custard. Avoid routinely offering packaged salted crackers or graham crackers. Individuals may prefer snacks that are soft and sweet, like ice cream. Nutritious snacks and foods should be set out at least four times a day: before, during, and after activities and during the night. Shakes should be given to those who eat less than 50% of their normal intake at a meal. They are a good alternative when meals are refused. Try a fruit smoothie, a milk shake with peanut butter (if peanut allergies are not present) and ice cream, or other supplemental products that the person will accept and swallow. Consider a beverage station that offers fruit juices, water, and other beverages 24 hours a day, or a 24-hour "comfort cart" with foods and beverages. The taste and textures of the food should be those that a person with advanced dementia will accept and swallow.

When developing a nutrition and dining program, consider using centralized dining services that can both provide general meal plans and accommodate individual preferences for food and food textures. Decentralized services can be used for specific unit nutrition programs (e.g., a beverage station, comfort cart). A trial-and-error approach on the unit can determine what the most desirable foods are.

Approaches to Monitoring Weights and Overall Interventions to Address Weight Loss

Weight loss is a significant challenge in advanced dementia. Because weight loss is a negative predictor of morbidity and mortality, it is important for facilities to implement procedures that militate against it. To begin with, residents should be weighed monthly to monitor for significant changes. If there has been a change in their weight, persons should be weighed daily or weekly. The interdisciplinary care team should review monthly weigh-ins for trends and should review all interventions that have been conducted to prevent weight loss. Any physical, mental, or physiological changes should be noted when reviewing weight trends.

There are several practical considerations for deciding who should be weighed more frequently than others. These include the following:

▦ If a person eats less than 75% of their usual meal consumption for 3 or more days, add them to the weekly weight schedule.
▦ If a person weighs less than 100 lb. and has a history of weight changes, weigh the person weekly.
▦ If a person is susceptible to fluid retention, weigh the person weekly or daily depending on the severity of edema.
▦ If a person has any physical, mental, or physiological change related to their condition, they should be weighed weekly.

Consider not weighing individuals who are on hospice, those actively dying, or those on bed rest. In these cases, comfort should be the focus. Weights must be taken under the same conditions each time to ensure accuracy.

Besides monitoring weight, other practices can help guard against weight loss. These include the following:

- Providing good mouth care can help ensure that foods continue to taste good. As soon as a person demonstrates trouble eating or stops altogether, a full assessment of their mouth is necessary to establish if disease or decay is present. If there is, seek appropriate medical or dental consultation and intervention (see chapter 10, on oral care, for more information). During team meetings, address challenges with individual food and fluid intake and with weight loss.
- Offer foods dense in calories or consider nutritional supplements for concentrated calories.
- Offer foods and beverages frequently throughout the day and especially when the person is most alert.
- Offer larger meals at breakfast and noon if the person generally eats poorly in the evening. Rearrange the normal eating schedule if the person eats larger amounts of food at certain meal times.
- Add condiments for flavor, if the person enjoys them.
- Try easily-handled foods such as finger foods; portable foods such as sandwiches cut into quarters, popovers, and ice cream cones; and assistive devices, such as cups with lids, to maintain independence and dignity.
- As a last resort, consider the use of orexigenic agents (medication that stimulates the appetite).

Feeding Considerations, Techniques, and Approaches

There are many challenges that caregivers can face when feeding a person with advanced dementia. These include pouching, dysphagia, refusing to eat, and the pacing of meals. Because of these challenges, it is important to monitor and provide assistance during meals. In general, encourage family members to become involved in assisting during meals and providing supportive care. What follows are some strategies to mitigate these challenges.

Pouching

Pouching is when the person being fed places food between the cheek and gum instead of swallowing it. Pouching can lead to poor oral hygiene. To reduce pouching, try giving small amounts of soft-textured foods, which are more easily swallowed.

Dysphagia

Dysphagia is the medical term for trouble swallowing. There are many causes. A medical evaluation might be indicated. For people with dysphagia, provide spoken or physical cues to stimulate swallowing. Check to see if the person is taking any medications that cause sedation. Note the specific food that the person has difficulty with and alter the texture (for example changing a raw food to a cooked one) or omit it altogether. Having the person sit upright can help with swallowing and strengthening the upper body. Make sure they are in a comfortable position.

Feeding Pace

The rate at which the meal is consumed should not exceed the person's swallowing and chewing capabilities. Monitor and document in the care plan the optimal pace for the person. Support self-feeding using hand-over-hand guidance at mealtime to reinforce the repetitive motion.

Refusing to Eat

Place a small amount of food on the lower lip to stimulate interest. The loss of major functions such as the ability to sit up or swallow necessitates high-calorie foods in liquid form, such as milk shakes, hot cereal, high-calorie soups, or other foods that can be pureed to a drinkable consistency. Fortified food can ensure improved nutritional content. Several very high-calorie supplements are available commercially. If agitation is present, refer to chapter 6, on behavior problems associated with advanced dementia. In extreme circumstances, refusing to eat can result in wasting.

Special care practices may need to be undertaken at the end of life. These include practicing good oral hygiene on the individual's behalf and providing calorie-enhanced foods so that no bite or sip is ever wasted on a noncaloric food or beverage—for instance, a beverage taken with medications. Above all, the focus should be on comfort care, which essentially means giving the person whatever they will accept and providing what is pleasurable for them.

Feeding the Person With Advanced Dementia: A Team Approach

Feeding a person with advanced dementia does not solely involve a nursing assistant with a spoon. It is a larger process that relies on multiple professionals to map out care planning strategies for eating difficulties and nutrition. The members of the interdisciplinary team include the primary care provider (physician or nurse practitioner), registered dietitian, nursing and direct care staff, occupational therapist, speech and language pathologist, dentist, and activity program coordinator.

Tube Feeding and Intravenous Hydration

When a person refuses or is no longer able to eat or drink, decisions may need to be made about artificial nutrition and hydration. Feeding tubes are sometimes used; however, there is no evidence that tube feeding extends life, prevents infection, or has any other benefits. Tube feeding is also associated with high levels of aspiration pneumonia, diarrhea, and physical restraint. Intravenous (IV) hydration may temporarily provide fluid, but cannot maintain nutritional requirements. Increased hydration may also decrease the person's comfort because hydration promotes excessive respiratory secretions, resulting in breathing difficulties. The absence of hydration is a normal part of the dying process and allows a more comfortable death over a period of days.

Advanced Care Planning

If artificial means are used, families will eventually be faced with the tough decision of whether or not to withdraw such treatments. For advance care planning, ensure that adequate documentation exists that specifies a person's advance directives related to IV therapy for hydration and the placement of feeding tubes (see chapter 16, on healthcare decisions for persons with advanced dementia, for more information).

EXHIBIT 9.1

Standards of Care for Providing Nutritional Support

A. The healthcare facility shall:
1. Develop and implement policies and procedures that address meals and dining considerations for persons with advanced dementia.
2. Provide food areas that limit noise and unnecessary distractions while offering a meaningful and pleasurable dining experience to persons with advanced dementia.
3. Provide comfort foods that are nutritious, combine taste with texture, and are readily accepted by the person with advanced dementia.
4. Provide a snack and beverage service throughout the day and during nighttime hours that is liberal and anticipates food and fluid requirements. Food should emphasize soft and sweet choices and comfort foods that the person will accept, eat, and tolerate.
5. Provide adequate direct care staffing to meet the dining needs of persons with advanced dementia.
6. Provide flexibility in mealtime schedules to meet individual preferences.
7. Provide resident seating arrangements that address the person's care needs, and appropriate healthcare staffing to meet the mealtime requirements of persons with advanced dementia.
8. If feeding difficulties arise, secure consultation from the members of interdisciplinary team: primary care provider, registered dietitian, nursing and direct care staff, occupational therapist, speech and language pathologist, dentist, and activity program coordinator.
9. Provide continuous training to healthcare staff in the principles of:
   a. Understanding the progression of dementia and palliative care approaches, and
   b. Nutrition principles, practices, and the dining process.

B. Healthcare staff shall:

1. Anticipate food and fluid needs 24 hours a day, 7 days a week.
2. Ensure a pleasant eating experience for persons with advanced dementia through specialized and/or individualized planning.
3. Use specialized dining considerations, when appropriate, such as:
   a. Positioning (i.e., moving immobile patients to avoid bedsores);
   b. Modifying the diet for chewing/swallowing;
   c. Offering frequent snacks and fluids; and
   d. Providing a supportive milieu that is both therapeutic and pleasant.
4. Conduct accurate monthly weigh-ins. Weigh individuals weekly or daily as recommended by interdisciplinary team members or if an individual's condition changes.
5. Notify healthcare team members when the person with advanced dementia experiences a change in eating habits, such as when they stop eating or have difficulty swallowing.
6. Document individual preferences, building in flexibility for changing food acceptance patterns and capabilities into the care plan.

C. Persons with advanced dementia shall expect:

1. Regular oral examinations to ascertain dental health status, as able.
2. No weight loss until the final and terminal stages of the disease process, after all other efforts have been maximized and exhausted. Members of the interdisciplinary team will be consulted about any weight loss.
3. Dining times customized to meet comfort and nutrition needs.
4. A mealtime setting and milieu that acknowledges environmental considerations, such as noise reduction, pleasant surroundings, and food presentation.
5. Specialized dining considerations to meet needs related to securing adequate nutrition during mealtimes and snacks best suited to their advancing disease state.
6. Special considerations related to advance care planning needs and advance directives, such as the use of feeding tubes or IV hydration.

■ REFERENCES

Alonzo, T. (2004). The comfort of food. In C. O. Long (Ed.), *Palliative care for advanced dementia: Train-the-trainer manual* (P6-Supp-1 to P6-Supp-8). Phoenix, AZ: Alzheimer's Association, Desert Southwest Chapter.

Alzbrain.org. (2004). *Nutrition*. Retrieved September 30, 2004, from http://www.alzbrain.org

Alzheimer's Association. (2006). Late-stage care: Providing care and comfort in the late stage of Alzheimer's disease. Retrieved January 24, 2010, from http://www.alz.org/national/documents/brochure_latestage.pdf

American Dietetic Association. (2005). Position of the American Dietetic Association: Liberalization of the diet prescription improves quality of life for older adults in long-term care. *Journal of the American Dietetic Association, 105*(12), 1955–1965.

Consultant Dietitians-Health Care Facilities. (2001). *Dining skills: Practical interventions for the caregivers of older adults with eating problems*. Chicago, IL: American Dietetic Association.

DiBartolo, M. C. (2006). Careful hand feeding: A reasonable alternative to PDG tube placement in individuals with dementia. *Journal of Gerontological Nursing, 32*(5), 25–33.

Dougherty, J. (2004). Comfort of food. In C. O. Long (Ed.), *Palliative care for advanced dementia: Train-the-trainer manual* (P6-Supp-1 to P6-Supp-8). Phoenix, AZ: Alzheimer's Association, Desert Southwest Chapter.

Dunne, T. (2004). Eating and Alzheimer's. *Clinical Nutrition, 23*, 533–538.

Frissoni, G. B., Franzoni, S., Bellelli, G., Morris, J., & Warden, V. (1998). Overcoming eating difficulties. In L. Volicer & L. Bloom-Charette (Eds.), *Enhancing the quality of life in advanced dementia* (pp. 80–90). Boston: Brunner/Mazel.

Gallagher, A. (2004). Undernutrition and causes of involuntary weight loss in long-term care. *Global Monitor: Special Meeting Reporter,* 5–9.

Kovach, C. R. (1997). Behaviors associated with late-stage dementia. In C. R. Kovach (Ed.), *Late-stage dementia care. A basic guide* (pp. 127–141). Washington, DC: Taylor & Francis.

Long, C. O. (2009). Palliative care for advanced dementia: Approaches that work. *Journal of Gerontological Nursing, 35*(11), 19–24.

Sampson, E. L., Candy, B., & Jones, L. (2009) Enteral tube feeding for older people with advanced dementia. *Cochrane Database System Review, Issue 2.* Retrieved January 24, 2010, from www.thecochranelibrary.com

Vailas, L. I., Nitzke, S. A., Becker, M., & Gast, J. (1998). Risk indicators for malnutrition are associated inversely with quality of life participants in meal programs for older adults. *Journal of the American Dietetic Association, 98*(5), 548–553.

Vogelzang, J. L. (2003). Dignity and dietary interventions for dementia. *Home Healthcare Nurse, 21*(1), 40–42.

Young, K. W., Binns, M. A., & Greenwood, C. E. (2001). Meal delivery practices do not meet needs of Alzheimer patients with increased cognitive and behavioral difficulties in long-term care facility. *The Journal of Gerontology Series A, Biological Sciences and Medical Sciences, 56*(10), M656–M661.

10

DRESSING AND GROOMING

Veronica Villafranca, Jan Dougherty, and Kathryn B. Lindstrom

INTRODUCTION

The ability to carry out basic personal care—putting on shoes, shaving, combing the hair—is important for independent living as people age. For someone with advancing dementia, however, dressing and grooming become a series of progressive challenges. In this chapter, we will examine the principles involved with dressing and grooming persons with advanced dementia.

GENERAL PRINCIPLES RELATED TO DRESSING AND GROOMING IN ADVANCED DEMENTIA

Dressing refers to the activity of putting on and taking off clothes and includes the consideration of footwear. Grooming refers to the activities related to an individual's personal hygiene and outward appearance.

Caregivers and persons with advanced dementia both face challenges in this area. The person with advanced dementia may resist the caregiver or exhibit aggressive verbal or physical behavior, or may experience grief and sadness stemming from their *loss* of independence. Aggressive behaviors may be based in global confusion, the nature of the caregiving situation, the infringement of privacy, the lack of dignity, generalized discomfort, or some specific discomfort or pain such as an arthritis or neuropathy. These behaviors should be seen as self-protective—related to an individual's need to protect himself or herself from perceived harm or physical discomfort.

Dressing and grooming activities promote personal hygiene and are essential components of the activities of daily living (ADLs). Caregivers who know the persons they are caring for will be better able to make these activities more enjoyable. The approach at all times should be respectful and, whenever possible, draw on the individual's preferences. Examples of preferences include knowing the person's favorite clothing based on the style and type of clothing they have enjoyed wearing in the past, or determining the shaving preferences of male residents.

As the disease progresses and total care becomes necessary, caregivers should think through practices that enhance dignity and ease the discomfort that dressing or grooming may cause. Caregivers can minimize frustration and discomfort for the person with advanced dementia by identifying what issues, if any, trigger dressing and grooming difficulties, such as shaving or brushing teeth, and then providing interventions that promote positive care.

Approaches to Care Related to Successful Dressing and Grooming

Basic Principles and Approaches to Dressing

By applying consistent principles, persons with advanced dementia are more likely to enjoy dressing and grooming activities. Try to accomplish dressing at the same time each day as part of the daily routine. Do not assume that the person with advanced dementia knows what you are doing. Provide a comfortable dressing or grooming experience. Always explain each step of the process as you proceed. Speak to the person at eye level and with good eye contact, adjusting the tone of voice to benefit the person. If they look uncomfortable at any time, look for sources of their discomfort and try to correct it. Check for any symptoms of pain. Do they resist care? Do they grimace or push caregivers away? Or are they unable to be consoled? These can all be symptoms. Stop caregiving tasks if the individual shows signs of pain and report it to the nurse or other personnel for intervention. If an individual routinely displays pain during grooming or dressing, administer pain medication an hour before beginning activities. Go slow during dressing and grooming, using a gentle and respectful approach. Rushing or pressure may cause anxiety and agitation. Discard approaches that are not effective and repeat approaches that work, but keep in mind that an approach that works one day may not work the next, which means caregivers must be flexible.

Whenever possible, incorporate the individual's past routine into the current one. Entertain or provide pleasant distractions during caregiving. Sing or speak kind words to them. Have them hold a comfortable object or consider giving them something pleasurable to eat or drink. Be mindful of the time it takes to dress or undress individuals and their willingness to be or get dressed. Determine the best order of dressing. Use one-step instructions and break down the task stage by stage. Persons may need to rest, so provide breaks as needed. If necessary, caregivers may have to segment a task, as the individual may only tolerate part of it. If the activity is overwhelming or distressing, break it down into segments so that it remains comfortable and meaningful connections are made. Use two caregivers whenever individuals cannot move their bodies on their own. Use two caregivers to dress a person if required. One can distract the person while the other dresses them. This allows one caregiver to concentrate on the task while the other can focus on the person. When necessary, use pillows to help position the individual to be comfortable. Acknowledge and praise them for allowing caregivers to participate in dressing or grooming activities. Provide positive reinforcement—validate them by complimenting how good they look afterwards. Change individuals immediately if they become wet or soiled. If briefs are used and they bother the individual, leave them open at the sides when the person is sitting or reclining.

During dressing, provide privacy to increase comfort and decrease embarrassment. Keep the room warm and well-lit. Avoid bright, glaring lights. Draw the blinds or close the door for more privacy. Make sure that the person with advanced dementia never feels cold or uncovered.

Considerations for Dressing and Footwear

Clothing choice will vary from individual to individual. It should not appear institutional. Encourage the family to bring clothes that can be easily removed. One size larger than an exact fit is best. Be on the alert for weight gain or loss, which can make clothes too big or too small. With increasing impairment, try easy-care clothing such as sweat suits and pants with elastic waistbands. Consider whether the individual will be able to easily sit. Pants should not be restrictive. Front-opening shirts are recommended, particularly if the person has difficulty with items that go over the head. Consider whether undergarments are providing comfort and support for women. If a bra is uncomfortable, try a camisole. If a person tugs at their clothes when idle, try to determine the cause. It may be the fit is too snug or a crease needs smoothing. Specialized catalogs are available geared to the dressing and grooming needs of persons with dementia (e.g., BuckandBuck.com). Consult these companies on the Web or inquire at specialty stores.

Footwear requires other considerations. When the person is able to ambulate short distances, it is important that shoes or slippers have a nonskid rubber sole. Inspect soles for grip and treads and avoid footwear with slippery soles. Check shoes periodically for fit, especially if the individual has gained or lost weight, has diabetes or a circulatory disease. Check feet, as well, for injuries. Footwear should not impede circulation. For persons who are no longer capable of walking, but who can self-propel in a wheelchair or are "transfers only," footwear is needed that can grip floor surfaces. Use nonskid slipper socks or booties as these provide needed traction for safe and effective movement and transfers. Consider tennis shoes with Velcro clasps or secure slip-on shoes (rather than tie shoes) for greater ease in dressing.

Basic Principles and Approaches to Grooming

Grooming activities include hair, mouth, and nail care; shaving for men; and makeup application for women. The following section outlines suggested approaches.

1. For hair care, determine the best time of day and approach. This will vary from resident to resident and should be reserved for time when the person is not agitated. Keep the person's hair in an easy-to-care-for style. Determine their preferred means of hair washing. Wash the hair using the techniques provided in chapter 13 if the individual is bedbound or unwilling to use the shower. Use no-rinse soap if the person is resistant to water and shampoo. If a visit to a barbershop or beauty parlor was an important part of the individual's former routine, consider incorporating one into their current one, if they are up to it.

2. With shaving, determine the best time of day and approach. Use the method of shaving (e.g., electric or safety razor) that the person is most used to. If uncertain about the method, contact the family or try trial and error to discover what works best. Consider an electric shaver if that is what the person used most of his life. If attempting an electric shaver for the first time, anticipate that the person may become frightened—have him feel the vibration on his hand first. With safety razors, use only high-quality disposable blades. Use shaving cream or other lubricants that moisten the face. Only shave when the face is wet and the beard softened. The best time is immediately after a shower or bath. Otherwise, make sure that the beard has been dampened with a warm and wet washcloth or that adequate shaving cream has been left on for at least 1 minute. Only shave in a downward direction, with the grain of the beard. If the person is prone to becoming combative, shave symmetrically: alternating a stroke on one side of the face with a stroke on the other. This will eliminate unevenness if shaving needs to be terminated. If the person resists, shaving can be accomplished in separate time segments throughout the day. Consider placing the individual's hand on the stem of the razor or on the shaver and providing hand-over-hand assistance to give a sense of participation.

3. When applying makeup, as with all ADLs, it is important to keep the individual's dignity and comfort in mind. Makeup can help female residents feel attractive. Determine if the individual prefers makeup routinely, only for special occasions, or not at all. Caregivers need to let the woman know what is being done to and for her, so as not to frighten her.

4. Nail care is often overlooked but needs to be addressed for both hygienic and aesthetic reasons. There are no established uniform standards here and, because of this, one should be familiar with any facility or agency policy. Overall, nails should be kept in good repair: clipped and perhaps filed, with no foreign particles underneath. Consider holding a beauty event featuring hand or foot massages along with nail care. Move slowly during the procedure and tell each individual what is going to happen each step of the way. Trim fingernails and toenails at least twice a month and as needed. Caregivers may get more cooperation if this is done while the person is watching television or listening to music.

5. Oral hygiene warrants significant attention. Mouth care is crucial to the health of people of all ages. For persons with advanced dementia, it is very important to continue the same habits the person had previously. To avoid tooth decay and problems with gums and infections, teeth, ideally, should be brushed twice or three times daily to remove the plaque that causes decay. Once a day is the minimum. Each person with advanced dementia reacts differently to tooth brushing and multiple techniques may be required, sometimes even day to day. The following are some practical approaches.

   a. Electric toothbrushes are acceptable, especially if the person has used one in the past. Consider using the kind of toothbrushes that are bent backward for easier access to the back of the mouth. (Note: Pink oral swab-type sponges do not remove food debris or plaque.) With people in wheelchairs or who are seated and who may have difficulty with brushing, it can be easier to assist from behind. By standing behind and gently cradling their head, one may be able to help them use the toothbrush themselves. Toothpaste is not necessary for decay removal. A brush with just water is fine. Use toothpaste sparingly to avoid producing large amounts of saliva. Children's toothpaste is less sudsy and may be better for this population. A towel around the neck can be helpful with drooling. If a person is receptive to tooth brushing and if they have used these items in their younger years, consider Stim-U-Dent or rubber tips to massage gums and for flossing. Floss gliders are easier to use than standard dental floss.

b. Persons with advanced dementia who wear dentures need regular checkups for gum and bone health. Remove the dentures at bedtime and place them in a cup with water or a cleaning solution. Poorly fitting dentures can contribute to poor nutrition and may result in weight loss, infections, constipation, and mouth sores. If nutritional problems occur, consult with the dietary staff to reevaluate the diet and food consistency. Also, consider a dental evaluation to ensure dentures fit properly.

c. Infection prevention will help avoid the pain of tooth decay. One way to prevent it is to encourage the drinking of water. Root decay and infections can be caused by dry mouth. If the person has offensive oral odor, they may have excess plaque and need extra brushing. If blood appears on the brush, the person probably has a gum infection and would benefit from a visit to the dentist. Consider using mobile dental services for regular checkups or any other dental concerns, as it will be easiest on these individuals.

EXHIBIT 10.1

Standards of Care for Dressing and Grooming Persons With Advanced Dementia

A. The healthcare facility shall:
1. Document in the care plan of the person his or her preferences on the means, time of day, distracters, comforters, and place for dressing and grooming to address personal hygiene needs, comfort, and enjoyment in the least restrictive manner.
2. Provide training to healthcare staff on dressing and grooming techniques that promote its importance as an activity versus a task to be performed.

B. Healthcare staff shall:
1. Provide guidance and care for persons with advanced dementia that respects human dignity and provides care in a comfortable, dignified, and respectful manner.
2. Provide education to families on measures that promote comfort while preserving dignity and functional performance for as long as possible.

Continued

Exhibit 10.1 *Continued*

  3. Use principles of dressing and grooming that promote comfort and independence:
     a. Be patient.
     b. Provide direction and assistance in a dignified manner.
     c. Consider likes, dislikes, and other personal preferences.
     d. Provide privacy during these tasks.
  4. Use pain assessment tools to document if a person looks uncomfortable. For example, if the person exhibits pain as indicated in the Pain Assessment in Advanced Dementia (PAINAD) scale or demonstrates verbal distress, combativeness, or a change in habits, look for the source and provide interventions to promote comfort.

C. Persons with advanced dementia shall expect:
  1. Maintenance of personal dignity and comfort during dressing and grooming.
  2. To be kept clean, neat, and presentable.

▒ REFERENCES

Alzheimer's Association. (n.d.). *Activity-based Alzheimer care: Building a therapeutic program.* Chicago, IL: Author.

Alzheimer's Association. (2004). *Dressing (topic sheet).* Retrieved January 24, 2010, from http://www.alz.org/national/documents/topicsheet_dressing.pdf

Alzheimer's Association. (2005). *Personal care: Assisting the person with dementia with daily changing needs.* Retrieved January 24, 2010, from http://www.alz.org/national/documents/brochure_personalcare.pdf

Buck and Buck. *Quality clothing for home health care and nursing home residents.* Retrieved January 24, 2010, from http://www.buckandbuck.com

Coleman, P., & Watson, N. M. (2006). Oral care provided by certified nursing assistants in nursing homes. *Journal of the American Geriatric Society, 54*(1), 138–143.

Dementia Care Learning Institute, Alzheimer's Association. (2004). *Dressing and grooming.* Retrieved October 23, 2004, from http://www.alz-sioux.org/dcli/dcli_tips12.pdf

Gaillot, S. L. (2002). *Caring for the patient.* Retrieved January 24, 2010, from http://studentweb.tulane.edu/~sgaillo/carepatient.html

Heacock, P. R., Beck, C. M., Souder, E., & Mercer, S. (1997). Assessing dressing ability in dementia. *Geriatric Nursing, 18*(3), 107–111.

National Institute of Aging. (2008, December). *Caregiver Guide* (NIH Publication No. 01-4013). Gaithersburg, MD: U.S. Department of Health and Human Services, National Institutes of Health. Retrieved January 24, 2010, from http://www.nia.nih.gov/Alzheimers/Publications/caregiverguide.htm

Pearson, A., & Chambers, J. (2004). Oral hygiene care for adults with dementia in residential aged care facilities. *Journal of Biomedical Informatics, 2*(4), 65–113 as cited in *Best Practice: Evidence-based Practice Information Sheets for Health Professionals, 8*(4), 1–6.

Rader, J., Barrick, A. L., Hoeffer, B., Sloane, P. D., McKenzie, D., Talerico, K. A., et al. (2006). The bathing of older adults with dementia. *American Journal of Nursing, 106*(4), 40–48.

11

BOWEL AND BLADDER MANAGEMENT

Marialorna Kerl and Jan Dougherty

INTRODUCTION

People with advanced dementia develop urinary incontinence, followed by fecal incontinence. A rapid onset of either urinary or fecal incontinence indicates that the individual has developed a new behavior or medical problem. It should never be suspected that persons with advanced dementia are using incontinence to manipulate caregivers, as they rarely do. Staff should always assume that the problem is beyond the individual's control.

Continence is usually lost once a person with dementia loses the ability to ambulate. Apraxia, the inability to perform remembered motor tasks, increases as dementia progresses and will greatly complicate toileting practices, especially because toileting requires a complex combination of motivation, visual recognition, and motor skills.

Because bodily functions are very personal and private matters, assistance with toileting becomes distressing for persons with advanced dementia and their caregivers. There are several key strategies to keep in mind when helping those with advanced dementia with toileting, including maintaining a matter-of-fact attitude and approach, offering reassurance, and maintaining a calm demeanor. It is important to help the individual retain a sense of dignity and privacy despite incontinence problems by conveying a supportive attitude to lessen feelings of embarrassment. In addition, evaluate each person with advanced dementia thoroughly and develop an individualized care plan to ensure that it supports the individual's needs.

GENERAL PRINCIPLES RELATING TO ASSESSMENT OF BLADDER AND BOWEL CONTINENCE

Loss of bladder and bowel continence are common complications as dementia becomes advanced. Incontinence is a leading cause of placement in care facilities outside the home and can be a cause of significant discomfort. Although incontinence is common, an evaluation of causes should always be undertaken. If incontinence is new, check with the person's primary care provider to determine if there are underlying medical reasons. Many causes can be controlled.

Assess potentially reversible causes using the DIAPPERS system:

Delirium, Dementia, Depression (the three Ds)
Infection (urinary tract infection)
Atrophic vaginitis
Pharmaceuticals
Psychological, Pain
Excess fluid (polyuria, edema)
Restricted mobility
Stool (constipation)

Measures such as bowel and bladder programs need to be implemented early to prevent complications. Bowel programs to prevent constipation need to be individualized to take into account body size and nutritional intake. A daily bowel movement is not a realistic goal for frail elderly persons with advanced dementia.

▩ GENERAL PRINCIPLES RELATED TO MANAGEMENT OF BLADDER AND BOWEL INCONTINENCE

Behavior Management of Urinary Incontinence

Strategies can be implemented to reduce urinary incontinence. These include timed voiding, habit retraining, and prompted voiding.

Timed voiding refers to toileting the person every 2–3 hours on a fixed schedule. The goal is to decrease bladder volume and the urge to void between toileting, as well as to lower volume wetting if incontinence does occur. Two studies found that with this technique, an 85%–91% improvement in incontinence occurred.

Habit retraining is patterned urge-response toileting. The individual's bladder-emptying pattern is determined through pant checks or electronic sensor monitoring systems (that monitor bladder activity), allowing the toileting schedule to be individualized. Not a lot of research has been done on this approach, although one study did find an overall 86% improvement in control, with one-third improving by 25% or better.

Prompted voiding combines routine toileting at a 1- to 2-hour frequency with verbal prompts from the caregiver and positive reinforcement to bladder cues (i.e., the feeling of urgency that is normal). Research has shown an overall 75% improvement, with about one-third of persons decreasing incontinence to less than once in 12 hours.

Additional behavior management for urinary incontinence includes setting a toileting schedule; leading the person to the bathroom or a bedside commode (BSC); assisting with disrobing; positioning the person to sit comfortably on the toilet or BSC; and monitoring to ensure that the person does not prematurely stand and leave the toilet. Include this information in a "bladder diary" that can be retained in the medical record or at the bedside or bathroom.

Keep a written record of when the person goes to the bathroom and when and how much he or she eats and drinks. Establishing such a record will help determine the person's natural toileting routine. If the person is unable to go to the toilet, use a BSC. Following completion of toileting, note whether the individual has had a bowel movement or has emptied his or her bladder. Ensure that good perineal care has been provided. Ensure that hygiene is complete by assisting him or her with hand washing. Commonly, toileting is encouraged every 2 waking hours, but toileting at longer intervals, such as every 3 or 4 hours, may be appropriate for some people. A bladder diary provides the best information for individualizing a program. If the bladder diary reveals that a person tends to urinate every 3 hours, encourage toileting every 2.5 hours to keep them dry. If the bladder diary reveals unusual frequency, investigate the possibility that an underlying medical cause may exist.

Behavior Management of Fecal Incontinence

Fecal incontinence can be a significant contributor to discomfort and poses an increased risk of decubitus. Another term that may be used to describe fecal incontinence is *fecal obstipation*. Although the terms may be used interchangeably, their definitions are different and their appropriate use in dementia is clarified here.

Fecal incontinence occurs late in advanced dementia. Loss of bowel control in the early stages of dementia suggests some other physical problem, such as damage to nerves that control the rectal sphincter, severe hemorrhoids, or rectal tumors.

Fecal obstipation is a massive accumulation of feces within the colon that occurs with dehydration, a low-fiber diet, and the use of anticholinergic medications. Long-term users of antipsychotic medications are at a higher risk for developing fecal obstipation. Assessment of whether there are copious amounts of hardened feces within the colon involves a rectal examination, and palpation of the colon and abdomen. Treatment consists of dietary monitoring, good hydration, and consistent bowel cleansing. Digging at the rectum may indicate hemorrhoids, impaction (severe obstipation that cannot be defecated and usually has to be removed), or skin problems in the perineal area. Women may dig at the rectal region because they have vaginal infections from antibiotics or because of thinning of the vulva resulting from estrogen deficiency. Any person digging at their rectal region should receive a perineal examination and females should receive a vaginal examination to exclude other potential causes of perineal discomfort.

Maintaining Bowel and Bladder Function

Many strategies can improve continence. Strategies to improve bladder function include the following:

- Avoid withholding fluids when the person starts to lose bladder control. This can cause dehydration, which can lead to urinary tract infections and further incontinence. Even minor dehydration can cause confusion.

▨ Ensure that the person is getting enough fluid to adequately stimulate the bladder and to avoid constipation. Address the person's preferences for fluids.

▨ Eliminate caffeinated drinks such as coffee, cola, and tea, because these are diuretics and can stimulate urination.

▨ Limit liquids at least 2 hours before bedtime but be sure to provide adequate hydration throughout the day.

▨ Use adult briefs and bed pads at night as a backup to the daytime toileting schedule.

Strategies to improve bowel function include the following:

▨ Monitor the frequency of bowel movements. Persons with advanced dementia need not have a bowel movement every day but if 3 days have passed without one, then the individual is in a state of constipation.

▨ Add natural laxatives to the diet to help soften the stool and improve bowel function. Foods that provide a natural laxative effect include prunes or fiber-rich foods such as bran or whole-grain breads.

▨ Incorporate stool softeners or mild laxatives into the plan of care, if necessary, to ensure regularity.

In general, to maintain bladder or bowel continence, watch for visible cues that may signal an individual's need to use the bathroom. These visible signs include restlessness, anxiety, agitation, pacing, unusual sounds, idiosyncratic facial expressions, sudden behavior changes with no evident cause, pulling at their clothes, dropping their pants, or suddenly stopping eating for no apparent reason.

Handling Incontinence

Experiencing incontinence is both embarrassing and uncomfortable. When working with people experiencing incontinence, be supportive by helping the person retain a sense of dignity. Some helpful strategies that help promote individual dignity include the following:

▨ Respect the individual's privacy by looking the other way if the person appears to be made uncomfortable by your presence.

▨ Provide clothing that is manageable and comfortable. Dress them in easy-to-remove and clean garments that are simple and practical.

▨ When possible, use adaptive clothes specially designed for impaired adults. These offer ease of care that is not always available in standard clothing and provide easier access to briefs.

▨ Select sleep clothes that are functional as well as comfortable. Nightgowns and nightshirts are easier to work with than pajamas. Do not use hospital gowns.

▨ Use disposable adult briefs and protective pads as needed. Adult briefs come in different levels of absorbency for day or overnight use.

▨ Use incontinence bedding. Disposable incontinence pads are made to protect bedding along with rubberized sheets and flannel sheets. A draw sheet combined with absorbent bed pads and rubber pad will keep the bed dry and promote comfort for the person.

Skin Care

Skin breakdown is inevitable if incontinence is left unattended. Caregiver vigilance is critical in preventing skin breakdown in the individual experiencing incontinence. Some suggestions for preventative skin care include the following:

- Pay attention to behavioral cues, because the person may be trying to communicate his or her need to be toileted or the need to change a wet or soiled brief.
- Never allow an individual to remain in wet or soiled briefs. Change briefs immediately to protect from skin breakdown. A person who remains in wet or soiled clothing can quickly develop irritations, sores, and painful rashes.
- Promptly clean the skin after each episode of incontinence. Provide scrupulous skin care to sensitive skin areas to keep the skin healthy. Clean the skin with mild soap and water or use cleaners designed to avoid excess dryness. Rinse skin thoroughly and gently pat dry.
- Consider using a sealant or moisture barrier to protect the skin if there is constant exposure to urine or stool.
- After toileting, aside from toilet paper, use adult or baby wipes that are free of chemicals, perfumes, and alcohol. Be sure to dry the skin afterward to avoid irritation and rashes.

Avoid skin rash occurrence through proper care. In addition to the strategies to maintain skin integrity, which are listed previously, there are additional cautions to keep in mind to avoid skin rashes. These additional tips include the following:

- Observe for behavioral cues that the person's brief needs to be changed.
- Use plain water with a soft cloth to wipe the person's perineal and rectal areas after toileting.
- Avoid wipes containing chemicals, perfumes, or alcohol.
- Expose the person's buttocks to air whenever possible.
- Avoid tight-fitting disposable briefs or plastic pants over cloth briefs.
- Apply petroleum jelly or barrier ointment (e.g., Desitin, A & D Ointment, or zinc oxide) after cleaning with a moist cloth to protect the person's skin.
- Interventions that should be avoided include talc powder, which, if inhaled, may irritate the lungs and cause pneumonia, and cornstarch because it may increase the yeast growth. Avoid unnecessary antibiotics—overuse may not only lead to skin rashes but also complications such as diarrhea.

Inspect skin daily, especially around vulnerable areas (e.g., the groin and buttocks), to identify potential problems early. Treat skin problems immediately. If sore spots occur, use moisturizing creams. Avoid products that contain alcohol. Apply topical moisturizers gently and without massage over bony prominences. Research has not shown that massage is helpful over bony prominences; in fact, it may be harmful. Consider allowing the perineal area to be left open to air in bed at night or any other time during the day. Use additional absorbent washable bed pads to adequately protect the person and promote comfort. Ensure that the person's dignity is maintained by the use of nighttime wear while taking into consideration physical constraints.

EXHIBIT 11.1

Standards of Care for Managing Bladder and Bowel Incontinence

A. The healthcare facility shall:
1. Develop and implement policies and procedures that address bowel and bladder management. This will include but should not be limited to issues of:
   a. Assessment of reversible causes of incontinence;
   b. An individualized toileting schedule; and
   c. Maintenance of individual dignity.
2. Provide adequate healthcare staffing to meet needs of all persons with advanced dementia who have moderate-to-maximum needs, such as:
   a. Daily frequent episodes of bladder incontinence;
   b. Assistance with changing brief or perineal care;
   c. Occasional bowel incontinence or assistance for continent bowel movement;
   d. Timed-toileting bladder schedule;
   e. Bowel care program in place or ostomy supervision;
   f. Totally incontinent of bladder;
   g. Daily ongoing toileting to minimize incontinence; and
   h. Total assistance for continent bowel care or requires total care with an ostomy.
3. Develop and implement policies that promote skin care related to bowel and bladder management. This includes considerations such as the:
   a. Frequency of toileting to promote urinary or fecal continence;
   b. Use of adult briefs and protective pads during the day and at night for those who are incontinent, with frequent changes to prevent the person sitting in a wet or soiled brief for prolonged periods; and
   c. Repositioning individuals who are not able to reposition themselves at a minimum of every 2 hours.
4. Ensure that the healthcare staff is trained and knowledgeable regarding continence and skin care strategies for persons with advanced dementia.

B. Healthcare staff shall:
1. Provide a sense of dignity and privacy despite incontinence problems by conveying a supportive attitude to help lessen feelings of embarrassment.

2. Use comfort measures that distract the person from the embarrassment and lack of dignity when perineal care is given.
3. Establish a primary caregiver whenever possible to ensure continuity of care and alleviate stress and anxiety.
4. Maintain a bladder diary or record to establish patterns for each person and to determine interventions to prevent incontinence episodes.
5. Provide clear access to toilets or BSCs at all times.
6. Conduct a skin assessment each time the person is cleaned after bladder or bowel incontinence.
7. Conduct daily inspection of skin and bony prominences for persons who sit and lie for long periods.

C. Persons with advanced dementia shall expect:
1. Maintenance of dignity by being kept dry and helped to avoid constipation.
2. Management of continence care that is individualized to a person's needs.
3. Maintenance of personal hygiene by using comfort measure for distraction.
4. Pressure relief, no matter what position that they are in.
5. Daily evaluation by healthcare staff for skin care and signs and symptoms of any skin disorder or breakdown.

▨ REFERENCES

AlzBrain.org. (n.d.). *Assessment and management of urinary or fecal incontinence.* Retrieved October 23, 2004, from http://www.alzbrain.org/modules.php

Alzheimer's Association (2004, October). *Incontinence (topic sheet).* Retrieved January 25, 2010, from http://www.alz.org/national/documents/topicsheet_incontinence.pdf

Lekan-Rutledge, D., & Colling, J. (2003). Urinary incontinence in the frail elderly: Even when it's too late to prevent a problem, you can still slow its progress. *American Journal of Nursing,* (Suppl.) 36–46.

Palmer, M. H. (2003). *Helping persons stay dry* (interview). Retrieved January 24, 2010, from http://www.findarticles.com/p/articles/mi_3830/is_6_52/ai_103194335/print

Volicer, L., Brandeis, G. H., & Hurley, A. C. (1998). Infections in advanced dementia. In L. Volicer & A. C. Hurley (Eds.), *Hospice care for patients with advanced progressive dementia* (pp. 29–47). New York: Springer Publishing Company.

Wells, T. (1997). Treatment approaches to common physical care needs. In C. R. Kovach (Ed.), *Late-stage dementia care: A basic guide* (pp. 73–84). Washington, DC: Taylor & Francis.

12

AMBULATION AND MOBILITY

Leslie Goin, Linda Duke, Deborah Hollawell, Antonia Horton, and Mary W. Voytek

▩ INTRODUCTION

In the advanced stages of dementia, people experience a progressive loss of ambulatory skills. Their gait deteriorates and becomes unsteady. However, because this is not always a result of dementia, if this kind of decline does occur, it is important to assess if other medical issues are involved. If other causes have been ruled out, caregivers then need to have an understanding of how dementia affects walking and mobility. What follows is an overview.

Once people with dementia lose the ability to walk, they require greater assistance. They will need ambulatory devices such as walkers and quad canes, help with wheelchair mobility, and help with positioning in wheelchairs to prevent pressure ulcers. They may display generalized rigidity and require two or more caregivers to transfer or ambulate. In addition, they will be at a much higher risk for falls. Between 40% and 60% of persons with advanced dementia fall each year, making them three times more likely to sustain a bone fracture than the population as a whole. The risk of soft tissue or brain injuries is also high.

There are major consequences related to extended immobility. Consequences can include the brain's failure to adequately communicate with the rest of the body; muscle atrophy; skeletal changes (e.g., osteoporosis and contractures); pressure ulcers, often from tissue ischemia; and systemic problems such as kidney stones, pneumonia, metabolic changes, and cardiovascular changes.

▩ GENERAL PRINCIPLES RELATED TO ASSESSING AMBULATION AND MOBILITY CAPACITY IN ADVANCED DEMENTIA

The maintenance of a person's ability to walk remains a significant challenge in advanced dementia. Persons with advanced dementia may have deficits in balance and judgment, or deficits related to coexisting medical conditions such as Parkinson's or neuropathies that can produce an unsteady gait and place them at a higher risk of falling.

Restorative care programming is necessary to promote and maintain upper and lower body mobility and to prevent premature and excess disability related to loss of upper or lower body mobility. Fall prevention programming is also necessary for persons with advanced dementia. These programs train caregivers to assess for fall risk, provide safeguards to prevent falls, monitor evaluation methods and address individual and community response to programming, and advocate for the minimum use of restraints.

All people with advanced dementia have the right to be free from unnecessary physical restraints. Although restraints may seem like a quick solution to prevent people from falling, studies show that they do not contribute to reducing falls. In fact, the use of restraints actually carry many risks that include falling with the wheelchair attached, strangulation, loss of muscle tone, pressure ulcers, depression, agitation, reduced bone mass, stiffness, frustration, loss of dignity, incontinence, constipation, injury from the restraint itself, skin breakdown, circulatory compromise, and decreased social contact.

With fall prevention programs, enlist skilled services or consultation, when appropriate. Involve the person in movement and exercise programs, if possible. Caregivers should be educated in strategies for anticipating needs, promoting mobility within a safe setting, and providing comfort with mobility difficulties. Always focus on quality of life.

▇ GENERAL PRINCIPLES FOR IMPLEMENTING AMBULATION AND MOBILITY SAFEGUARDS

There are many practices and safeguards that may improve and preserve mobility and ambulation in persons with advanced dementia. Assessing the person's level of mobility as well as identifying the cause of change in mobility and ambulation with the help of an interdisciplinary team is an important first step. An assessment will determine whether the person has:

A. Experienced a recent and acute change in ambulatory status (within the last month). This is often the result of acute infection and immobility from short-term bed rest, orthopedic injury, or an acute cerebrovascular accident (with resulting acute weakness or numbness). In these cases, restorative potential is generally relatively good. Or:

B. Suffered from long-term immobility. This may be a result of prolonged bed rest or confinement in a chair. The restorative potential is greatly influenced by the individual's motivation and mental status; these aspects, unfortunately, are limited in persons with advanced dementia.

With long-term immobility, professional and family caregivers should be educated regarding the typical progression in function loss with advanced dementia. The Functional Assessment Staging Tool (FAST) scale may help to anticipate future needs (see chapter 1 on determining and defining advanced dementia). Once the typical progression is learned and the myriad of exceptions identified, it can be easier to determine which kinds of functional decline are likely to respond to specific programs and the intervention of trained therapists. All caregivers, however, must guard against a tendency to attribute changes solely to the progression of the disease. It is important to be on the alert for signs that a new or different problem may have started.

After the assessment, establish ambulation practices. Evaluate abilities such as balance, distances walked, frequency, endurance, any safety concerns, and any personal routines that should be considered when developing a care plan. If indicated, have a medical professional evaluate cardiac, respiratory, or other possible physical causes of limitations. Consider physical therapy consultations for specific issues, such as the use of adaptive devices to assist with transfers. Assess fall risks using an objective measurement. The Functional Reach Test, for instance, can determine the potential for recurrent falls because it is a measure of balance and is the difference, in inches, between arm's length and maximal forward reach, using a fixed base of support. The test can be used to detect balance impairment and change in balance performance over time. The test measures functional abilities. A reach of less than or equal to six is predictive of falls.

Consider adaptive clothing and other assistive devices (although, often, persons with dementia can do well without numerous assistive devices, if provided with a safe and controlled environment). Use rubber-soled shoes or nonskid footwear. Consider using protective devices to reduce the potential for injury from a fall (e.g., padded garments that include hip protectors) or lowering the bed so that it is low to the ground. Use a gait belt, when appropriate, for ambulation and safe transfers. Always have the individual's comfort be the primary goal.

If a person with advanced dementia tries to rise from the chair, assess what he or she may be trying to communicate through this action; for example, the person may be trying to tell the caregiver that he or she needs toileting. Anticipate needs to prevent the individual's attempt at unsafe ambulation. The caregiver can then incorporate interventions into a care plan to meet these anticipated needs, which include a regulated schedule to:

- Initiate frequent toileting
- Change a person's position at least every 2 hours to increase comfort and decrease the chance of pressure ulcers
- Conduct a pain assessment
- Engage in activities with the individual that prevent boredom

If there appears to be a need for movement, encourage the attempt with guided assistance. Often this may be just enough to satisfy a person's desire to move. As the disease progresses, people will need physical assistance to perform basic mobility tasks. The anticipation of needs becomes even more important then, because a person with advanced dementia will no longer be able to use words to express their needs.

Persons with advanced dementia often need assistance with transfers (e.g., from bed to chair or wheelchair to car). Efforts should be made to keep this skill in place for as long as possible. To start, assess the person's coordination and balance. The person may need the assistance of one or two persons. Sufficient personnel or mechanical resources must be available. When preparing for a transfer, reassure the person and use the soft approach. This will minimize his or her desire to struggle (see chapter 6 on behavior problems associated with advanced dementia). Use a gait belt to lighten the required caregiver effort and to ensure safety for the persons involved.

In planning a program, it is crucial to consult with the interdisciplinary team. The following are the practice scope, experience, and contribution of the interdisciplinary team to the program plan.

Direct care staff might observe the ways the person moves and help him or her use these movements while assisting them with hygiene, dressing, grooming, and toileting. They can encourage persons with advanced dementia to use any skills they still possess, such as raising their arms or standing while dressing or grooming. Direct care staff can assist with mobility and stretching by performing range of motion exercises with them (e.g., passive movement of limbs). If individuals are able to ambulate with assistance, caregivers can develop a routine of walking them into the dining room for each meal. Because of the risk of falls, direct care staff should be required to have knowledge of proper body mechanics and how to use a gait belt for safe transfers.

Nursing staff can assess for infection or other medical condition that might be causing changes in ambulation, notify the primary care provider if infection is present, and initiate appropriate wound management interventions related to skin breakdown. While providing nursing care or giving medications, nursing staff should look for ways to incorporate movement. Nursing staff will be involved with providing care related to skin breakdown problems or to treating injuries from a fall.

Restorative therapy can help by performing range of motion routines, assisting with walking, and providing positioning devices and adaptive equipment.

Activity professionals and recreation therapists can assist persons with advanced dementia by instituting activities that provide opportunities for movement and decrease boredom. Some gratifying experiences that incorporate movement for persons with advanced dementia include sitting in a circle for a game of balloon toss, kicking an oversized beach ball, reaching for bubbles, moving hands or arms by holding on to a string of tied scarves or a parachute, holding hands with a caregiver and moving to music, or shaking a percussion instrument while music plays (see chapter 14, on activity programming, for more information). Social services can advise caregivers on the need to obtain necessary medical equipment or adaptive aids and can recommend helpful community resources.

Physical therapists can assist with proper positioning to keep a person comfortable, recommend environmental adaptations and restraint reduction, provide caregiver training in areas such as safe transfer and assistance with walking, preventing loss of bed mobility (to prevent contractures or bed sores), the identification of restorative needs for range of motion, and the incorporation of strategies to improve or maintain general fitness.

Occupational therapists can identify remaining abilities the individual may have that caregivers can engage during guided mobility. Special attention is paid to the upper extremities: hand placement, mobility of the shoulder, the ability to grasp or pinch, and so forth. These skills can make a difference for caregivers when it comes to transfers, proper seating, or the use of adaptive equipment.

Implementing a Fall Protection Program

A fall protection program will involve conducting a complete risk assessment upon admission into a long-term care or assisted-living facility. Both intrinsic and extrinsic factors need to be included in the risk assessment.

Intrinsic Factors

Intrinsic factors, many of which involve age-related changes, relate to the body. Conducting a risk assessment involving intrinsic factors includes the investigation of the following:

- *History of falls.* Secure a history of falls, if possible. Studies have shown that a history of falls is a predictor of future falls.
- *Acute illness.* Assess for presence of acute illness. Determine if there has been a recent rapid onset of symptoms associated with other disorders including seizures, urinary track infections, upper respiratory infections, delirium, stroke-related manifestations, orthostatic hypotension, and febrile conditions with or without associated dehydration.
- *Pain or chronic disease.* Complete a medical history to determine the person's history of pain or chronic diseases that might place them at a high risk for falls. These could include arthritis, cataracts, glaucoma, hypotension, diabetes. Check the person's musculoskeletal system for muscle atrophy, including the calcification of tendons and ligaments, contractures, curvature of the spine, the effects of osteoporosis, and the ability to maintain balance and proper posture.
- *Reduced vision.* Test vision, including decreased night vision or visual acuity, altered depth perception, decline in peripheral vision, or glare intolerance. Make sure that the person has the right glasses. Residents often switch with others. Determine how well the person's vision state will allow them to function in the environment.
- *Mobility and ambulation.* Finally, while evaluating these intrinsic factors, complete the previously described therapeutic recommendations and direct caregiver assessments related to mobility and ambulation. Integrate the documented findings into the overall assessment.

Extrinsic Factors

In addition to evaluating intrinsic factors, it is important to consider extrinsic factors, or factors related to the physical environment. In this category, conduct a risk assessment involving extrinsic factors that includes the investigation of the following:

- *Bathtubs and toilets.* Examine the individual's bathtubs and toilets to determine if proper support is available for the caregiver to safely assist with the use of bathroom facilities.

▇ *Furniture design.* Examine the furnishings to ensure that they are at a good height for easier transfers.

▇ *Ground surfaces.* Examine the condition of the ground surfaces. Clear the area of potentially hazardous obstacles (e.g., scattered rugs or small objects that might impede the patient's pathway). Ensure that there is proper lighting. Ensure that walking surfaces are even and that the person is wearing nonskid shoes or treaded socks.

▇ *Assistive devices.* Ensure an ample supply of assistive devices required by patients. An inadequate number of assistive devices may contribute to falls.

▇ *Caregiver training in the proper use of assistive devices.* Improper caregiver use of assistive devices, such as bedrails or mechanical restraining devices, can raise the risk of falls for patients. It is important to develop an individualized care plan that incorporates the use of these devices and provides caregiver training in their proper and safe use.

▇ *Medications.* Review the individual's list of medications to determine if the effect of the medication, alone or in combination with another, might contribute to the risk of patient falls. This list would include a review of sedatives, tranquilizers, benzodiazepines, antipsychotics, anticholinergics, and antihypertensives.

Use a dementia-specific fall risk factors assessment tool to identify individuals at risk (see Table 12.1). *Know* the person with advanced dementia—how do they communicate their needs? Why do they attempt to get out of a chair or bed when unattended and how can mobility be enhanced rather than restrained? Anticipating needs is the primary emphasis of fall prevention programming.

Intrinsic interventions can prevent falls. Intrinsic interventions relate to the assessment of intrinsic risks. The interventions are intended to accommodate the risks identified, including accommodating failing mobility, vision, pain, and disease. Anticipate the primary care needs of a person with advanced dementia related to positioning, the need for toileting, or pain relief. Implement a scheduled toileting program to decrease the discomfort that may prompt the person to walk when it is not safe. Do not leave the person unattended during toileting sessions. Assist with transfer when the person attempts to rise from a sitting position. This may be his or her way of telling the caregiver that he or she prefers to be mobile, if only for a short while, or that he or she may have other needs. Be aware of any declining medical condition that may require additional assistance.

Use the least restrictive enabling device to maintain safety. Table 12.2 gives examples of extrinsic interventions that can help prevent falls or be useful with positioning. Use devices *not* as restraints but for comfort and safety. Employ key healthcare team members—certified nursing assistants (CNAs) or other direct care staff; nurses; occupational, physical, and recreational therapists; and activities and social service personnel—to implement an individual care plan for the person at risk for falls. Equip the primary care provider and family with copies of the individualized fall prevention program. Educate the family about what the advancing disease process entails and the fact that there is an increased risk for falls.

TABLE 12.1

Dementia-Specific Fall Risk Factors Assessment

General	Mobility

▓ New admission or transfer to another unit
▓ Fall(s) within last 30 days
▓ No trauma
▓ Injury _____
▓ Bladder and/or bowel incontinence
▓ Low body mass
▓ Seizures
 	
   Episode of acute illness
	▓ Ambulatory and active
	▓ Ambulatory but weak or debilitated
	▓ Using assistive device: walker, cane, other _____
	▓ Unable to use assistive devices properly
	▓ Nonambulatory
	   ☐ Self-propelled wheelchair
	▓ Increase reliance on proprioception to maintain balance (i.e., as evidenced by removing footwear when ambulating)

Cognition	**Neuromotor Changes**

▓ Depression
▓ GDS Stage 6
▓ GDS Stage 7
▓ Change in cognitive level from GDS/FAST stage _____ to _____
▓ Poor reasoning or judgment that places self in unsafe situations
▓ Unable to recognize ambulation deficits
▓ Unable to tolerate wearing eyeglasses
▓ Unable to tolerate wearing hearing aid(s)
▓ Unable to verbally communicate needs
▓ Unable to comprehend bed or chair alarm
	▓ Rigidity present:
	   _____ Arms
	   _____ Legs
	   _____ Neck
	   _____ Torso
	▓ Rigidity induced by bed or chair alarm sounds
	▓ Decreased grip strength
	▓ Loss of protective reflexes
	▓ Impaired recovery balance
	▓ Impaired arm outstretching or extension

Altered Gait and Balance	**Vision Changes**
▓ Start hesitancy and freezing ▓ Shuffling ▓ Scissoring ▓ Noncontinual walk with hesitation ▓ Deviated from straight path ▓ Difficulty making turns ▓ One or both feet scrape ground surface ▓ Unable to step over obstacle ▓ Unable to navigate around obstacles ▓ Reduced walking speed ▓ Unsteady standing balance ▓ Uses furniture to maintain standing or walking balance ▓ Sinks to feet when ambulating ▓ Postural sway ___ Forward ___ Backward ___ Left side ___ Right side	▓ Decreased depth perception ▓ Decreased peripheral vision ▓ One-sided visual neglect ___ Left ___ Right **Behavior Changes** ▓ Self-stimulating wandering ▓ Restless pacing ▓ Resistive to ADL care ▓ Anxiety, agitation ▓ Sleep disturbance

Abbreviations: ADL = activities of daily living; GDS = Global Deterioration Scale; FAST = Functional Assessment Staging Tool.

Continued

Table 12.1 *Continued*

▨ Unstable rising from seated positions
▨ Unstable getting out of bed
▨ Unstable sitting balance
▨ Unable to sit up
▨ Unable to perform unassisted chair/bed
   transfers
▨ Feet slide away on ground during transfers

Source: Data from Lucero, 2004. Adapted with permission.

It may be appropriate to reassess fall risk when the following occurs: there has been a change in a person's physiological, functional, or cognitive status; when a person falls; when there is a transfer between healthcare settings or disruption in normal routine; or every 3 months or at other specified times according to facility policy. Document the findings and interventions on the person's plan of care. Ensure that the evaluations are communicated among team members and integrated into the care plan. Conduct regular system-atic evaluations to determine effectiveness of the fall intervention program. Use members of the interdisciplinary team to determine both the individual's response to the program and the facility's progress in minimizing falls. Imple-ment a fall follow-up plan.

TABLE 12.2

Progressive Fall Interventions and Positioning Options

Fall Intervention and Purpose	Consent Needed if Outside of Private Home	Precautions	Release from Restraint	Reposition Every 2 Hours	Least Restrictive Device to Try Prior
Color-coded identification bands to assist with easy recognition of people at risk for falls.	No	N/A	N/A	N/A	N/A

Fall Intervention and Purpose	Consent Needed if Outside of Private Home	Precautions	Release from Restraint	Reposition Every 2 Hours	Least Restrictive Device to Try Prior
Merry Walkers (see Fig. 12.1) allow a person to walk safely while having the security of a seat behind him or her in case of fatigue and a bar to hold on to if feeling unsteady. Because the Merry Walker surrounds him or her on all sides, it is impossible for a person to forget to use it. A Merry Walker works well for people who have a tendency to rise and then sit, or who still ambulate on their own, but have poor safety awareness that leads to falls.	Yes, in addition, the Merry Walker company's guidelines come with a specific assessment that should be completed by a physical therapist.	If no longer ambulating in Merry Walker, use it instead as a chair for a more comfortable alternative. It may be used in conjunction with other interventions based on the individual's energy level.	Yes, if a person is too sedentary, assess for a transfer to a chair or bed with a clip alarm. Release while being directly supervised by staff such as during meals, care, and activities (if ambulation is not required).	No	Safe and independent ambulation.
Standard wheelchair and/or custom wheelchairs.	No	Some people find wheelchairs uncomfortable and may do better with a combination of a wheelchair for mobility and a soft and comfortable chair while sitting.	N/A	Yes	Merry Walker or combination of wheelchair and comfortable furniture.

Continued

TABLE 12.2   *Continued*

Fall Intervention and Purpose	Consent Needed if Outside of Private Home	Precautions	Release from Restraint	Reposition Every 2 Hours	Least Restrictive Device to Try Prior
Clip alarm for chairs, wheel-chairs, or bed. These items clip a string to a person's clothing while connecting to a sounding device. When a person gets up, the string pulls free from the sounding device and sets off an alarm.	No	When a person gets up, an alarm will sound alerting others that someone who is unsafe to ambulate on his or her own is doing so. Assess for thirst, hunger, pain, toileting needs, range of motion, bore-dom, or other unmet needs.	N/A	Yes	Merry Walker or combina-tion of wheel-chair and comfortable furniture. A clip alarm may be attached to a chair to allow for vari-ous seating positions.
Pressure pad alarms are similar to clip alarms, except that the alarm is sounded once someone gets up from the pressure pad.	No	Same as clip alarm.	N/A	Yes	Same as clip alarm.
Wheelchair with wedge cushion helps to relieve pressure and prevents slid-ing down.	Yes, unless used for positioning.	Monitor that the cushion does not slip out; use nonslip rubber material to hold in place if appropriate.	If used for positioning you would not want to alter; if used as a restraint, you may want to consider other alter-natives for seating when supervised such as during meals and activities.	Yes	Wheelchair with clip alarm.

Fall Intervention and Purpose	Consent Needed if Outside of Private Home	Precautions	Release from Restraint	Reposition Every 2 Hours	Least Restrictive Device to Try Prior
Wheelchair with pummel wedge cushion helps to properly position someone in a wheelchair who has poor balance, trunk control, or slides out easily. This can be used to prevent people from standing in an unsafe manner.	Yes, unless used for positioning.	Same as with wedge cushion; monitor for comfort, some people do not like the feel of the pummel; assess for increased agitation.	If used for positioning, you would not want to alter; if used as a restraint, you may want to consider other alternatives for seating when supervised, such as during meals and activities.	Yes	Wheelchair with wedge cushion.
Lap Buddy in wheelchair is typically a soft foam material that is placed in the arms of a wheelchair and goes across a person's lap. People with late-stage dementia may benefit from one that has tactile items attached to it.	Yes	Same as listed for clip belt. If the individual enjoys holding things, provide a Lap Buddy with tactile items.	Yes, same as for clip belt.	Yes	Self-releasing clip belt in some cases.
Self-release clip belt on wheelchair.	Yes, unless used for positioning and person can demonstrate that he or she can release the belt when asked to.	Assess for same concerns as listed for clip alarm. Also, assess for increased agitation caused by restriction. People with advanced stage dementia may not know how to release the clip belt.	Yes, release while being directly supervised by staff such as during meals, care, and activities.	Yes	Clip alarm, Lap Buddy in some cases especially if the person is unable to self-release the clip belt, but is able to remove a Lap Buddy.

Continued

TABLE 12.2 *Continued*

Fall Intervention and Purpose	Consent Needed if Outside of Private Home	Precautions	Release from Restraint	Reposition Every 2 Hours	Least Restrictive Device to Try Prior
Geriatric chair (a soft reclining chair on wheels).	Yes	This restricts independent movement, requiring others to propel geriatric chair.	N/A	Yes	A wheelchair is less restrictive if a person is able to propel the chair independently.
Bean bag chairs.	No	This works well for people who have poor trunk control. They often slip out of wheel and geriatric chairs. The bean bag conforms to the person, providing a comfortable and safe sitting position. Because he or she is difficult to get out of, it can limit a person's movement. It also may be difficult for caregivers to get a person out of the chair.	N/A	Yes	Wheelchair or geriatric chair.
Low beds are beds that can be lowered closer to the floor or a stationary bed that is permanently closer to the floor. This shorter distance (approximately 7 in. from the floor) limits the risk of injury if a person rolls out of bed.	No	Use a mat on the floor next to the bed. If the bed does not have an electronic means of raising and lowering, the caregiver may have a difficult time transferring a person in and out. Proper transfer techniques should be used.	N/A	N/A	N/A

FIGURE 12.1

Merry Walker

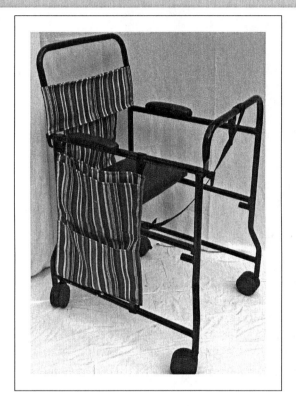

EXHIBIT 12.1

Standards of Care for Evaluating and Managing Ambulation and Mobility

A. The healthcare facility shall:
   1. Develop policies and procedures that:
      a. Identify and specify the ambulation and mobility needs of persons with advanced dementia.
      b. Schedule screening of individuals for their fall risk.
      c. Identify prevention, restoration, or preservation programs that maintain mobility and/or freedom of movement while maintaining safety, such as minimizing fall risks.
      d. Incorporate healthcare team members, such as physical, occupational, recreational, and activities personnel, in the evaluation and care planning for individuals who have limited mobility and are at risk for falls.

Continued

Exhibit 12.1 *Continued*

     e. Use healthcare team members, such as CNAs and other caregivers, activities and recreation therapy staff that can assist in providing appropriate exercise and adapted programs. Use the guidance of physical and occupation therapists in care planning, as appropriate.

     f. Use restraint-reduction programs that periodically assess for the least restrictive devices. Advocate for a restraint-free or restraint-appropriate environment.

  2. Provide an environment with clear pathways that offers familiarity and a sense of security, while maximizing mobility and minimizing falls.

  3. Provide regular training to healthcare staff that includes:

     a. Information on mobility, restorative, and fall prevention programming;

     b. Interventions to reduce falls;

     c. Interventions that promote comfort and anticipate the person's needs;

     d. Instruction on safe transfers and ambulation, gait, balance, strength training, and the proper use of positioning or assistive devices;

     e. Techniques to integrate mobility interventions into the usual activities of daily living;

     f. Instruction on proper body mechanics and transfer techniques;

     g. Instruction on the proper use of mechanical lifts; and

     h. Instruction on scheduled bowel and bladder programs.

  4. Calculate the monthly fall rate for all persons in the facility and specifically for persons with advanced dementia. Examine these indicators over time with the goal of reducing preventable falls.

B. Healthcare staff shall:

  1. Institute mobility and restorative care programming for persons with advanced dementia who show signs of difficulty with movement or seek comfort in positioning.

     a. Regularly provide ambulation or other forms of movement for those who are able to move.

     b. Incorporate physical activity into the activities of daily living and to the general activity programs that focus on upper and lower extremity mobility (see chapter 14 for more information).

     c. Encourage freedom of movement in the least restrictive fashion.

  2. Institute and adhere to a fall prevention program that uses a fall-risk assessment and programming to minimize opportunities for falls while maximizing mobility for persons with advanced dementia. Include all interdisciplinary team members in this program.

C. Persons with advanced dementia shall expect:

  1. A safe, therapeutic, and restraint-free or restraint-appropriate environment that promotes mobility and the reduction of fall risks.

  2. An assessment and plan during the course of an ambulation and mobility program that maximizes movement while meeting safety needs and promoting comfort and palliative care.

3. The recognition that other comorbidities may influence function, mobility, and ambulation and that attention to these conditions will be that of comfort care.
4. Opportunities for safe ambulation that use appropriate assistive devices and enablers.
5. Recognition that when medical and functional decline is occurring, healthcare staff will accommodate this changing condition and make the appropriate modifications in the care plan that use other measures and modalities to preserve mobility and diminish other potential health risks related to the specific and systemic effects of immobility.

■ REFERENCES

Alzbrain.org. (n.d.). *Falls (factsheet)*. Retrieved January 24, 2010, from http://www.alzbrain.org/pdf/handouts/2031.%20FALLS%20FACT%20SHEET.pdf

Alzbrain.org. (n.d.). *Transfers (factsheet)*. Retrieved January 24, 2010, from http://www.alzbrain.org/pdf/handouts/2040.%20FACT%20SHEET%20ON%20TRANSFERS.pdf

Alzheimer's Association, Desert Southwest Chapter. (2004). *Fall prevention program*. Phoenix, AZ: Author.

Beatitudes Campus. (2001). *Vermilion Cliffs fall risk policy and procedure*. Phoenix, AZ: Author.

Cotter, V. T., Evans, L. K., & Hartford Institute for Geriatric Nursing. (2003). Avoiding restraints in patients with dementia. *Try This: Best Practices in Nursing Care for Hospitalized Older Adults with Dementia, 1*. Retrieved March 25, 2005, from http://www.hartfordign.org/uploads/File/Fulmer_EM_dementia.pdf

Glencroft Care Center. (2003). *Falls protocol*. Glendale, AZ: Author.

Gray-Miceli, D. (2007). Fall risk assessment. *Try This: Best Practices in Nursing Care for Hospitalized Older Adults, (8)*. Retrieved January 24, 2010, from http://consultgerirn.org/uploads/File/trythis/issue08.pdf

Lucero, M. (2004). *Dementia-specific fall risk factors assessment*. Radium Springs, NM: Geriatric Resources, Inc.

Premier Incorporated. (n.d.) *Fall prevention*. Retrieved January 24, 2010, from http://www.premierinc.com/quality-safety/tools-services/safety/topics/falls/

Tideiksaar, R. (2002). *Falls in older people: Prevention and management* (3rd ed.). Baltimore, MD: Health Professions Press.

Trudeau, S. (1999). Prevention of physical impairment in persons with advanced Alzheimer's disease. In L. Volicer & L. Bloom-Charette (Eds.), *Enhancing the quality of life in advanced dementia* (pp. 80–90). Boston, MA: Brunner/Mazel Publishers, Inc.

Weiner, D. K., Duncan, P. W., Chandler, J., & Studenski, S. A. (1992). Functional reach: A marker of physical frailty. *Journal of the American Geriatrics Society, 40*(3), 203–207.

BATHING

Jan Dougherty

■ INTRODUCTION

Bathing can be a pleasurable experience for persons with advanced dementia. There are methods that caregivers can incorporate into their care plan to make the bathing experience more enjoyable for the individual. It is helpful to take into consideration the fact that traditional bathing schedules and showers may work for some individuals but not for others. Various options can be considered for those who balk at the prospect of traditional bathing schedules and showers, such as the towel bath, which can be used as an alternative bathing approach. This chapter will examine some of these options.

■ GENERAL PRINCIPLES RELATED TO BATHING A PERSON WITH ADVANCED DEMENTIA

As dementia progresses, bathing requires increasing care and supervision. As a result, unwanted behaviors may occur. The person with advanced dementia may resist by pushing the caregiver away, striking out, biting, kicking, yelling, swearing, moaning, or crying. These behaviors may be a result of global confusion, the infringement of their privacy, generalized discomfort or pain, or simply not wanting to bathe. The unwanted behaviors often are self-protective—the person's attempt to assert control over the situation or to protect himself or herself from perceived harm.

Practice Guidelines for Successful Bathing in Advanced Dementia

Bathing can be performed without excessive challenge by rethinking one's approach. Determine the person's preferences, such as favorite time of day and type of bathing experience. Identify bathing rituals that promote comfort and control for the person, such as listening to music, taking a bubble bath, or watching television. Create a pleasurable experience by not rushing, making the room temperature comfortable, and playing music.

Use a soft approach when introducing the idea of taking a bath. Smile, be pleasant, and avoid sounding rushed. Do not ask the person if he or she wants a bath or shower if you are not willing to accept the possibility that he or she will say no. If the person refuses, come back later—usually 2–5 minutes will give the person time to forget. Think about rephrasing—instead of saying "You need to get a shower," try saying, "Let's get freshened up."

Try employing the following steps to successful bathing: First, be organized. Have the room ready to go and set up for bathing. Have bathing supplies ready. Ensure that a person with pain has been medicated 1 hour prior to bathing. Position the person comfortably. Pad any bony prominences (e.g., hip, coccyx) using a padded insert or towels on the shower chair. Make sure the person's legs are not left dangling but rather are supported by a stool. Keep the person covered at all times using large towels or blankets to promote dignity and warmth. Begin by washing the person in the least intrusive place—usually beginning at the feet and then working up, saving the face and perineal area until the very last. Wash the hair last or separate it from the bath completely. Alternatively, consider using the beauty or barber shop for hair. Use distraction techniques liberally, such as singing, giving treats, talking about a favorite topic, or giving the person an object to hold.

Consider a towel bath in lieu of a shower or tub bath for persons who are resistant to the shower or tub. This procedure allows the person to be bathed in bed. Caregivers should use warm and wet towels that are premoistened with warm water and no-rinse soap. Bathing is done via massage (it is important not to massage over bony areas). Think of the towel bath as a spa experience. This method promotes safety, dignity, and comfort. Follow the procedure outlined here for performing a towel bath.

Towel Bath Procedure

This procedure should be considered as a primary method to keep clean those persons who are frail, nonambulatory, experiencing pain on transfer, fearful of lifts, acutely ill, afraid or overstimulated in the shower, or those persons who request this method. Many persons with advanced dementia fit this description.

Equipment:

- Two or more bath blankets
- One large plastic bag containing:
  - One large (5′ 6″ × 3′) lightweight and fan-folded towel (you may use a bath blanket if large towels are not available)
  - One standard bath towel
  - Two or more washcloths
- Two 3-qt. plastic pitchers filled with water (~105°F–110°F), to which you have added 1–1.5 oz. of no-rinse soap

Procedure:

1. Prepare the person by explaining the bath process.
2. Prepare the room so that it is quiet (or consider using music) and ensure privacy.

3. Undress the person, keeping him or her covered with a bed linen or bath blanket.
4. Prepare the bath solution and pour it into the plastic bag directly over the towels and washcloths until they are uniformly damp but not soggy. If necessary, wring out the excess solution. Twist the top of the bag to retain the heat.
5. Expose the person's feet and lower legs and immediately cover the area with the warm, moist towel. Then, gradually uncover the person while simultaneously unfolding the wet towel to re-cover him or her.
6. Place the covers at the end of the bed. You may wish to cover the person with a bath blanket over the warm moistened towels to keep the heat in longer.
7. Start washing any part of the body that is least distressing to the person by massaging directly through the towel, avoiding bony areas.
8. Bathe the back of the person's legs by bending his or her knee and going underneath.
9. Bathe the face, neck, and ears with one of the washcloths—you may also encourage the person to wash his or her own face.
10. Turn the person to the side and use the smaller towel from the plastic bag to wash the back, massaging in a similar manner. No rinsing or drying is required.
11. Use the washcloth from the plastic bag to wash the genital and rectal areas.
12. After the bath, the person can be left unclothed and covered with a bath blanket or bed linens, then dressing will follow.
13. Place used linen back into the plastic bag and afterward into a hamper.

Modifications to the Towel Bath. Remove the moist towel before turning the person to wash his or her back. Do not use a moist towel. Cover the person with a large dry towel and wash under the towel with washcloths that are wet with no-rinse soap. Stand to wash the back, perineal area, and rectum. Double bag the towels with the no-rinse soap mixture. Moisten disposable wipes (ones without perfume or alcohol) with warm water to wash rectum if it is very soiled.

Use other helpful bathing strategies during the bathing experience to reduce resistance and agitation related to the bathing experience. These strategies include the following techniques:

- Use verbal and nonverbal responses that fit the person's capabilities. Use verbal interventions with persons who can still talk and pay attention to nonverbal behaviors of those who cannot talk.
- Follow the person's lead. Talk if the person responds and is not overwhelmed. Sing if the person likes it.
- Use topics of conversation or songs that are favorites of the person. Know the names of family members, food preferences, and choice of music.
- Avoid the word *bath* with persons who do not like to bathe. Use an expression that is acceptable like *wash up* or *freshen up*.
- Speak calmly, slowly, and simply while facing the person.
- Use the person's name.
- Tell the person what you are going to do at all times and avoid surprises.
- Praise and reassure often.

- Consider bathing the person before he or she is dressed for the day.
- Wash one area at a time and then cover to keep the person warm.
- Time the bath to fit the person's history, preferences, and mood.
- Apologize any time the person expresses discomfort.
- Use distractions, such as candy or other food that the person likes, to soothe him or her or to give him or her something else to do or to hold on to.
- For those who are most resistant, consider dividing the body into seven parts and washing one part of the body over the next 7 days.
- Separate the bath from hair washing.
- For hair, consider using cloths that have been moistened with diluted no-rinse soap.
- If washing hair in bed, use the shampoo rinse tray along with no-rinse soap or shampoo. Be careful not to splash water on the person's face or in their ears as this may cause agitation. (Dougherty, 2004)

Finally, never force the bath when the person has indicated "No!" either through actions or words. Document what works for successful bathing—best time of day, frequency, type of bath experience, comfort measures (for instance, distractions) needed. Direct care staffs need to be flexible and creative to get the person clean. There are no state licensure requirements that dictate bathing frequency, but you must document on the care plan how the person is kept clean. When bathing does not occur, document the alternative approaches that were offered and refused.

EXHIBIT 13.1

Standards of Care for Providing Individualized Personal Hygiene

A. The healthcare facility shall:
  1. Have a policy or procedure that provides the person a choice on the means, time of day, place, and venue for bathing while acknowledging the need for meeting personal hygiene needs and to promote comfort and enjoyment in the least restrictive manner.
  2. Institute a policy and procedure on the towel bath.
  3. Provide training to healthcare staff on successful bathing strategies for persons with dementia, including the towel bath.
  4. Provide physical resources to healthcare staff to use for successful bathing. This includes sufficient towels, blankets, washcloths, no-rinse soap, padded inserts for shower chairs, other adaptive equipment, and distracting items.

B. Healthcare staff shall:
  1. Identify the preferred method of bathing and the desired schedule and frequency for those persons with advanced dementia.
  2. Provide daily hygiene needs through the least restrictive means while preserving dignity.

3. Use basic principles of bathing that promote comfort:
   a. Assemble the supplies in advance to expedite the bathing experience.
   b. Position the person comfortably by using adaptive equipment as needed.
   c. Keep the person warm and covered as the bathing progresses.
   d. Incorporate fall-prevention techniques if a shower or bathtub is used.
   e. Identify bathing modalities that promote comfort and cause the least consternation during bathing, such as the use of appropriate cleansing supplies (e.g., nonrinse soap).
4. Use the behavioral techniques of approaching the person gently, anticipating the needs for a positive bathing experience, and distracting and engaging with identified strategies (e.g., music, food, topics, etc.) for persons who may resist the bathing experience.

C. Persons with advanced dementia shall expect:
   1. Maintenance of personal hygiene without threats or humiliation.
   2. Maintenance of personal dignity and comfort during the bathing process.
   3. The provision of hygiene needs in the least restrictive setting possible.
   4. To be free from chemical and physical restraints when receiving care for personal hygiene needs.

▥ REFERENCES

Alzheimer's Association (n.d.). *Tips on personal care: Bathing.* Retrieved January 24, 2010, from http://www.alz.org/professionals_and_researchers_tips_on_personal_care.asp#bathing

Barrick, A., Rader, J., Hoeffer, B., Sloane, P., & Biddle, S. (2008). *Bathing without a battle: Person-directed care of individuals with dementia* (2nd ed.). New York: Springer Publishing Company.

Dougherty, J. (2004). The comfort of bathing. In C.O. Long (Ed.), *Palliative care for advanced dementia: Train-the-trainer manual* (P5-Supp-5 to P5-Supp-7). Phoenix, AZ: Alzheimer's Association, Desert Southwest Chapter.

Dougherty, J., & Long, C. O. (2003). Techniques for bathing without a battle. *Home Healthcare Nurse, 21*(1), 38–39.

Long, C. O. (2009). Palliative care for advanced dementia. *Journal of Gerontological Nursing, 35*(11), 19–24.

Perlmutter, J. S., & Camberg, L. (2004). Better bathing for residents with Alzheimer's. *Nursing Homes Long-Term Care Management, 53*(4), 40–43.

Rader, J., & Barrick, A. L. (2000). Ways that work: Bathing without a battle. *Alzheimer's Care Quarterly, 1*(4), 35–49.

Rader, J., Barrick, A. L., Hoeffer, B., Sloane, P. D., McKenzie, D., Talerico, K. A., et al. (2006). The bathing of older adults with dementia. *American Journal of Nursing, 106*(4), 40–49.

SECTION IV

PROVIDING FOR OTHER
HEALTHCARE NEEDS

14

ACTIVITIES PROGRAMMING

Gary A. Martin, Diane Mockbee, Tena Alonzo, Kathleen Deyo, Jan Dougherty, and Antonia Horton

INTRODUCTION

"First, throw out everything you know." That is what we tell caregivers and activity professionals when we begin their training in advanced-dementia care. That is because traditional approaches to caregiving and activity programming are just not relevant and do not work when it comes to caring for persons who have advanced dementia. This chapter focuses on activity programming for persons with advanced dementia. In some ways, the philosophies, principles, and practices discussed here are extensions and adaptations of those that can be found in the general dementia care literature, especially coming from the person-centered care model.

However, in many ways, what is discussed here reflects a paradigm shift. Gone are the large groups and structured classes. Gone are the old standby activities like bingo, cards, and crafts. Moreover, gone are the rigid month-long activity calendars. We discard and reinvent caregivers' roles, titles, and job descriptions. And we completely redefine what an activity is and how it is done—activities are no longer big bold events, but rather, a series of small intimate interactions. Business as usual no longer applies when considering the needs and care of persons with advanced dementia, especially when it comes to activities.

Most persons with advanced dementia live in care settings that include a large number of residents who do not have dementia. Some are in special care programs where every resident has dementia, which includes persons from the mild-to-moderate stages and beyond. Unfortunately, only a few live in settings that are designed specifically and exclusively for persons with advanced dementia, because so few of those programs exist. One of the problems with living with mixed populations is that persons with advanced dementia often get lost in the shuffle, and this is especially true when it comes to activity programming. Even in special care programs, activities tend to be geared to the higher-functioning residents who can walk, talk, follow directions, and actively participate. Rarely are those activities adapted to the special needs and abilities of persons with advanced dementia and, as a result, they are left behind.

Traditional activity programming emphasizes recreational and social events that are prescheduled in 30- and 60-minute time blocks. Anywhere from two to six activities occur each day. Activities are scheduled at least 1 month ahead of time, and monthly calendars are posted at the beginning of each month. Many activities are put on a weekly rotation where they are repeated the same time, same day each week (e.g., bingo every Tuesday at 2:00 p.m.). One-time or occasional special events, such as holiday celebrations, outings, and special entertainment programs, are also posted on the calendar. A typical activity calendar might include an exercise class, coffee social, and arts and crafts in the morning, with game playing (e.g., bingo, cards), sing-alongs, and happy hour in the afternoon. Some popular activities, such as exercise class and bingo, might be repeated during the week, and church services are often scheduled on Sundays.

One should note that, with the possible exception of church services, none of these activities are geared for persons with advanced dementia. Even so, it is common practice for caregivers to bring their advanced-dementia residents to these activities, believing that they might somehow benefit from being there. A cynic might say that this is done to get residents out of the way and to babysit them for a while; or maybe to meet the documentation requirements so they can show that the residents "participated" in the activity program. However, even under the best of circumstances, there is no benefit to persons with advanced dementia attending activities that are not geared for them and, as a result, they often fall asleep or become restless and agitated.

The challenge in programming for persons with advanced dementia is that they are severely confused, functionally incapacitated, cannot walk, and have severely impaired language and communication skills. Traditional activities, like arts and crafts and bingo, require somewhat clearer thinking, more intact perceptual and motor skills, longer attention spans, and greater social awareness than persons with advanced dementia possess. It is difficult, if not impossible, for them to enjoy or appreciate an activity if they cannot do it and do not understand it, and attending these types of activities is more likely to bore, distract, or distress them than anything else.

Unfortunately, activity programming is often considered a low priority in many care settings. Administrators, doctors, and caregivers tend to focus on the importance of addressing medical and care needs, often at the expense of the person's activity-based needs (e.g., social, cultural, spiritual, and recreational). For example, it is not uncommon for a nursing home resident to be taken out of an activity because it was in conflict with his or her shower schedule. In contrast, proponents of the person-centered care model would argue that activity needs are just as important as care needs and should be prioritized accordingly. In making this argument, they would point out that the individual's sense of self and personhood derive from activity-driven issues like family, friends, jobs, culture, religion, hobbies, and interests, and that maintaining a sense of self and personhood depends almost entirely on the nature and quality of the activities in which he or she engages.

Chapter 4 maintains that "the most important challenge for caregivers of persons with dementia is to help maintain and enhance their personhood despite all the losses and changes that they are and will be experiencing." In this chapter, we contend that one of the most critical factors in maintaining and enhancing the personhood of individuals with advanced dementia is the activity program and how well it reaches and affects them. In this regard, traditional activity programs generally fail. It is our contention that, structured correctly, activity programs can be made meaningful, therapeutic, and rewarding for persons with advanced dementia and can be instrumental in promoting their personal comfort, personhood, quality of life, and human dignity.

This chapter is a reconsideration of activity programming's more traditional notions used in care settings today. Much of it will go against the grain of what is currently practiced in facilities throughout the United States. The bottom line is that most care settings do a poor job of meeting the activity needs of persons with advanced dementia, and business as usual is not acceptable anymore. In this chapter we will focus on six guiding principles:

1. The goal of all activities is to make positive *meaningful connections* between caregivers and the persons with advanced dementia.
2. Activities need to be *individualized* and customized for persons with advanced dementia.
3. Activities must be done in a *one-to-one format* or in small and targeted groups.
4. *Sensory stimulation* and *sensory calming* are key concepts in doing activities with persons with advanced dementia.
5. *Activities of daily living* (ADLs) are meaningful activities and, as such, are opportunities to engage in meaningful connections and should be considered an important part of activity programming.
6. *Activity calendars* should reflect tremendous flexibility in scheduling around-the-clock activities for persons with advanced dementia.

GUIDING PRINCIPLES IN ACTIVITY PROGRAMMING FOR PERSONS WITH ADVANCED DEMENTIA

Meaningful Connections

Dementia causes a decline in many cognitive and functional abilities, including those that affect the capacity to remember, understand, and maintain normal interpersonal relationships. By the time persons reach the advanced stages of dementia, they have lost their ability to remember significant others' names, as well as the details and nature of those relationships, and they may not be able to recognize or remember close family members, friends, and caregivers. However, that does not mean they have no feelings or do not benefit from their relationships with others. Most persons with advanced dementia still have a great capacity for affection and warm human contact and are quite receptive to expressions of affection offered by others. We refer to the often brief and subtle exchanges of warmth and personal contact between caregivers and residents as *meaningful connections*, and they are the single most critical aspect of good activity programming for persons with advanced dementia.

Meaningful connections are what caregivers should always be striving for in their interactions with persons with advanced dementia. Rather than focus on the tasks at hand, caregivers should instead attend to the quality of their interactions by being open, warm, accepting, and giving. The measure of caregivers' success is not how many showers they give or how many residents attended an activity; the measure of their success is the number and quality of meaningful connections they make throughout the day while caring for their residents. The goal is for residents to experience a continuous stream of these meaningful connections, each one of which helps to reaffirm the individual's sense of self, maintain his or her sense of personhood, and enhance the quality of his or her life.

In accomplishing this goal, there are a few factors to consider. First, the milieu must be comfortable and comforting. It is virtually impossible to have meaningful connections when the situation is loud, distracting, or uncomfortable. Second, the caregiver must be situated close to the individual and in a position to give direct, focused attention. Meaningful connections cannot be made in large-group activities and cannot be made from across a room. Third, the individual's comfort needs must be met so that he or she is physically and emotionally comfortable. It is unlikely that meaningful connections can be made when residents are wet, hungry, distressed, or in pain; so before initiating an activity, caregivers should make sure that all comfort needs have been addressed and the resident is indeed comfortable. It should also be noted that providing this kind of care to a resident is a wonderful opportunity to engage in meaningful connections. Fourth, if the person begins to fall asleep, becomes agitated or restless, or begins to yell, cry, or moan, no connection can be made. In fact, such behaviors mean that the activity is missing the mark, or that the individual has become uncomfortable in some way. It is the caregiver's responsibility to immediately address the situation then try to reestablish a meaningful connection.

The deficits associated with advanced dementia sometimes cloud our ability to recognize when a meaningful connection is being made. A rule of thumb is to "look for the light in their eyes" and watch for clear signs of comfort, affection, and happiness in the individual's gestures and expressions. These can be evidenced by the following:

- Open eyes, eye contact, visual tracking
- Orienting or attending to others
- Smiling, laughing
- Pleasant verbalizations, talking, singing
- Positive changes in facial expression, changes in body language
- Positive changes in behavior (e.g., calmer demeanor, slowed breathing, relaxed muscles, yawning)
- Improved level of alertness
- Improved awareness of surroundings

Individualized Activities

Activity programming for persons with advanced dementia should be individualized according to each person's unique abilities, past and current interests, pace, and level of participation. All persons with advanced dementia are not alike and, in fact, have a wide range of individual differences. Activity programming must therefore be strategically planned and specifically targeted to the individual.

For example, music activities are often very effective at making meaningful connections. Even well into the advanced stages of dementia, musical perceptions, musical memory, and emotional sensitivity to music seem to survive long after other cognitive abilities have waned and disappeared. Those of us in the field of advanced dementia care have seen many cases in which persons with severely impaired language skills could sing all the verses to a familiar song. However, music activities for persons with advanced dementia must account for personal taste. Just like everyone else, persons with advanced dementia like certain songs and genres and do not like others, so the music played in any activity must be customized to the tastes and preferences of the individual. Similarly, food-oriented activities can also be effective in making meaningful connections. However, everyone has their own taste in foods—they like some foods and do not like others. Although soft and sweet (e.g., ice cream, pudding, sweetened yogurt, pureed fruit, soft cookies) is a rule of thumb for persons with advanced dementia, that rule does not apply to everyone. We have certainly seen our share of cases where individuals preferred potatoes, cheese, pasta, or even spicy foods or foods smothered in gravy, over sweets.

The key here is for caregivers to *know* their residents and know them well. Knowledge about residents' preferences, routines, and histories is the door through which caregivers make meaningful connections. As we see described in chapters 3, 5, 6, 7, 9, and 11, knowing and understanding the resident is one of the most critical factors in maintaining personhood, addressing behavior problems, and giving good care. It is also the key to successful activity programming. That does not mean just knowing their name, age, marital status, and past occupations. It also means knowing the details about their cultural and religious histories, educational background, and family history.

Unfortunately, persons with advanced dementia cannot tell caregivers about themselves, so it is up to their caregivers to gather that information. This means putting together a life history—information that goes well beyond what is noted on a traditional social history form, including details and insights on past interests, personal preferences, established routines, favorite foods, musical tastes, sleeping habits, hobbies, leisure time, and travels.

Several models and formats of life histories (also called biosketches and life stories) are available. Here are a few examples:

- In *The Best Friends Approach to Alzheimer's Care*, Bell and Troxel (2003) spelled out in great detail the gathering and use of information for the life story.
- In chapter 9 of Kovach's *Late-Stage Dementia Care: A Basic Guide*, Hellen (1997) described making a comprehensive life story book for persons with advanced dementia.
- Habib (2002) reported on place-biosketches that were designed for use with dementia residents in care facilities.
- Dougherty, Gallagher, Cabral, Long, and McLean (2007) developed a tool specifically for persons with advanced dementia called About Me, which is a written document that is posted in residents' bedrooms to help hospice staff and caregivers gain a greater understanding of the individual.

Life history information need periodic review and updating to take into account changes in the individual's abilities and interests as time passes. Informants should include anyone who has knowledge or information about the person, past or present, including family, friends, and past and current caregivers. Personal records and documents may also be helpful. In addition, trial and error should be used as a means of continuously developing, shaping, and individualizing this personal database for activity planning. In using a trial-and-error strategy, caregivers should try various approaches to a given activity to determine which approaches are successful in making meaningful connections. Over time, a list of successful approaches will be developed, which can then be incorporated into an overall activity plan. Approaches that are unsuccessful should be discarded. As the plan grows and changes, it should be continually documented and communicated to all caregivers so that everyone, not just activity staff, know and use it.

Customizing and individualizing each person's activity plan takes time and effort. It requires input from many sources, good communication among caregivers, and a flexible, trial-and-error approach to planning. Although time-consuming in practice, the concept is a simple one: figure out what the person likes to do, then do it with him or her as often as possible.

Formats that Promote Connections

A few years ago, we conducted an informal survey of several experienced and highly skilled certified nursing assistants that were based in skilled nursing facilities and asked them about their ability to make meaningful connections while doing activities with residents who have advanced dementia. When asked whether they could connect with an individual on a one-to-one basis, they unanimously and emphatically said, yes, they could. They also agreed that they could fairly easily make simultaneous connections with a 2:1 resident-to-staff ratio. When asked about resident-to-staff ratio of 3:1 situations, they hesitated before deciding it usually can be done, but can be challenging. However, when it came to 4:1 resident-to-staff ratio, they admitted that three was the limit and that they usually could not make meaningful connections with four residents at a time.

This raises an important point in activity programming. Because the single most critical aspect of good activity programming for persons with advanced dementia is making meaningful connections, caregivers must be sure that the activities formats are conducive to making those connections. Obviously, a one-to-one format is more conducive for making meaningful connections than group formats, which means that caregivers should strive to use a one-to-one format as much as possible. However, because a one-to-one approach to activities is not always possible, there are times when other formats can be effective. The following is a discussion of those formats and the circumstances under which they might be used.

One-to-One Activities

Most activities should be done on a one-to-one basis to make the necessary meaningful connections between the caregivers and person with advanced dementia. Examples include massages, personal grooming, ADL care, walks, going outside, and having snacks.

Small Groups With Two to Three Participants

Sometimes small groups are appropriate and desirable because of the social aspect of the group and the potential for contact and emotional intimacy between residents. The challenge of small group activities is to establish and maintain meaningful connections with all group members at the same time. Activity groups of this nature should have no more than three participants; otherwise, meaningful connections cannot be made or maintained. Examples include reading aloud, praying and reading scriptures, playing or listening to rhythm instruments, pet visits, going outside, tactile activities, and snacks and other food-related activities.

Small Groups With Four to Six Participants

Some small group activities are designed to establish a brief connection with only one person at a time. This type of group should include no more than six participants—any more would too severely dilute the attention given to any one participant. Each person gets individualized attention while the others wait. Those waiting get only indirect attention, and meaningful connections with them are generally lost until it is their turn. All persons in the group get their fair share of attention on a rotating basis. Examples include massages, personal grooming (e.g., brushing hair, manicures), showing photographs, eating snacks, praying and reading scriptures. Most one-to-one activities can be adapted to this kind of group.

Large Groups With Six or More Participants

Large groups of six or more participants are rarely effective with persons who have advanced dementia and should be done on a very limited basis. It is extremely difficult to establish meaningful connections with a large number of persons all at the same time. To be effective, such groups must be bold and attention grabbing. Group leaders must be loud enough to gain the group's attention, but not so loud as to scare, upset, agitate, or otherwise overstimulate the individuals in the group. With large groups, it is helpful to have additional caregivers present to individually attend to participants to make connections (e.g., sing-alongs and other musical entertainment).

It is important to note that because persons with advanced dementia usually reside in care settings with mixed populations (e.g., nondementia or milder stages of dementia), they are often brought to large-group activities that include people who do not have dementia, or those who are in the earlier stages of dementia. This practice should be discouraged. However, we always yield to the principle that, *if they like it they can do it*. Therefore, if, through trial and error, it is obvious that an individual with advanced dementia truly enjoys or benefits from mixed group activities, as evidenced by clear signs of meaningful connections, then that individual should be included in those activities.

Sensory Stimulation and Calming

Many of the most effective activities for persons with advanced dementia involve simple sensory acts. For example, a gentle hand massage, using a pleasantly scented lotion or oil, is a wonderfully soothing activity that involves touch and smell, and will usually elicit a meaningful connection between the individual and the caregiver. Other gently handled personal care tasks can have the same affect, such as manicures, applying makeup, brushing hair, and smoothing lotion onto dry skin. Warm, personal, and pleasurable sensory events such as these are important in helping persons with advanced dementia to maintain contact with their milieu while enhancing their sense of comfort. Such events also help individuals to maintain a heightened awareness of the people around them while supporting and enhancing their sense of personhood and self.

Sensory-oriented activities can be either stimulating or calming. Stimulating sensory events are generally designed to help heighten an individual's awareness and to help him or her be more attuned to his or her surroundings. These types of activities can be especially therapeutic for persons who tend to be lethargic or who otherwise do not easily orient to their environment or respond to others. Potentially effective sensory stimulation activities include the following:

- Massages (emphasis on gently stimulating rather than calming)
- Personal grooming (e.g., trimming nails, combing or brushing hair, applying scented lotion)
- Food and drink
- Walks
- Going outdoors
- Pets
- Babies and young children (also baby dolls)
- Lively music (e.g., listening, singing, moving)
- Dance or rhythmic movement
- Simple rhythm instruments
- Spiritual activities (e.g., lively hymns)
- Aromatherapy
- Tactile activities (e.g., touching familiar items, textures)
- Adaptive sports (e.g., ball toss, balloon volleyball, etc.)

Calming sensory events are generally to relax and soothe the individual. These types of activities are therapeutic in calming individuals who are restless or agitated, or to simply help the person relax or go to sleep. Potentially effective sensory-calming activities include the following:

- Soothing music (e.g., listening)
- Reading to
- Spiritual activities (e.g., prayers, scriptures, soothing hymns)
- Aromatherapy
- Massages (emphasis on calming rather than stimulating)

An interesting example of a serendipitous sensory-calming event occurred several years ago when a woman with advanced dementia was referred for a behavioral consult because of problems with agitation and loud screaming. When initially seen by the psychologist, she was seated alone at the far end of a nursing home dining hall where she was observed loudly screaming while rapidly rocking back and forth in her wheelchair. On the other side of the dining hall was a small group of residents who had convened for a Catholic service conducted by a visiting nun. The nun began the service by leading the group in reciting the Rosary. The instant the recitation began the agitated woman bowed her head, made the sign of the cross, and recited the Rosary along with the others—even though she was at least 50 ft. across the room from the others. Throughout the remainder of the service, she remained calm and quiet. Later, the psychologist found a recording of recitation of the Rosary and instructed caregivers to play the recording whenever she became agitated, which was found to be highly effective on calming her and eliminating her bouts of agitation and yelling.

It should be noted that various multisensory activity programs have proven effective for persons with advanced dementia, as well. Five published examples of this sort of programming include Snoezelen, Simple Pleasures, Gentle Care, Caring Connections, and Bright Eyes. The notion behind these programs is that two or more sensory events are combined and coordinated in a strategic and therapeutic fashion to stimulate or calm persons with advanced dementia. These programs may be used individually or in groups, although we always recommend that activity groups of any sort be limited to very small numbers.

ADLs as Meaningful Activities

ADLs are just that: *activities*. These are the things we do to take care of ourselves during the course of a day. When applied to persons in care settings, ADLs typically refer to care issues like bathing, grooming, dressing, feeding, incontinence care, and all other issues relating to maintaining personal hygiene. Because persons with advanced dementia are unable to do their own ADLs, they are entirely dependent on caregivers to do their ADLs for them.

Resisting and fighting ADL care is one of the most common behavior problems exhibited by persons with advanced dementia. That is because every aspect of ADL care requires caregivers to intimately touch and handle the persons they are assisting, which, for many severely confused persons, can be distressing and upsetting. Most books on dementia care include lengthy discussions about this phenomenon, including advice on how to diminish the sense of violation persons with dementia feel during caregiving. For example, in chapter 6, a soft approach is recommended, which emphasizes being warm, friendly, gentle, and respectful when providing care for persons with advanced dementia. In this section, we take this issue one step further by suggesting that caregivers treat ADLs the same way they treat other activities—as sensory-based activities that provide the opportunity to make pleasant meaningful connections.

Caring for persons with advanced dementia involves much more than just keeping them dry, clean, and fed. It also involves issues concerning respect, integrity, self, and personhood. Advocates of the person-centered care model emphasize the importance of caring *about* persons with dementia, not just *for* them. They go on to suggest that ADL care provides caregivers an opportunity to have a deeper level of involvement with persons with dementia, which includes elements of empathy, nurturing, and validation. In effect, every caregiving situation is an opportunity to make a positive, meaningful, and sensory-based connection with the person with advanced dementia. Because individuals with advanced dementia are totally dependent on caregivers for all of their ADL care, these situations occur dozens of times each day. By using the right techniques, the gentlest of approaches, and an attitude of compassion, warmth, and empathy, and by treating ADLs in the same way they treat all other activities, caregivers are in a position to repeatedly make meaningful connections throughout the day.

Several years ago, the Alzheimer's Association designed and developed a national training program called Activity-Based Alzheimer Care (ABAC), which is still offered in local chapters throughout the nation. The program teaches that activities are the foundation of care, and that every event and interaction the person has throughout the day, scheduled or not, is an activity. The model further says that all activities must be made meaningful to the individuals involved by giving them a sense of belonging, helping them to feel useful, bringing them sense of enjoyment, and reflecting their interests and lifestyle. Although not necessarily designed for persons with advanced dementia, the ABAC philosophy and care model may be a good fit because it treats ADLs as meaningful activities, rather than as mere tasks to be completed. In this way, ADLs become truly therapeutic and supportive in nature.

Activity Calendars

Traditional facility-based activity calendars are written a month at a time and are posted on walls for all to see. They tend to use a weekly rotation, with the same activities occurring at the same time on the same day of the week, week after week. Activities are blocked off in 30- and 60-minute increments and are interspersed with occasional special events. This type of activity calendar is universally accepted and is often state mandated. It is also completely irrelevant and even antitherapeutic when applied to activity programs that include persons with advanced dementia.

Individuals with advanced dementia have limited stamina, short attention spans, and diminished cognitive and functional skills. They do poorly in large-group activities where it is virtually impossible for caregivers to make the necessary meaningful connections with them. They require individualized approaches to activity programming and do best in one-to-one situations that focus on personalized sensory-oriented activities. Traditional activity calendars are not designed to address these issues and, as a result, should not be used in activity planning for persons with advanced dementia.

As we have come to see, activity programming for persons with advanced dementia must be fluid and flexible, allowing for individual preferences and differences, and accounting for each individual's special needs. Activity calendars must reflect all of these issues and should therefore be considered a flexible guideline, rather than set in stone. Short attention spans and limited stamina means that activities should be no longer than 20 minutes, with adequate rest time between activities. Individual differences and the need for one-to-one attention require that several alternative activities be simultaneously scheduled on the calendar, with consideration for last minute changes that fit the situation as they unfold. This approach requires that all caregivers participate in activity programming (not just the traditional one activity assistant), and that ADLs, meals and snacks, and downtime be included in the activity calendar.

None of this fits well on a traditional calendar format, so we suggest revising the way activity calendars are written. Instead of trying to preschedule all activities on a single monthly calendar, with one activity listed for each time block, we suggest the use of two different types of calendars simultaneously:

Daily Calendar

The first is a daily calendar that lists time blocks starting at the very beginning of the day and extending all the way to the very end of the day. Each time block includes a list of several alternative activities that could be considered for that block of time, and allows caregivers to choose what would be the best alternative given the unique needs and preferences of the residents they are serving at that moment in time. ADLs, meals and snacks, and rest times are included in the daily calendar because those activities are just as important in activity planning as social, recreational, and sensory events. This sort of daily calendar gives caregivers a structure and guidelines for activity planning, while at the same time offers the flexibility needed to account for each individual's needs. It also allows staff to engage many residents at once on a one-to-one or small group basis, and gives them the latitude to change course as the situation changes. Because it is designed to be flexible, this daily calendar can be written on a single sheet of paper (distributed or posted) and does not need to change from day to day. It is repeated day in and day out, flexibly using new combinations of activity options each day, so there is no need to print new calendars unless revisions are made while fine-tuning the format.

Special Events Calendar

The second written calendar is more like the traditional calendars used today and is designed to list special events that go beyond the activities listed on the daily calendar. This is where holiday celebrations, birthday parties, and one-time entertainment programs are listed, and it also includes important once-a-week activities like religious services. Special events calendars can be drafted on a weekly or monthly basis and need to be rewritten and reposted accordingly.

■ STAFF ISSUES

Facility-based activity programming for persons with advanced dementia, if it is to be done right, requires on everyone's part a somewhat radical change in policies, practices, attitudes, and culture. This sort of change starts at the top. Owners and administrators need to be educated so that they can understand, institute, and support the types of activity programming needed to care for, *and about*, persons with advanced dementia. Regulators need to infuse flexibility and understanding into their regulatory roles and responsibilities, including the drafting and enforcement of activity-specific regulations and policies that allow for the special activity needs of persons with advanced dementia. Managers and supervisors need to draft and support new policies and procedures. Job descriptions need to be rewritten, caregivers need to be retrained, and families need to be brought into the loop. Much needs to be done if we are to develop activity programs that truly benefit persons with advanced dementia.

At the ground level, hands-on caregivers need to be cross-trained in activity programming, taking into account the special needs and issues of persons with advanced dementia. They should be expected to be involved in all phases of activity programming, including organizing, overseeing, running, encouraging, and participating in activities. They also need to be trained in how to make meaningful connections with their residents, and the specifics on how to make ADLs meaningful activities. In this regard, each caregiver is important and meaningful and has a moral obligation to make activity programming a number one priority for all their residents with advanced dementia.

Finally, activity programming should include everyone who surrounds the person, including all of the caregivers and family members who are involved in the person's care and well-being. Whenever possible, family-oriented programming should be included in the activity plan that encourage and help maintain close family contacts. The family can be especially important to the process, and it is up to caregivers to work with the families so that they can better understand their loved ones and participate meaningfully in their care.

PROGRAM EVALUATION

All activity programs should be periodically assessed for appropriateness and effectiveness, including those designed for persons with advanced dementia. Minimally, activity program must comply with federal and state regulations, using the terminology set forth by regulatory agencies. Although this may be challenging, in no way does the type of activity programming discussed in this chapter violate federal and state regulations, as long as the facility is conscientious in how the program is executed, monitored, and documented.

In designing an appropriate format for program evaluation, facilities should consider using nontraditional outcome measures that are specifically relevant to the advanced dementia population. Persons with advanced dementia do not register complaints, offer praise, or fill out satisfaction surveys. Instead, their responses to activities and the effectiveness of the program must be measured by more subtle behavioral indicators. A brief list of such indicators includes, but is not limited to the following:

- *Nonverbal connections:* Eye contact, open eyes, eyebrows raised, head turns toward voice, nods, claps to music, taps fingers or toes to music, smiles, laughs.
- *Verbal connections:* Mumbles, repeats sounds or phrases, hums, sings, shares positive words or comments.

▨ *Mimicking behaviors:* Laughs, smiles, smiles when others laugh, tries to sing, prays.
▨ *Physiological indicators:* Slowed breathing, relaxed muscles, yawning.
▨ *Making physical connections* (e.g., giving back): Strokes a caregiver's hand, leans over to kiss a caregiver.

The following is a list of activities, conceptual and specific, that should be included in activity programming for persons with advanced dementia. These should, therefore, be included in any program evaluation assessment. The list includes, but is not limited to the following:

▨ Sensory stimulation activities
▨ Sensory-calming activities
▨ Physical activities
▨ Cognitive activities
▨ Emotional activities
▨ Self-esteem activities
▨ Gender-oriented activities
▨ Task segmentation
▨ Seasonal activities and special events
▨ Outdoor activities
▨ Activities that are sensitive to individual's culture and ethnicity
▨ Activities that are sensitive to individual's spiritual heritage
▨ Adaptation and special needs
▨ In-room activities

▨ TIPS: DOs AND DON'Ts

Finally, we offer some tips, using the ubiquitous dos and don'ts format. We have found them helpful in working with persons with advanced dementia, and especially in retraining caregivers in doing activities with persons who have advanced dementia.

DOs

▨ Play music from CDs or tapes that fit the person's taste and that elicits a positive reaction.
▨ Play tried-and-true movies and television programs on VCRs or DVDs that fit the person's taste and that elicit positive reactions.
▨ Use a trial-and-error approach to radio and television programming; play only those programs/styles that elicit a positive response from persons (when in doubt, turn it off).
▨ Consider that person's work history in developing and customizing activity plans.
▨ Pay attention to sounds and how they affect persons.
▨ Activities throughout all waking hours.

- Incorporate rest into activity plans.
- Go slow.
- Smile and laugh a lot.
- Approach from the front and establish eye contact.
- Take the person outside for short periods whenever possible.
- Physically touch persons in a loving manner (as long as touch elicits a positive response).
- Use praise and kind words.
- Let the person know you are there.

DON'Ts

- Play network or cable television (unless the person shows a clear and consistent positive response to specific television programs).
- Overstimulate or exhaust persons with activities.
- Approach suddenly or startle the person.
- Rush or go too fast.
- Take the person on car trips or other travel trips.
- Talk past the person as if he or she is not there.
- Mock or mimic persons.
- Laugh at persons.
- Grab and pull person's hands.
- Pull wheelchairs backwards.
- Talk to persons in childlike tones or baby talk.
- Approach from behind.

EXHIBIT 14.1

Standards of Care for Activities Programming

A. The healthcare facility shall:
 1. Adopt a care philosophy that acknowledges activities programming as an essential part of caregiving, especially in enhancing quality of life of persons with advanced dementia by making frequent and meaningful connections.
 2. Establish a policy and procedure that specifies purposeful and balanced around-the-clock activities for persons with advanced dementia.
 3. Incorporate all direct care staff in the planning and execution of the activities program.
 4. Provide activities around the clock, as noted in the facility activity calendar.
 5. Acknowledge and address the need for one-to-one and flexible activity programming in lieu of activities programs that are geared to large-group activities.

B. Healthcare staff shall:
1. Attend initial and ongoing training in activities programming.
2. Use the life story as a means to identify and plan for a meaningful activities program.
3. Use a format that is most appropriate for those with advanced dementia, such as one-to-one and small group activities.
4. Incorporate purposeful activities into the everyday ADLs.
5. Demonstrate evidence of the balance of sensory-stimulating and sensory-calming activities for persons with advanced dementia.
6. Document in the service plan or care plan the interventions that provide meaningful connections for the person with advanced dementia.
7. Document in the service record the outcomes or results of the activity program.

C. Persons with advanced dementia shall expect:
1. An enhanced quality of life from purposeful and meaningful activities programming.
2. The appropriate assessment and plan related to an individualized activities program that is flexible and continually evaluated.
3. Multiple daily opportunities to make meaningful connections with others through activities programming.
4. Purposeful interventions that balance sensory-stimulating with sensory-calming activities.
5. The most appropriate and therapeutic program that takes into account the format, type of activity, and indicators of making meaningful connections.

▥ REFERENCES

Alzheimer's Association. (n.d.). *Activity-based Alzheimer care: Building a therapeutic program.* Chicago, IL: Author. Retrieved January 25, 2010, from http://www.alz.org/professionals_and_researchers_activity_based_care.asp

Bell, V., & Troxel, D. (2003). *The best friends approach to Alzheimer's care (revised).* Baltimore, MD: Health Professions Press.

Brattico, E., & Jacobsen, T. (2009). Subjective appraisal of music: Neuroimaging evidence. *Annals of the New York Academy of Sciences, 1169,* 308–317.

Brown, E. J. (1999). Snoezelen. In L. Volicer & L. Bloom-Charette (Eds.), *Enhancing the quality of life in advanced dementia* (pp. 168–185). Philadelphia: Brunner/Mazel Publishers, Inc.

Buettner, L. L., & Greenstein, D. B. (2000). *Simple pleasures: A multi-level sensorimotor intervention for nursing home residents with dementia.* Alexandria, VA: American Therapeutic Association.

Chaudhury, H. (2002). Place-biosketch as a tool in caring for residents with dementia. *Alzheimer's Care Quarterly, 3*(1), 42–45.

Clair, A. A. (2002a). Dance for emotional intimacy: Simple one-to-one interventions for family caregivers with loved ones in late-stage dementia. *Activities Directors' Quarterly for Alzheimer's & Other Dementia Patients, 3*(3), 33–41.

Clair, A. A. (2002b). Practical ways to use music to manage agitated behaviors in late stage dementia. *Activities Directors' Quarterly for Alzheimer's & Other Dementia Patients, 3*(1), 41–48.

Cuddy, L. L., & Duffin, J. (2005). Music, memory, and Alzheimer's disease: Is music recognition spared in dementia, and how can be assessed? *Medical Hypotheses, 64*(2), 229–235.

Dougherty, J., Gallagher, M., Cabral, D., Long, C. O., & McLean, A. (2007). About me: Knowing the person with advanced dementia. *Alzheimer's Care Quarterly, 8*(1), 12–16.

Ennis, K., & Paul, M. (1997). *Pets in long term care settings. A practical guide*. West St. Paul, MB, Canada: Middlechurch Home of Winnipeg.

Filan, S. L., & Llewellyn-Jones, R. H. (2006). Animal-assisted therapy for dementia: A review of the literature. *Journal of International Psychogeriatrics, 18*(4), 597–611.

Geboy, L. (2009). Linking person-centered care and activity programming. *Alzheimer's Care Today, 10*(3), 156–171.

Habib, C. (2002). Place-biosketch as a tool for caring for residents with dementia. *Alzheimer's Care Quarterly, 3*(1), 43–45.

Hellen, C. (1997). Communications and fundamentals of care: Bathing, grooming, and dressing. In C. R. Kovach (Ed.), *Late-dementia care: A basic guide* (pp. 113–123). Washington, DC: Taylor & Francis.

Jones, M. (1999). *Gentlecare: Changing the experience of Alzheimer's disease in a positive way*. Point Roberts, WA: Hartley & Marks.

Kovach, C. R., & Magliocco, J. S. (1998). Late-stage dementia and participation in therapeutic activities. *Applied Nursing Research, 11*(4), 167–173.

Kuhn, D., Fulton, B. R., & Edelman, P. (2004). Factors influencing participation in activities in dementia care settings. *Alzheimer's Care Quarterly, 5*(2), 144–152.

Lucero, M. (2001). Caring connections: A sensory stimulation program for late stage dementia. *Activities Director's Quarterly for Alzheimer's and other Dementia, 3*(1), 33–40.

Lucero, M. (2004). Enhancing the visits of loved ones of people in late-stage dementia. *Alzheimer's Care Quarterly, 5*(2), 173–177.

Nolta, M. M., & Hall, B. A., (2005). *The dementia care plan directory. A behavior-based careplan idea book*. San Diego, CA: Recreation Therapy Consultants.

Sherratt, K., Thornton, A., & Hatton, C. (2004). Music intervention for people with dementia: A review of the literature. *Aging & Mental Health, 8*(1), 3–12.

Trudeau, S. (1999). Bright eyes: A structured sensory-stimulation intervention. In L. Volicer & L. Bloom-Charette (Eds.), *Enhancing the quality of life in advanced dementia* (pp. 93–106). Boston, MA: Brunner/Mazel Publishers, Inc.

Volicer, L., Simard, J., Pupa, J., Medrek, R., & Riordan, M. (2006). Effects of continuous activity programming on behavioral symptoms of dementia. *Journal of the American Medical Directors Association, 7*(7), 426–431.

Wexler, M. (2004). Getting to know you: Making the connection. *Alzheimer's Care Quarterly, 5*(1), 81–87.

Witzke, J., Rhone, R. A., Backhaus, D., & Shaver, N. A. (2008). How sweet the sound: Research evidence for the use of music in Alzheimer's disease. *Journal of Gerontological Nursing, 34*(10), 45–52.

CULTURAL DIVERSITY

Noemi de Vera, Melissa Beardsley, Hong Chartrand, Dan Lawler,
Kathryn Elliot-Hudson, Minnie Jim, Mika Kondo, Bianca Martinez,
Susana Marquez, Yen Nguyen, Niela Redford, and Onetta Revere

INTRODUCTION

America has never been more of a melting pot—or perhaps, more accurately, more
of a mosaic—than it is today. An enormous range of cultures now exists in the
United States. Many of these cultures have particular beliefs about physical and
mental health, the way a family should care for its elderly people, and what dementia really is. Caregivers who work with people from other cultures will need to
become educated about their patients' and their patients' families' cultural beliefs
in order to provide maximum levels of care.

Table 15.1 shows how diverse the mosaic has become.

A COMPENDIUM OF CULTURES

This section will examine some of the core beliefs held by various ethnic and
racial groups and their members about health care, illness in general, and
Alzheimer's disease (AD), in particular. The listing is by no means all-inclusive
but will present some helpful information that has been within the space limitations. In addition, it is important to note that attitudes described here pertain to
people within these groups *in general*. Groups, however, consist of individuals,
and not every individual will subscribe to the attitudes and beliefs of the larger
culture to which he or she belongs. Caregivers should use this section to get a
sense of how a person might think or respond, given his or her cultural background. Learning about normative general beliefs does not substitute for getting
to know a person as an individual. On the one hand, it is important not to make
assumptions that the person with whom you are working automatically holds
to the beliefs of the culture from which he or she comes. On the other hand,
getting to know what these beliefs are will help caregivers to better understand
each person (see the Appendixes at the end of the book, which provide national
guidelines for delivering culturally appropriate care and Web links to sites that
can offer more information, to learn more about ethnic and racial groups not
described here).

TABLE 15.1

Percentage and Numbers of Minority Populations in the United States

Population	U.S. #	U.S. %
Two or more races	4,339,831	1.2
Native Americans/ Aleutians/Eskimos	1,578,684	0.5
Asian Americans/ Pacific Islanders	12,311,914	4.3
Blacks or African Americans	34,809,867	12.1
Hispanic	40,322,931	14.0

What is Culture?

In the broadest sense, a culture is a system of shared symbols and beliefs that guide its members on how to interact with each other. People who belong to a culture absorb its particular beliefs as children, through the language. These beliefs can change over time, as a culture is not a fixed entity, but more like a living organism. It is continually evolving, made different by changes that occur in the environment, within the social system, and during personal interactions.

Any number of factors influences a culture's character. Race or ethnicity is perhaps the most obvious of these. However, a culture is also shaped by its members' average age, the predominant religions, the general financial and educational levels, and various outside forces that exist in the global society.

People's cultures permeate much of their lives. It is central to their worldview. The common practices can provide them with a sense of safety, security, integrity, and belonging. A culture's numerous domains can influence their attitudes about everything, from food and spirituality, to how high-risk behaviors should be defined. Because we take a lot of these attitudes for granted, it is important for caregivers who work with people from other cultures to gain self-awareness about their own culture. Until they do, they run the risk of assuming that their own practices are just how it is done. Once they have, they begin to acquire cultural competence.

Cultural competence means demonstrating an understanding of each patient's culture, accepting and respecting cultural differences, and adapting accordingly. It is an important approach to take when caring for persons with AD who are from other cultures, for Alzheimer's does not respect the boundaries of ethnicity and culture. Sometimes, however, this practice can be a challenge. Until recently, there has been minimal research into what the prevalence and risk of contracting Alzheimer's are for many minorities—Native Americans, African Americans, and

Hispanics, to name a few. In reviewing the 2000 U.S. census, the Alzheimer's Association (2006) concluded the following:

> There are significant information and data deficits about ethnic and cultural minority groups in most major research areas in Alzheimer's disease, including screening and neuropsychological testing instruments; diagnostic procedures; recruitment and retention in research protocols and clinical trials; clinical and neuropathological correlative studies; caregiving and family studies; basic laboratory investigations; genetics projects; development of new models of long-term care and management of these services; epidemiological and health services research; and the economics of care.

The following sections are designed to provide information about the beliefs and traditions of various cultural groups living within the United States. Information about each cultural tradition is presented consistently using the following categories for each group: overview and heritage, communication and language, family roles and relationships, nutrition, religion and spirituality, death rituals, and healthcare practices and practitioners. This compilation of information is intended to provide caregivers information about cultural traditions that are unfamiliar to them and to help them begin to overcome some of the challenges to providing culturally sensitive care.

CHINESE AMERICANS

Hong Chartrand

Overview and Heritage

The Chinese in the United States may share some attitudes and beliefs, but they do not comprise one culture. They come from numerous countries, including mainland China, Jamaica by way of mainland China, Taiwan, and Hong Kong, and each of these places has its own culture, languages or dialects, values, and beliefs. In mainland China alone, for instance, there are 56 separate nationalities and ethnic groups.

The Chinese have been living in the United States since 1785. They were the first Asians to immigrate to America, and today, they constitute the largest group of Asians in the country. The large Chinese communities are in metropolitan areas, with scatterings in almost every community in the country. Approximately 50% live on the West coast.

The Chinese initially migrated in the United States for economic reasons. Later, they came for political reasons and the chance for better education. Overall, there have been five large immigration waves, beginning with what are called the pioneer families and continuing through to the so-called astronaut families (1850–1919); the small business families (1920–1942); the reunited families (1943–1964); the Chinatown and dual-worker families (1965–1977); and the new immigrant, refugee, and astronaut families (1978 to the present).

Many people think the Chinese are limited to working in restaurants, the service sector, and the garment industry. Historically, that might be the case. However, more recently, highly educated Chinese have come to the United States for professional and managerial positions and, today, it is possible to find Chinese with PhDs or those with only a few years of education, who are very rich, and who are very poor.

Communication and Language

The early Chinese immigrants spoke Cantonese, a dialect from Southeast China and Hong Kong. Since the 1950s, more and more Mandarin-speaking Chinese immigrants have arrived from Taiwan and mainland China. Mandarin, China's official language, is becoming the dominant language in Chinese communities. People who grew up in the United States and those who are acculturated may speak English or their native dialect, depending on the situation. Although the Chinese use different dialects, they all use the same written characters, in either a simplified form or the more elaborate traditional style.

Caregivers who are working with Chinese patients will benefit from getting acquainted with their cultural conventions. For instance, traditionally, if asked whether they understood what was just said, Chinese say "yes," even if they have not. To answer "no" would mean losing face or being impolite. Nodding does not always mean the person is giving consent. It may simply be a polite gesture. In conversation, Chinese often speak loudly. This can be misinterpreted as anger or impoliteness, but actually, it is just the way Chinese communicate with each other. Of course, they also speak in moderate and low voices, depending on the circumstance.

When engaged in conversation, many Chinese maintain a certain distance from each other to show respect. They may avoid eye contact, also as a sign of respect, especially with the authority and people who are older. Emphatic facial expressions are commonly used among family members and close friends. Greetings often include asking about the whole family. Chinese usually do not express their emotions openly. However, in front of family members and close friends, it is different. Emotional expression is more readily accepted in women than in men. Crying out loud is acceptable for women. Men are expected to be more stoic and strong.

In meeting someone the first time, it is not uncommon for Chinese to ask personal questions, including the person's income, age, or children. However, the topic of sex and anything related to sex (e.g., homosexuality, premarital living arrangements, etc.) is a taboo.

Two entirely opposite views of time can be found in the Chinese community. For many people, lateness for appointments is expected and acceptable; it is perfectly normal for friends and family to knock on someone's door without an appointment. However, some consider lateness as a sign of disrespect and unprofessionalism.

The order of names in Chinese is opposite from what is commonly used in the West. The family name comes first, followed by the given name (e.g., Smith Jamie, if the custom were used in English). It is impolite to call a person by any name but his or her family name, unless that person is a family member or close friend. Titles are important to the Chinese. It is proper to use a person's title whenever possible. In modern times, women in mainland China do not use their husband's last name after marriage, but women from Taiwan, Hong Kong, or those who have lived in a Western country for a long time might. Some Chinese take another name that is English, on the belief it may be difficult for Westerners to pronounce their Chinese name. Most Chinese do not use middle names, unless they have adapted to U.S. culture. It is best to ask someone who is Chinese how they would like to be addressed.

In the distant past, Chinese bowed to each other in greeting. Today, shaking hands is an accepted social gesture. It is common for members of the same gender to walk hand in hand or arm in arm, or to put their arms around each other's shoulders if they are friends. This carries no sexual connotations (but because of the influence of Western culture, fewer Chinese practice this custom now). Men and woman usually do not touch each other. Couples usually do not hold hands, kiss, hug, or observe other intimate behaviors in public, nor do other family members. Affection between family members is rarely exhibited in public.

Family Roles and Relationships

Among the Chinese, the head of household or the decision maker and spokesperson is typically the eldest male in the house, although this changed for some in mainland China during the reign of Chair Mao, when the saying "women can hold up half the sky" was common. Today, women who work can be decision makers in the family. The traditional patriarchal family has transformed in many cases to a biarchal system. Families from Taiwan and Hong Kong, however, are more traditional. More women from mainland China work, but they are also supposed to take responsibility for the housework. However, increasingly, their husbands try to help with this.

Chinese are raised to pursue family harmony and unity and to pass family traditions down from one generation to the next. Children, especially boys, are highly valued; and so is education. Typical Chinese parents want their children to become medical doctors and lawyers rather than pursue other occupations. Parents usually try their best to find a good area to live so they can send their children to the best school district. They want their children to receive training in music or art and, also, not to forget the Chinese culture and language. They may enroll their children in local Chinese schools to learn Chinese.

Reverence is shown to older people. Filial loyalty is essential. "Respect the elder and love the younger," as an old saying goes. Grandparents take care of grandchildren when there is a need. Women are expected to be part of their husbands' families and to play the traditional role as caregivers, whereas Chinese children are expected to take care of their parents when they grow up. The extended family is important. Chinese like to build and maintain relationships among family members, including ones in the extended family. Each person is part of the family and works toward common goals. For each family member, including the extended family members, there may be a descriptive name that indicates order and rank in the family. All these complicated names can confuse the younger generation!

Economics determines social status. Traditionally, marriage was used to reinforce a family's position in society. One old saying advises, "Be well matched in social and economic status." Marriages extend the complicated webs of relationships that are important to the Chinese and on which they depend to work and live. Divorce is legal but not encouraged, although the divorce rate among Chinese has begun to increase.

Nutrition

Anyone who spends time with Chinese people will soon realize how important food is in their culture. People will conduct business at a dining table; otherwise, it is difficult to achieve goals. One common greeting is *"Ni Chi le Ma?"* ("Have you eaten?"). A literal response is not necessarily expected; the question is routine. The Chinese always treat guests with food. They want every guest to eat as much as they can. They like to hear their guests praise the food and hope that they will have leftovers. If guests do not offer such praise, a Chinese host will feel they have not provided enough and will lose face. Nearly all events and activities involve food preparation. Traditional Chinese medicine often uses food to treat diseases and increase the strength of older and weak persons.

It is difficult to describe what typical Chinese foods are. People from different regions of China have their own preferred dishes. However, in general, people from northern China prefer wheat-based food, whereas people from southern China prefer rice. Pork, chicken, and fish are commonly consumed, although in some areas, people prefer other seafood, beef, duck, or lamb. Then again, many Buddhists do not eat any meat or eggs at all, but instead get their protein from bean-related products such as tofu. Chinese chefs place a lot of emphasis on including many ingredients in one dish. Soup is a favorite with all Chinese, especially people from Guangdong Province and Hong Kong.

Toasts are made before the meal or during the meal with or without a speech to family, friends, or business associates. It is better not to leave chopsticks in a way that they are standing vertically in the food, because it is considered bad luck. It is considered a sign of appreciation to make noises, such as slurping or burping while eating. Traditionally, a Chinese dining table is round, symbolizing union. Foods are placed in the center of the table. It is common that the host holds up the food for the guests to see. The host serves the most important guests or signals everyone to start. The Chinese hope that all the guests try their best to eat as much as they can and they like to hear the guests praising the food or say they had a wonderful meal. On special days, such as that of the Qingming Festival, food is displayed to honor and remember the dead. Chinese believe many foods can prevent and/or treat diseases and enhances body strengthening.

Religion and Spirituality

The Chinese practice Buddhism, Christianity, Catholicism, Taoism, and Islam. Although, from 1949 through 1977 everyone in mainland China was officially an atheist. When the Communist party took over in 1949, all religions were declared superstitions and banned. Since the end of the 1970s, more and more Chinese in China and the United States have become believers of one faith or another. Often, Chinese follow a combination of religions. Many also adhere to Confucianism, which is an ethical belief system that focuses on right action, although some scholars believe it is a religion. It originated in China in the 4th century B.C. and has a strong influence in China, Korea, and Vietnam. Prayer and folk remedies are common, as is the use of religious incense. Even those who do not belong to any religious group may pray or burn incense as a source of comfort and for an improved life.

The Chinese derive meaning in life in terms of cycles and interrelationships, believing that life gets its meaning from the context in which it is lived. When they attempt to explain life and what it means, they speak not only of the importance of the current phenomena but also about the importance of what occurred many years, maybe even centuries, before their lives. Individuals get financial, physical, emotional, and spiritual strength from family, friends, and even their ancestors. They also hope to receive it from society. The cyclical explanation of life is manifested in their healthcare practices in which everything is connected to health.

Death Rituals

The Chinese think of death as a natural part of life. Caregivers, however, will find many Chinese hesitant to discuss end-of-life issues. This is because of a belief that if you talk about something bad, it might occur. There are also some taboos regarding death. The number *four*, for example, is regarded as unlucky, because the word for it in Chinese is pronounced the same way as the word for death.

Extended family members become involved in end-of-life care. After a death occurs, most families will not agree to an autopsy or organ donation—procedures that alter the body. They may place special clothes or amulets on the body. The home will be kept open to mourners. Family members wear white and black with black armbands and white strips of cloth tied around their heads, whereas other mourners wear white or black. Vocal expressions of grief are acceptable and expected. The body may be cremated or buried.

There is a strong belief in the afterlife and eventual resurrection of the dead. Chinese worship their ancestors. During the Qingming Festival, which takes place every April, families bring food (real or artificial) and paper money for the spirits to the gravesites of the deceased. Others establish altars in their homes and decorate them with flowers and food.

Healthcare Practices and Practitioners

Traditional Chinese medicine teaches that certain foods and herbs have healing properties. "When radishes are available in the market, no pharmacy needs to be open," an old saying goes. Chinese medicine emphasizes balance: physically, emotionally, and spiritually. The Chinese believe that their yin and yang must be balanced for them to have a healthy body, mind, and spirit (see section on "Korean Americans" later in this chapter, for more on yin and yang). They practice tai chi, qi gong and other soft-technique martial arts to enhance health and spiritual balance.

The major illnesses Chinese suffer from are hepatitis B, cardiovascular disease, diabetes, osteoporosis, and tobacco-related diseases. Depression is widespread, especially among new immigrants and refugees.

Many Chinese are not familiar with the healthcare system in the United States. Younger Chinese Americans are usually more likely to seek a healthcare provider's help when they are sick and, if that does not work, try traditional medicine. Older Chinese tend to do the opposite: consult a traditional specialist first. In recent years, there has been a growing trend in the Chinese community toward combining traditional Chinese and Western medicine to treat diseases. Often, a Chinese person will not tell their healthcare provider about other kinds of treatment they have used, out of a fear of losing face.

If a family member is terminally ill, other family members will often keep them in the dark about the diagnosis, or give them only selective bits of information. The fear is that the person might grow despondent. Many individuals, in fact, would not want to discuss the matter. At the end of life, many Chinese prefer to take a passive role and allow family members to make decisions.

CASE EXAMPLE

The article "Health and Health Care for Chinese-American Elders" provides the following example of end-of-life care issues that arise in Chinese families.

A 65-year-old Chinese woman, who immigrated to the US in 1995 to live with her eldest son and his American wife, is brought in after a one week history of malaise, nausea and vomiting, and sudden jaundice. She is admitted to the hospital where diagnostic studies reveal an obstructive mass in the liver. Biopsy reveals hepatocellular carcinoma. Serologies show chronic active hepatitis B status. The son is asked to help translate and break the news to his mother that she has cancer. He is very concerned about his mother's diagnosis and prognosis, but asks the physician not to tell his mother that she has cancer. The physician feels that it is important that the patient know her diagnosis, but the son is firm that he does not wish his mother to know this. Despite his wife's recommending that she be told, he refuses. The physician tries to discuss end-of-life issues such as hospice care and "do-not-resuscitate" (DNR) orders, but when the physician brings up these subjects, the son tries to discuss other issues such as when can she go home. (Tom, 2006)

The Chinese believe in practicing *yang bing*, loosely, taking time to rest and get nourishment to regain one's health.

Usually, when a person is sick, family members are the caregivers. However, when a person needs long-term care, this can create problems within the family. As one saying goes, "there are no filial children when a person has been sick for a long time."

Many Chinese treat their diseases by themselves, based on their own judgment. Another old saying says, "One becomes a medical doctor after being sick for a long time." Many new immigrants and students worry about the high cost of medical treatment in the United States and so they bring their medicine here and take it when they are sick. They also share their healing experiences with their family members and friends.

The Chinese, in general, tend not to complain of pain, although complaints of pain are more culturally acceptable for women. When they do describe pain or sickness, they attempt to describe not only direct symptoms but also more general ones. They are more accustomed to medical treatments that minimize discomfort. Sickness is considered an unavoidable part of life and payback for past misbehaviors. For this reason, many Chinese will bear a lot of physical pain before deciding to look for treatment or respite.

Mental disorders are thought of as a private issue and have shame attached to them. They stay within the family and often are not shared with outsiders, including healthcare providers. Chinese are also reluctant to report or admit depression.

CASE EXAMPLE

Here is another example of issues related to end-of-life care for Chinese Americans from the article "Health and Health Care for Chinese-American Elders."

Mr. W. is a 75-year-old Chinese-American male who presents with vague and multiple physical complaints that he reports he has had for several weeks. Prior to this he had been in good health and would come in only for periodic physical exams. His son tells the physician that his father has been complaining of "heart pain," indigestion, and weakness. He had been seeing an herbalist, but has continued to complain to his son. The patient does not speak much English, and his son interprets for him. During the interview the physician finds out that Mrs. W., his wife of 50 years, died last year. His son is busy and sees him about once a month and will be moving to a job in another state. The exam, laboratory and diagnostic tests are normal. On a return visit, the physician brings up the possibility that Mr. W. may be depressed. The son and the patient get very upset and vehemently deny any depression. The patient states that he is sick, not crazy. (Tom, 2006)

There are several factors in the Chinese culture that can become barriers to their receiving effective medical treatment, including lack of healthcare coverage, family reluctance to disclose the diagnosis to the person, reluctance to go to a hospital, belief by many people that they know their health better than any healthcare providers, discontinuing treatment after the initial treatment, unfamiliarity with services available, and reluctance to disclose information that might be private or embarrassing. The discussion of sexually transmitted diseases and drug use are taboo, for instance. Often, Chinese will not look for services because they believe older persons should be taken care of at home by their families.

AD is considered, variously, a part of the normal aging process, a form of mental illness, and a result of fate. It is not clear how prevalent Alzheimer's is among

Chinese Americans, because no large-scale population-based studies have been done. One study of 125 Chinese Americans older than the age of 60 did find that nearly 75% demonstrated significant cognitive impairment. Another study indicated that vascular dementia was prevalent among Chinese American elders, possibly more so than Alzheimer's is.

KOREAN AMERICANS

Melissa Beardsley and Dan Lawler

Overview and Heritage

After China, the United States is home to the second-largest Korean community in the world, with more than 1 million ethnic Koreans living in the United States. Most of them live in metropolitan areas. The country that they, their parents, or grandparents come from is a mountainous peninsula that is bordered by China to the north and the Sea of Japan to the west, east, and south. It has a monsoon climate with cold winters.

Many Koreans practice Confucianism. Confucianism emphasizes family, frugality, hard work, and education. Education is the way one raises one's status in Korea. College entrance exams there are highly competitive. One extremely strong reason people migrate here is to enroll their children in the best U.S. schools.

Communication and Language

About 78 million people throughout the world speak Korean or one of its dialects. Korean is thought to be distantly related to Japanese. Its distinctive alphabet dates to the 15th century and is believed to be the first phonetic alphabet used in East Asia. In Korea, there are only 274 family names. *Kim*, *Lee*, and *Park* account for nearly half of them. A wide range of first names is used. Some people in Korea believe that a person's fate is influenced by his or her name and will go to a "name picker" when they have a child. The name order in Korea is the same as in China: family name first, then the given name.

There are seven different levels of speech in Korean. Each one has its own verb endings to indicate degree of intimacy. Inappropriate language is highly shocking and shameful. Whether someone shares their thoughts and feelings with you will depend on your relative age, gender, and status. Koreans are more comfortable with social silences than Americans are. Confucianism teaches that "silence is golden." Small talk may come across as disrespectful.

Koreans have a different sense of personal space when it comes to touching strangers. In a store, a Korean merchant will feel more at ease placing the change on the counter than in someone's hand. Their sense of personal space is different from Americans'. Koreans stand in proximity to one another and do not excuse themselves if they bump into someone. If an elderly person touches a younger person, they are extending permission to reciprocate. Koreans show respect by bowing on meeting and by not looking a person in a position of seniority in the eye. If you are a caregiver, do not expect a Korean American patient to hold your gaze at first. Facial expressions can be taken as a lack of intellect. A Korean may strike an American as less animated for that reason.

Family Roles and Relationships

Confucianism exalts yang, which represents heaven, male superiority, and active principles. Ying, the opposite, is represented by the earth and female and passive principles. The idea of equality between the sexes is alien to Confucianism. Men are highly regarded and Korean women have long been considered inferior. Women are expected to be submissive and take care of all household tasks.

Society accords a lot of respect to those who work in valued professions; these include teachers, professors, and doctors. Social status is inherited but may be improved through education and profession. It can also become diminished if one's children are involved in anything scandalous. Alternative lifestyles are not accepted. Women who are divorced are frowned on, homosexuality is not accepted, and mixed marriages are very much looked down on.

The family system is seen as a safety net in Korea. Children are expected to care for their parents in their old age, which, according to the Chinese lunar calendar, begins at 60 years of age. The elderly are well respected. If you are older, it is assumed you have worked hard your whole life and have earned this level of respect.

When a caregiver is making decisions for the person with dementia, it is important that the family be consulted.

Many Koreans believe that it is their familial duty and responsibility to take care of loved ones rather than moving them into a long-term care facility. At one time, in Korea, women never worked outside the home. Now, Korean women, both in Korea and in the United States, have outside jobs that put them in conflict with the caregiving tradition. One study found that Korean American caregivers in America were more likely to be depressed and anxious than European American caregivers, because of the stresses of acculturation. The Korean government emphasizes the importance of traditional family ethics, which require family caregivers to assume the entire responsibility for their older population with dementia. "Insufficient health and social infrastructures supporting home health care or long-term care for demented elders in Korea impose a heavy burden and distress on family caregivers" (Youn, Knight, Jeong, & Benton, 1999).

CASE EXAMPLE

Most Korean women in Korea were able to stay home and take care of their parents; however, the new generation's women are working outside of their home and that brings a lot of issues of taking care of their elderly parents. It also brings the same issues here in America because most Korean couples are working outside of their home. (Sun Wright, personal communication, December 1, 2005)

Traditionally, Korean society values a woman who followed her husband and took care of the family. Owing to the rapid economic growth and influx of Western culture, Korean people, too, are experiencing internal conflicts. Another study determined that many people in Korea now value someone who earns money over someone who stays home and takes care of the family. In Korean tradition, the eldest son and his wife were obligated to take care of their parents. Westernization and urbanization are challenges for Korean Americans who face difficulties in practicing the traditional expectations of filial piety and in their changing life situations in the United States. In the United States, most Korean American immigrant wives are employed, disrupting the practice of Korean family traditions.

CASE EXAMPLE

When I visited the home of a Korean family, I first had to be introduced to the elders before being introduced to their daughter, even though I had many phone conversations already with the daughter. But since I was entering their home, it was proper for me to meet the elders before anyone else. (Melissa Beardsley, family care consultant)

Nutrition

Food is at the center of Korean life. It plays a major role in special events and festivals. Particular dishes are served at a child's first birthday, as part of a marriage ceremony, or during ancestral rites. Regional specialties include raw fish in Busan, beef ribs in Suwon, and mixed vegetables with rice in Jeonju. The traditional Korean diet is spicy and high in salt. Numerous small dishes are served during a meal. These foods have often been pickled in brine or packed in salt and lightly rinsed. This high-salt diet predisposes Koreans to hypertension. In the healthcare setting, one problematic situation that crops up in relation to the diet is that Korean patients with congestive heart failure sometimes have trouble giving up their customary foods.

CASE EXAMPLE

In the home of one Korean family I worked with, the wife insisted that, before we started talking, I have a glass of her homemade mango juice. She wanted to be sure that I was comfortable and refreshed before our talk. Throughout the meeting, she offered me refills of juice and food. Although I was not thirsty and I do not like mango juice, I accepted the juice with a show of gratitude so as not to offend her. Another Korean family insisted I have a full meal with them before we discussed their mother. (Melissa Beardsley, family care consultant)

Religion and Spirituality

Korean elderly people place strong emphasis on active participation in the church. Involvement in the church is not only for religious activities but also for social and cultural activities. Buddhism, Confucianism, and Christianity are practiced in Korea. However, Korean Americans historically have a strong conservative Christian heritage. In the United States in 2005, there were approximately 2,800 Korean Christian churches, compared to only 89 Korean Buddhist temples. In current Korean society, these three heterogeneous religions coexist under the support and protection of democratization and industrialization.

Traditional healing is common where shamans, who practice sorcery for healing and divination, are used in healing rituals to ward off restless spirits. The Korean government has discouraged the belief in shamanism, yet the shaman is still present today, seen as a professional who is consulted, when needed, by clients. Koreans use multiple options for healing: ceremonies, prayers, herbs, acupuncture, acupressure, and other integrative modalities. Using an American physician for someone who has dementia may not be the first choice for someone who is of Korean descent. Their preference might be to first go to their spiritual leader.

Death Rituals

The funeral ritual is vitally important in Korean culture, because it is thought to ensure safe passage of the loved one's spirit to the afterlife. It is considered bad luck to bring the deceased back home if the person died in a hospital. A viewing occurs where the person died, whether it was at home or in the hospital. If in the hospital, it occurs in a place that can be set aside for a viewing; not necessarily in the hospital room. The eldest son sits by the body of the parent (or more often nowadays, next to a photograph of the parent) and holds a cane to show he needs support. Several days are set aside for the viewing. Guests at the home are offered the deceased's favorite foods. For burial, both religious and cultural rituals are taken into consideration. Considerations would include positioning of the body, the place of burial, and whether the decedent adhered to Christian or non-Christian beliefs. In general, moaning and crying are part of the funeral rituals.

CASE EXAMPLE

My sisters and I discussed sometime ago who will take care of my mother if she became seriously ill and needed 24-hour care. We decided we will rotate her care so we do not have to send her to a nursing home and this is one reason we are all living within few miles of each other. I think most Korean people will do same way. (Sun Wright, Korean caregiver in Arizona)

Healthcare Practices

Some Koreans are stoic and therefore slow to express emotional or physical distress if they are in pain. Korean elders may find it hard to ask for help from home care or case management workers. Blood transfusions are acceptable among Korean Americans. Organ donation and transplant are rare, reflecting the traditional reverence held for the integrity and purity of the body. Korean Americans may avoid seeking healthcare because of the language barrier. They will often prefer to see a Korean physician. The ideal doctor is an old man with gray hair.

Dementia is becoming a more common problem in Korea and is associated with increased morbidity and mortality, functional loss, caregiver burden, and institutionalization. The rate of vascular dementia caused by cerebrovascular disease is much higher among Korean Americans than among other groups in the United States. This has been attributed to insufficient prevention, diagnosis, and treatment of hypertension, diabetes, and hyperlipidemia (elevated lipids in the bloodstream). The most common diseases for Koreans include schistosomiasis, liver cancer, tuberculosis, hepatitis, hypertension, lactose intolerance, vascular dementia, and gum disease. In older Korean Americans, diabetes, hypertension, hepatitis B, and nutritional deficiency are common. Care providers should note that in general, all Asians generally require lower dosages of psychotropic drugs.

FILIPINO AMERICANS

Noemi de Vera

Overview and Heritage

Asian Americans today form 4.3% of the U.S. population—a figure that is 63% more from what it was in the 1990 census. Asian Americans are currently the fastest growing of all the major racial or ethnic groups. The Filipinos are the second-largest subgroup, behind the Chinese. Filipinos have settled in all 50 states, with the largest concentrations in California, Hawaii, Illinois, New York, and New Jersey.

The Philippines is an independent nation located in the western Pacific, 500 mi. off the coast of Southeast Asia, with Taiwan to the north and Borneo to the south. It has a total land area of 115,600 sq. mi. divided among 7,100 islands. The first inhabitants of the Philippines were the *aetas*, considered to be Negritos, who are small statured. Later, it was populated by waves of Indonesian and Malay migrants.

Communication and Language

There are 11 languages and 87 dialects spoken in the Philippines. Eight of these dialects—Tagalog, Cebuano, Ilocano, Hiligaynon, Bicolano, Waray-Waray, Pampangan, and Pangasinan—are used by about 90% of the population. Filipinos greet each other by bowing or shaking hands. People are expected to recognize older persons first.

Filipinos avoid direct critical remarks and are sensitive to implied insults or criticism. A third party may propose a solution if two people cannot resolve or smooth over a conflict. Like the Chinese, Filipinos put great emphasis on saving face and looking good. Filipinos go to great lengths to avoid being shamed (*hiya*), and to try to save other people's face.

Filipinos maintain a smile when disagreeing or feeling embarrassed to diffuse difficult situations. Prolonged eye contact is considered rude and provocative, especially if it involves people of different status or occurs between a man and woman. *Passing and crossing* is an etiquette that recommends lowering the head and lightly holding together extended hands when passing or crossing a room where people are talking. Filipinos have a highly developed sensitivity to the nonverbal aspects of communication. They watch their listeners carefully and identify body language cues to assess what the person is feeling. The Philippines have been characterized as a touch-oriented society.

Family Roles and Relationships

The husband is traditionally the acknowledged head of the household and expected to be the economic provider for the family. Conversely, the wife is credited primarily for her ability to have children, take good care of them and her husband, and manage the finances. In recent times, however, she can work to help support the family. The mother plays an equal role in decisions about healthcare, welfare, and family finances. Either spouse can engage in a profession without the consent of the other.

Family comes before the individual and older persons are respected. Older children are expected to sacrifice their personal goals to help put their younger siblings through college. Adult children take care of all their parents' needs. The respect for authority is based on the special honor paid to elder members of the family and by extension to anyone in a position of power. This characteristic is generally conducive to the smooth relationships that frequently exist among members of the family and the smooth running of society.

In relationships, Filipinos strive to be agreeable, even under difficult circumstances; sensitive to what others are feeling; and willing to adjust their behavior accordingly. Smooth relations are maintained through *pakikisama* (giving in, following the lead or suggestion of others). Smooth relations are highly valued by all Filipinos but more so by men and individuals with less education, lower social class, and more rural backgrounds.

CASE EXAMPLE

My mother always said to me that in order to maintain harmony and smooth relations with other people, I should just be quiet and not say anything even if I disagree because I am highly educated. (Noemi de Vera)

Nutrition

Dishes served in a Filipino home often incorporate the fruits and vegetables that are in season. Food is regarded a symbol of social life and a means by which people communicate. Food also provides a way of staying connected to ethnic values. Filipinos have a strong sense of obligation to share food. Anybody who arrives at mealtime or any other time will be served something to eat. If a guest is allowed to help in the kitchen, it indicates acceptance and inclusion into the insider's circle, something that is known as *hindi ibang tao*, or one of us.

Fish and seafood are a central part of the diet. Frozen fish is bought only if live fish is unavailable. Filipinos believe in moderation and adherence to the idea that too much of anything has a negative effect on health. Filipino households may keep potted medicinal plants in the backyard to treat colds, stomach upsets, urinary tract infections, and other minor health problems. Garlic and ginger are thought to have healthful properties.

Religion and Spirituality

Religion holds a central place in most Filipinos' lives. Religious rituals, ceremonies, and adjurations provide them with continuity in life, cohesion in the community, and a moral purpose for existence. In one study, approximately 82% of the population was Roman Catholic; Muslims accounted for only 5%. The remaining population was mostly affiliated with other Christian churches, although there were also a small number of Buddhists, Taoists, and tribal people who believe in supernatural beings. Most Filipino Americans are Roman Catholic.

The spiritual side of life pervades every aspect of daily life. Omens are constantly watched for, especially before long journeys or at the start of important enterprises. The stars are consulted for auspicious times. Women in both rural and urban settings may seek treatment from both traditional healers and modern health centers even in the United States.

Death Rituals

A wake is held when someone dies. It can last from 3 days to 1 week, depending on how long it takes family members to arrive at the home. Food and entertainment (e.g., card playing, music, etc.) are provided throughout the wake and after the burial.

Funeral rites are consistent with the family's religious traditions, which may be Roman Catholic, Muslim, Buddhist, or another belief. Nine days of novena (*pabasa*) are held in the home or in the church. Food is offered after each prayer. Families in the United States follow variations of this ritual according to their social and economic circumstances.

Mourners are reunited on the first year anniversary of the death. The family holds a mass and serves food. On All Souls' Day, families gather to remember loved ones and to decorate their graves. Many Filipinos do not believe in cremation, preferring the body to remain whole, although some now accept cremation for economic and practical reasons.

Healthcare Practices and Practitioners

Health is construed as a general sense of well-being, rather than the absence of illness. Rural Filipinos are more knowledgeable about home remedies, traditional healing techniques, and supernatural ailments, whereas those from urban areas rely more on Western medical interventions and over-the-counter drugs. Filipino Americans tend to rely more on Western medical interventions. The more traditional forms of self-medication include certain Chinese oils or ointments, which serve as cure-alls in relaxing, heating, and comforting the muscles or providing relief for dizziness, colds, headaches, sore throats, and other maladies. Self-medication may include the use of folk healing techniques consistent with the Chinese hot or cold classification system of disease.

CASE EXAMPLE

When I asked one of our Filipino friends whom he would see first regarding his wife's abdominal pain, he said, "I would go to an albularyo [folk healer] first before consulting a medical practitioner." (Noemi de Vera)

It is possible to buy all types of medications without prescriptions in the Philippines. Filipinos consult medical healthcare providers informally, learn the brand names of drugs that are supposed to be effective, and purchase them. Self-diagnosing and self-medication is common. Filipinos from the United States ask their relatives in the Philippines to purchase medicine for them. Their relatives will either mail these or arrange for someone who is going over to bring the medications with them.

Filipinos generally do not seek healthcare until a medical condition is quite advanced and serious. Some Filipinos consider minor aliments as natural imbalances that run their course and eventually disappear. Many do not seek medical advice because of economic reasons, distrust of the healthcare system, limited access to healthcare centers, poor transportation to facilities, religious beliefs and practices, lack of knowledge of disease processes, and inability to articulate their healthcare needs.

Traditional Filipinos emphasize balance and moderation in all areas of their lives: in activities, diet, and temperature. The ideal environment for them is one that is warm, moderate, and balanced. Changes in any area need to be introduced gradually, because it is thought that a sudden shift from hot to cold or inactivity to activity will create imbalance, undue bodily stress, and illness.

Western medicine is acceptable to most Filipinos. However, those Filipinos who live in rural areas of the Philippines still believe in traditional approaches to healing. Immigrants may combine both traditional folk medicine and Western methods of healing. Although folk healers are less commonly found in the United States, when they are, they can contribute to facilitating rapport between Western healthcare providers and clients and encourage patients to use Western health resources.

With an illness, Filipinos may do several things before setting up an appointment with a physician. They may begin by monitoring their symptoms to ascertain possible causes, severity, threat to their functional capacity, and possible economic and emotional inconvenience to the family. They may discuss the concern with a trusted family member, friend, or spiritual healer, or self-administer natural and commercial remedies (e.g., herbs, food, teas, nonprescription medicines, nutritional supplements, etc.). When they do go to a doctor, many prefer physicians from the same region they come from, although some will look for one who has a good bedside manner and is knowledgeable and competent.

CASE EXAMPLE

My sister-in-law came to me first for her back pain because I am a nurse and, at the same time, her sister-in-law, before setting an appointment with her doctor. (Noemi de Vera)

Filipino immigrants are at high risk for developing cardiovascular diseases, hypertension, and diabetes. HIV, tuberculosis, and cancer are also common. In intergenerational Filipino households, consultations with screening services may be delayed or rejected by adult family members who feel an obligation to protect relatives from external forces. Diet and weight are rarely studied in this population, but the prevalence of fried foods in the diet has been connected to overall weight gain. In addition, poor diet and lack of physical activity have been implicated in various diseases, such as cancer. Little has been done to look into what health-promotion behaviors Filipino Americans do practice.

According to a recent study, Filipinos and other Asian Americans believe that dementia is a natural consequence of aging rather than a medical illness with no known cure. It is considered shameful or embarrassing to talk about a family member's senility problems. Families believe these should be solved within the family. A diagnosis of dementia can be difficult to obtain because of the reluctance of patients and family to report symptoms. Some experts cite a need for vigorous case finding for Filipinos with dementia. One study of Alzheimer's centers in California revealed that a very small number of Filipino Americans (0.7% of all patients) screened for dementia during an 8-year period were found to have dementia.

■ JAPANESE AMERICANS

Mika Kondo

Overview and Heritage

Japan is an island in East Asia, located between the North Pacific Ocean and the Sea of Japan, consisting of 245,586 sq. mi. of land. The climate varies significantly, because the island runs 1,860 mi. northeast to southwest. The original Japanese most likely came from the region of the Korean Peninsula. The culture has been influenced by China since the late 400s. This influence can be seen in many areas of Japanese culture, including religions, lettering, and rituals. All in all, 99% of the population is Japanese. The other 1% is made up of Koreans, Chinese, Brazilians, and Filipinos.

Japanese immigration to the United States started around the mid-1800s, with most people coming for better education and employment opportunities. The majority settled in Hawaii and the Pacific Coast area. Education in Japan is valued and emphasized. School systems teach students to respect and obey elderly people and authority figures. Recent Japanese immigrants, too, have come for education and business opportunities, although these more recent arrivals tend to be highly educated and have fewer language barriers. Interracial marriages are increasingly common in the younger immigrant population, whereas older generations still place importance on cultural and racial purity and so oppose that trend. Older generations, such as the *issei* (first generations) and the *nisei* (the second generations), had limited access to education because of the internment during World War II and might not be as well off.

Communication and Language

The official language of Japan, Japanese, uses Chinese characters, as well as two separate sets of Japanese characters, *hiragana* and *katakana*. People tend to judge one's intelligence and educational attainment based on how many Chinese characters they know.

Many dialects exist in Japanese. The dialect spoken in Tokyo is considered standard Japanese. People use different word choices and tones, depending on whether their conversational partner is younger or older, or socially lower or higher in status. Higher status individuals might include an employer, doctor, professor, or teacher.

When people meet, younger people are expected to first greet and then bow. Older people are called by their last name, whereas with younger ones and close friends, first names are used. Japanese Americans appreciate more personal space than Anglo-Americans do. Touching is considered very personal—hugging or kissing on the cheek is not practiced even among close friends or family. Always ask for permission before skin contact occurs between you and your care receivers. When communicating with each other, Japanese Americans are highly aware of saving each other's face.

Japanese Americans are raised to control emotional expressions; therefore, obvious facial expressions are often discouraged. Showing too much emotion is viewed as a lack of self-discipline and self-control. Paying lip service is socially acceptable as long as it keeps situations peaceful. People might not share their true feelings so as not to offend others. This is particularly true when they do not know each other well. Women tend to be passive in communication and often choose to listen. People are expected to take hidden meanings from the conversation's context—to understand that "yes" might mean "no" and "no" can mean "yes." Direct eye contact is discouraged, especially with older people and authority figures, because it can be taken as being challenging.

Japanese Americans tend not to disagree with their doctors or ask them questions, because doctors are viewed as authority figures. There is a stigma attached to receiving assistance from nonfamily members. Dementia brings shame not only to the person but also to the whole family. Thus, the family might minimize or deny any problems. For this reason, Western medical practitioners might find it difficult initially to interview and assess Japanese American clients' needs.

Family Roles and Relationships

There is a strong emphasis on family values and traditions. Traditional Japanese families include extended family members, but this concept of family is gradually disappearing. The oldest members of the family, especially males, are considered heads of households. Every family member is responsible for maintaining harmony within the family so as not to bother others. Family members try to solve problems from within rather than seeking assistance from outsiders. Patience may be necessary before they open up.

Women who marry the oldest son are expected to move in with his parents after marriage and look after them until their death. It is common for children, regardless of age, to live with their parents until they get married. In return, children take care of their parents later in life. Women tend to stay close to their parents even after marriage and consult with them about day-to-day matters. Elderly parents often volunteer to watch their grandchildren while their children work during the day. The elderly are considered a source of wisdom and receive respect. It is not unusual for elderly parents to provide financial assistance to their grown-up children so they do not have to receive help from outsiders.

In Japan, more women are pursuing higher education. Nevertheless, most quit work and stay home after marriage because they are expected to look after their family and elderly parents. Traditionally, men are the breadwinners and major decision makers. Women are involved with decision making, but usually agree with their husband and/or parents. When the wife is the primary caretaker for her husband with advanced dementia, any decision making or completing advanced directives might take a long time, because she will likely consult with all family members. The majority of elderly Japanese Americans choose to stay home rather than move into an institution, unless this is medically unavoidable. Some Japanese Americans choose to die at home. Cremation is commonly accepted. The oldest son and his wife will arrange the funeral.

Nutrition

Food has significant meaning for family, social, and business occasions. Much attention will be paid to presentation, how the food is arranged on the plate, and to the texture of the dishes. People enjoy conversation during meals.

When a Japanese American is in an institution, it is important to be sensitive to how they are used to eating. A typical meal consists of rice, miso soup, vegetables, and grilled fish. Japanese Americans consume much less meat than in the typical American diet. Most use chopsticks instead of a knife and fork, so chopsticks should be made available. Japanese foods are traditionally salty but not spicy. Caution should be taken not to automatically serve someone spicy food. They might not be used to it. There is a high rate of lactose intolerance among Japanese Americans. Attention to these special nutritional needs will be a source of comfort to persons in the advanced stage of dementia.

People usually drink green tea with meals. Chinese tea accompanies heavier meals, such as with steaks. Both men and women commonly consume alcohol. Some men prefer beer to tea at the dinner table. Sake is used for purification and celebration—on New Year's Day to purify the mind and spirit, or at a wedding ceremony to celebrate. Alcoholism exists among Japanese Americans. Awareness of it, however, is low and denial is common.

CASE EXAMPLE

A 72-year-old nisei (second generation) Japanese woman was admitted to a skilled nursing facility because of dementia. She had raised four children with her husband, who had died not long before, and had maintained a Japanese lifestyle throughout her life, preparing food and practicing rituals the way her parents taught her. Her children had their own families and lived out of state. After the death of her husband, her health had gradually begun to deteriorate. At a family conference, her children decided that it would be best to place her in a skilled nursing facility, as none of them was able to relocate to care for her. She was polite and pleasant, and soon became acquainted with other residents and staff members. A few days later, the nursing staff noticed she was not eating much, but when she was asked about it, she said she was fine and just not very hungry. This continued day after day. She continued to deny anything was wrong. A social worker finally contacted one of her children. After interviewing him, the social worker realized that the trouble lay with the foods she was being served—mostly American food and spicy southwestern. These were foreign to her, because she had eaten Japanese food her whole life. She had apparently felt too embarrassed to tell staff members about her traditional diet, not wanting to bother them or make them lose face. After the social worker talked to her and staff members, she felt comfortable voicing her preferences. The kitchen staff now serves Japanese or some type of Asian cuisine. Her appetite has returned to normal. (Mika Kondo)

Religion and Spirituality

Religion and rituals play important roles in daily routines, culture, ethics, and morals. Buddhism and Shinto are the most commonly practiced religions (although in the United States, some Japanese Americans are Protestant or Catholic.). Practitioners celebrate special events such as weddings, anniversaries, or funerals at temples or shrines. They might carry small amulets, called *omamori* to keep evil spirits away. You might also find a small shelf in the corner of the house. It is called *kamidana* and is a way to worship Shinto deities. It is best not to touch any religious articles without asking permission first.

In mid-August, during the festival of Obon, it is believed that ancestors' spirits return for a visit. This is also a time for family reunions. New Year's Day is the most important holiday for Japanese Americans. Special ceremonies are held at temples or shrines at midnight to celebrate the new year. Family members come to worship together and monks serve sake to visitors.

In child rearing, parents may invoke reincarnation as a way of making children behave and do well at school. Japanese Americans use spiritual healing methods such as reiki and prayer beads. The numbers *four* and *nine* are considered unlucky, because four symbolizes death and nine indicates suffering. It is best to avoid placing a Japanese American person in a room with either of these numbers on the door.

Death Rituals

End-of-life discussions involve all family members. The oldest son and not the mother makes final decisions regarding the father. Japanese Americans find virtue in self-control and discipline, which might lead them to decline pain medication and be stoic about discomfort. They might decline hospice service. The concept of an advanced directive might be foreign to them.

Traditional Japanese funerals are held at a temple. After the ceremony, the family purifies the entrance of their home with salt before entering. People gather and discuss memories of the deceased. Japanese Americans see body and mind as equally holy. They tend to oppose organ donation or autopsy because of their beliefs that a body should remain intact. Japanese Americans, especially males, are raised not to show emotions openly. When a loved one dies, the family might not cry or display anger in front of others. Give them time to themselves.

Healthcare Practices and Practitioners

Japanese enjoy some of the longest life expectancies in the world; for men, age 77, for women, 84. This is largely because of people's engagement in daily disease and illness prevention including regular exercise, restriction of obesity, and adherence to stringent diets. Shinto teaches that one becomes sick from contact with evil spirits.

When someone in the family does become sick, the wife of the oldest son or daughter typically becomes the primary caretaker. Because of cultural expectations, caregivers might overburden themselves and decline assistance from nonfamily members. Provide them with information on community and government resources, including material on respite programs and support groups. Family members might deny or minimize the problem. With this in mind, it is important for caregivers to concentrate on retaining a sense of objectivity in order to make an accurate assessment.

In addition to cultural factors, language barriers can prevent Japanese Americans from seeking professional assistance. A professional translator may be needed to maintain objectivity. Family members should be used in this capacity only when professional translation is unavailable. Traditional herbal remedies and spiritual healing methods are commonly practiced and people accept Western medicines. Physicians are viewed as absolute authority figures and have an enormous influence on the decisions that families make. A family might refrain from asking questions or discussing alternatives once a doctor has made a recommendation. Mental disorders are still viewed as a source of shame. Do-not-resuscitate orders might go against religious beliefs.

Vascular dementia is three times more common than AD among Japanese Americans. Some Japanese Americans see dementia as an unavoidable part of aging, whereas others believe it is a mental illness and shameful. People with dementia and their families try to hide the illness and postpone seeking help because of the stigma.

Regardless of the dementia level, always address the person by their last name (e.g., Mr. Yamada or Mrs. Saito). It might take a while for people to open up and discuss issues with you because you are a nonfamily member. Prepare to take more time to establish rapport.

▉ VIETNAMESE AMERICANS

Yen Nguyen, MPH

Overview and Heritage

Vietnam is an S-shaped country that encompasses some 200,000 sq. mi. China lies to the north, Laos and Cambodia to the west, and the South China Sea to the east. The Pacific Ocean curves around the east and south. Vietnam is a verdant tapestry of mountains, deltas, forests, and beaches. The climate in the south is tropical and in the north, rainy, hot, and humid during the monsoon. Of the 75 million people who live in Vietnam, 80% are Vietnamese. The rest belong to any of more than 50 different ethnic groups.

Vietnam has a rich but turbulent history. Between 207 B.C. and the 10th century, it was under the rule of successive Chinese dynasties. The country was colonized by France from the mid-19th century through World War II, when it was invaded by Japan. After the war, the predominantly Communist Viet Minh declared Vietnamese independence. France attempted to reestablish control through the French Indochina War in 1954 but failed. That same year, the Geneva Accords left the country divided into two parts: a Communist north and an anti-Communist south. In 1964, a war began between them. The conflict lasted 8 years and involved hundreds of thousands of troops from the United States and other countries. In 1973, after a temporary cease-fire, the United States withdrew, leaving South Vietnam to fight on its own. In 1975, Saigon, the capital of southern Vietnam, fell to the North Vietnamese Army. Many South Vietnamese and opponents of Communism escaped by boat. Many drowned or encountered hunger, illness, or pirates. An international outcry went up, which set the United Nations refugee policy for the next decade.

Since the fall of Saigon, the number of Vietnamese living in the United States has changed dramatically. The 2000 census estimated the population at 1.2 million, nearly double the number that was counted in 1990. The largest concentrations are in California, followed by Washington, Virginia, and Massachusetts. Vietnamese Americans today are sponsoring their relatives, just as American families and organizations sponsored them when they first arrived in the United States.

Communication and Language

Among the many languages spoken in Vietnam are Vietnamese, Chinese, English, French, and Russian. There are three basic Vietnamese dialects; all are understood by most Vietnamese people. Vietnamese is very different from English. Verbs do not change form, articles are not used, and nouns do not have plural endings. Many Vietnamese who live in the United States are bilingual in English and Vietnamese; the older generations may also speak French.

Family Roles and Relationships

Vietnamese culture has been influenced by Buddhism and by Confucian philosophies, which emphasizes respect for authority, social order, loyalty, and filial piety. Family values have a great influence on adolescents. Young people are expected to contribute to family goals and care for their elders. Vietnamese children often live with their parents until marriage and even after, along with their spouse.

In the old days, families always arranged marriages, but sons and daughters were usually consulted on the choice. The typical engagement lasted 6 months, with little contact between the bride and groom. As the influence of Western tradition continues to grow, parents have begun to play more of an advisor role than a matchmaker. Now in the United States, most young Vietnamese Americans date.

By tradition and culture, Vietnamese women are loyal and respectful to their husband. They reside with their spouse's family after marriage. For the older generations, the husband continues to be the head of the household and family spokesperson. The wife is responsible for everything inside the house; however, this no longer necessarily holds true, as more Vietnamese American women receive higher education and enter the workforce. Both husband and wife now share responsibility for housework and decision making, although the women are generally still in charge of healthcare decisions.

Nutrition

The country's cuisine is greatly influenced by the cuisines of France, China, India, and Thailand. For instance, dishes in the north reflect Chinese cooking styles, with stir-fries and noodle-based soups being popular. Rice is a dietary staple. It can be served for breakfast, lunch, and dinner. Fresh herbs are often used, including lemongrass, basil, coriander, lime, and chili. Soup is served at almost every meal.

Appetizers include spring rolls; crepes filled with pork, shrimp, and onions; and rice pancakes. One of the most popular is a noodle soup called *pho*, made of rice noodles, thinly sliced beef or chicken, mint, and scallions. The national condiments are fish sauce (*nuoc mam*) and soy sauce. These are added for flavor.

Religion and Spirituality

Spiritual life in Vietnam is a panoply of belief systems, including Confucianism, Taoism, Buddhism, Christianity, and Tam Giao, or "triple religion," which is a blend of Taoism, popular Chinese beliefs, and ancient Vietnamese animism. Most Vietnamese, including Catholics, worship their ancestors. The predominant religion is Buddhism, which was introduced in 2 B.C. by Chinese immigrants and Indian preachers who came by sea.

Traditional Vietnamese ascribe illnesses to several different causes, including imbalances in one's yin (*am*) and yang (*duong*), a dysfunction of the nervous system, or supernatural phenomenon. The yin and yang beliefs are based on Chinese traditional medicine, which explains physiological imbalances as being brought on by high emotional states or external influences such as sudden climatic changes that block the circulation of vital energy (*chi*) or blood. Climatic changes may produce common colds, mild fever, or headache. Treatments may be herbal, dietary, hygienic, or acupuncture. The Vietnamese also believe that illnesses can be caused by improper functioning of the nervous system. Neuroses are believed to come from weakness of the nerves, and psychoses from turmoil of the nerves. Anxiety, depression, and mental deterioration may signal weak nerves and be treated by a nerve tonic or tranquilizer. Another explanation for illness places the blame on gods, spirits, or demons. The Vietnamese believe that illness may be a punishment for violating some religious or moral code. To treat this form of illness, Buddhist priests and lay monks provide amulets and medicines for physical ailments, as well as conducting exorcisms.

Death Rituals

Vietnamese believe that the soul does not vanish at death but is reincarnated. Cremation, although not widely practiced in the past, has become more common in Vietnamese American communities. Traditional mourning practices include wearing white clothes for 14 days. After this, men wear black armbands and women, white hand bands. Yellow daisies are set out during the rites for the dead and at the traditional yearly celebration of the anniversary of a person's death. During this celebration, which is held at home or in a temple, the family places fruits and traditional foods on an altar and burns incense and fake money for the deceased. Burning incense signifies messages delivered by their ancestors that can protect them and their family from danger or harm. Traditional mourning is no longer observed, however, by many Vietnamese Americans and the younger generation in Vietnam. They have adopted the American custom of wearing black to the funeral and no longer celebrate anniversaries of a death.

Healthcare Practices and Practitioners

Common mental health problems among Vietnamese and other Southeast Asian immigrants (e.g., Cambodians and Laotians) include posttraumatic stress disorder, depression, and anxiety. Southeast Asians often report having pain and sleep disorders. These symptoms are associated with disruptions, which refugees have suffered because of the war, loss of family, low socioeconomic status, underemployment, and poor English skills.

Many Vietnamese immigrants will not seek care for health conditions until they become symptomatic. The appointment system can be a deterrent, as can the language barrier. They may instead try various home remedies, including herbs, coin rubbing, cupping, therapeutic burning, and acupuncture.

A lack of knowledge and awareness about dementia exists in this community. One study of Vietnamese Americans in Hawaii found that older people considered dementia-related symptoms to be a natural part of aging. Dementia is rarely discussed by Vietnamese Americans. Most of them would not think to seek medical treatment for it, and even if they did, very few would have the slightest idea where to look for help. When a healthcare provider is working with a Vietnamese patient who has dementia, it is important to educate the family as well as the individual.

CASE EXAMPLE

I grew up in Vietnam, surrounded with many older relatives who often used excuses like being lam cam *or* lu lan *(confused or forgetful) as a result of aging if they forgot to do something.* (Yen Nguyen)

Vietnamese are not accustomed to discussing personal feelings openly. A healthcare provider might try the following techniques to help clients avoid feeling uncomfortable: Use simple sentences, paraphrase words with multiple meanings, avoid metaphors and idiomatic expressions, and pay close attention to behavioral cues. With new clients, approach in a quiet and unhurried manner and do not interrupt while they are talking.

▥ AFRICAN AMERICANS

Onetta Revere and Kathryn Elliott-Hudson

Introduction and Overview

At 12% of the population, African Americans are the largest minority in the country. They are also the largest minority group among people older than 65 years of age. In 2005, 2.7 million African Americans were 65 years of age or older—a figure that, by the year 2050, is expected to reach 8.6 million.

Most African American ancestors came here after they were forced out of Africa by European slave traders, who sold them to slave owners in the northern, central, and southern United States and the Caribbean. In the United States, in 1861, the North went to war with the South to have slavery abolished. In 1865, after the Civil War ended, a 13th Amendment to the U.S. Constitution was passed, making slavery illegal. Since the early part of the 20th century, African American leaders have led a fight for equal treatment for all.

Today, African American culture is not one monolithic bloc. Many African Americans are of mixed ancestry or migrated from parts of South America and the Caribbean (e.g., Jamaica, Haiti). People who came here from Jamaica will have different attitudes and beliefs than people whose families have lived here for six generations. Nonetheless, broad common traits do exist. Education, for instance, is highly valued by many, although historically, it was difficult for African Americans to obtain educational and employment opportunities because of segregation and discrimination. Various court decisions and legislations have improved this situation.

Communication and Language

Most African Americans speak English, of course, although people who have come here from Haiti or Africa may speak French or an African language. Many speak formal English as well as a dialect, Black English, also called *jive*. Black English reflects the history of Black America. In addition, a few people still speak Gullah, a Creole found among African Americans who have lived for generations on coastal islands of Georgia or South Carolina. Gullah is thought to have originated with slaves from Angola and Sierra Leone. The dominant language spoken among African Americans is Standard English; however, various dialects or informal languages have emerged in different parts of the United States. Others may have a language that is connected with their own religion or region of the country from which they have immigrated and where they currently live. The English spoken by African Americans is highly varied—as varied as the English spoken by any other racial or ethnic group.

Black English refers to informal English spoken by some African Americans. Linguists prefer the term *African American Vernacular English* or *Black Vernacular*. It is a social dialect reflecting the history of Black America.

African Americans, in the main, are highly verbal and open about conveying feelings with family and friends. Speech, intonations, and gestures tend to be expressive, which can be misinterpreted as overly assertive. Examples of this expressiveness are found in storytelling about ancestry and family, which is a large part of the African American culture. Formality is expected in salutations and conversation with strangers. It is important to address older persons as *Mrs.* or *Sir*. Handshakes and direct eye contact are fine, although direct eye contact with non-African Americans may be difficult for elderly African Americans who were conditioned to avoid such encounters. African Americans are acutely aware and protective of their personal space.

Family Roles and Relationships

A single head-of-household is acceptable in the Black community and is often the norm. Families, whether they consist of two parents or one, are typically very private, not sharing concerns with strangers. There is a belief among many that what is discussed within the family stays within the family. African American families, as do many families throughout the United States, aspire to the American Dream.

In times of illness, the extended family usually provides care, which can include networks of friends, or several generations living in the same home. African Americans value taking responsibility within both the nuclear and extended family. Traditionally, elders are respected, obeyed, and considered a source of wisdom. Caregivers are typically women, although men do step up to the plate as well. Long-term care from outside sources is a last resort for most families, although help from social service agencies is acceptable. Family members may be reluctant to attend support groups on the assumption that most people there will be White and will not have the same views toward illness and caregiving.

Nutrition

If an African American offers you a meal, never reject it. If you do, you have rejected the giver. Food in this community is a symbol of health and wealth. As one saying goes, the ideal weight is "having enough meat on your bones." Soul food includes a lot of greens, pork, ham hocks, and smoked turkey. African American diets in general tend to be higher in fat, with less fiber and fruit, a fact that may be rooted in the scarcity of available food during slavery.

Care providers who have African American patients should check to be sure that they do not belong to a religious affiliation, such as Muslim or Seventh-day Adventist, which has dietary prescriptions.

Religion and Spirituality

Many African Americans believe that one's inner strengths come from trusting in God. They tend to have strong affiliations with their faith community. In times of illness, many rely on prayer and the informal support that their church family offers. Spirituality and prayer are the Black caregivers' most common form of coping. Some of the most popular denominations include African Methodist Episcopal, Apostolic, Baptist, Jehovah's Witnesses, Nation of Islam, Pentecostal, and Roman Catholic. The most frequently used coping strategy is prayer. Songs are sung with emotion and as a testimony to one's faith. One's inner strengths come from trusting in God. Families frequently seek support from their faith community, including ministers and church groups.

Death Rituals

African Americans are likely to rally for life-sustaining measures. The length of time life is extended is taken as a measure of how successful the treatments are. Black Americans are less likely to have advance directives in place, although there is general support for planning for healthcare decisions. They tend to believe that the body must be kept intact after death. Cremation is unacceptable for many older adults. Reverence and respect are shown toward the dead. African Americans are highly expressive of grief at a funeral. People may "fall out"—suddenly go paralyzed and collapse, become temporarily unable to speak or see. Funerals are referred to as *going home* or a *homecoming*. After a death, the community often turns out to support the family and to celebrate the life of the person who has died.

Healthcare Practices and Practitioners

Many African Americans face certain obstacles, both internal and external, when it comes to obtaining care. Typically, they will not seek outside services, either because they are unaware that the services exist or because they believe elders should be cared for at home by family. Others may distrust American healthcare, owing to several historical cases of mistreatment of Blacks by the system. In one well-known incident, the Tuskegee Syphilis Experiment, the U.S. Public Health Service made guinea pigs of 399 Black men with syphilis, withheld treatment, and neglected to disclose their diagnoses to them to observe what would happen as their disease progressed.

African Americans may use home remedies and folk healers in addition to Western medicine. Information about herbal healing is passed around within the community. Caregivers should determine if alternative practices are being used, to rule out potential conflicts with standard medicine.

The person or persons closest to the family member who is ill will discuss the prognosis with the healthcare provider and family members. Medical information is considered a private matter. Obtaining consent and information may be difficult at times, if there is distrust that has been engendered by personal and group history.

African Americans are generally open about pain. Pain-rating scales will be helpful. However, some individuals may not want to take pain medication because of fear of addiction, of losing control, or because they have used home remedies all their lives. Others will refuse it from the belief that pain and suffering is inevitable in life and must be tolerated.

It is important for caregivers to understand the historical context that shapes African American hesitancy to enlist outside care providers. In some ways, it is a legacy of slavery and African traditions. The institution of slavery provided few vehicles for individuals and families to receive support for survival outside the slave community. The availability of social support was internal to the slave community—survival was a group effort, an attitude that has come down to the present day. For this reason, and because of significant disparities in the health-care system resulting in unequal access to hospice and palliative care—research shows that African Americans are more likely to be undertreated for pain of all types and are less likely to have regular medical care.

African Americans are at an increased risk for several diseases, including heart disease, stroke, kidney disease, diabetes, vascular dementia, and possibly even AD from the little research that has been done. This can mean that adult children who are caring for a parent may be themselves at high risk for these diseases. Although Alzheimer's is more prevalent among African Americans than among Whites (estimates range from 14% to 100% and higher), there is an overall lack of knowledge about AD among African Americans. Few African Americans participate in dementia research studies, so very little research has addressed the subject of African Americans and the disease. The result has been a lack of community awareness. Symptoms are often attributed to normal aging, which can result in situations where individuals do not receive necessary treatments and wider support. Black Americans have a greater familial risk of contracting Alzheimer's. In addition, research into the causes of Alzheimer's in African Americans is underway to determine if they may be different from that in Caucasians.

■ NATIVE AMERICANS

Niela Redford and Minnie Jim

Overview and Heritage

The basic numbers give a sense of how varied Native Americans are as a group. Although Native Americans comprise less than 2% of the U.S. population, there are 569 federally recognized Native American tribes and 200 unofficially recognized groups living on 275 federally recognized reservations. Tribal groups may be related linguistically, by the region they inhabit, or by their origins as described in oral histories and creation stories, but together, all Native Americans share a history of having been uprooted, disenfranchised, and subjugated within the society. Because of this, a widespread distrust of mainstream institutions exists. It is important for a caregiver to acknowledge this history in order to build trust with a client.

Native American cultures are very complex. What holds true for one tribe or clan may not for another. Professional caregivers should educate themselves, with the help of family caregivers, about tribal beliefs, traditions, and preferences, and perhaps more importantly, individual preferences.

The various creation stories different tribes tell illustrate how different the clans' belief systems are. In the Hopi creation story, the Hopi people emerged into this world, called the *Fourth World*, through the *sipapu,* the earth's navel. "Hopi knew that life in this fourth world would be difficult and that we must learn a way of life from the corn plant," one Hopi Web site says (The Hopi Tribe, 2006). "Cultivating corn has therefore been a profound experience for us and has shaped our lifeway, which is based on humility, cooperation, respect and earth stewardship" (The Hopi Tribe, 2006). Through the suffering they had experienced in the first, second, and third underground worlds, they learned the values necessary to live an honorable life. The Hopi poet Lomatewama (1998) refers to these values when he writes, "One will be Hopi when one possesses these virtues: knowing thyself; having respect for all, for all things; being self directed and motivated; being industrious; and sharing the fruits of these virtues with others."

The Desert People, Tohono O'odham, tell a very different story of their origins. *I'itoi* (Elder Brother), Spirit of Goodness, and another brother, Earth Medicine Man, created themselves. "I'itoi created himself from the foam that you see on the water," tribal leader Felix Antone says (Beal, 2004). "The other man created himself from the mud that was under the ocean." The brothers then created the Tohono O'odham from clay. "I'itoi told the Tohono O'odham to remain where they were, in that land of the Crimson Evening, which is the center of all things," Felix Antone relates. "And there the desert people have always lived."

CASE EXAMPLE

The O'odham believe that the hindac, *or the way of life, is a guiding force for the way we conduct our lives on this Earth today. Certainly, it dictates how we are to interact with the other people. And when O'odham talk about people, in general terms, they are talking about plants, animals, and humans, and that there is no hierarchy here, we are all equal, and so we have to take care of each other, we have to respect each other.* (Angelo Joaquin, Southwest Indian Art Coordinator, Arizona State University)

The complex Navajo creation story tells how the *Diné*, the Navajo people, passed through three underworlds before entering the Fourth World, the Glittering World, which is the one we inhabit. The people became prepared for existence in the Fourth World as they ascended through the tiers of the underworld. Four sacred Western mountains define the four cardinal directions for the Navajos: at the east, Mount Blanca (associated with the color white), representing the beginning of life and thought; at the south, Mount Taylor (blue), representing the process of planning and the development of physical abilities and health; at the west, San Francisco Peaks (yellow), representing life, the development of social competence, and the importance of relationships; and at the north, Mount Hesperus (black), representing hope.

In all tribes, a strong elder population contributes to the preservation and practice of traditional ways. Elders are respected for their wisdom, experience, and knowledge. They are the teachers, caretakers of the young, and the keepers of oral history and ceremonies. Tribal leaders who exemplify traditional values are vital in upholding traditions. Many Native Americans are concerned that the absorption of non-Indian behaviors and ways of thinking into the tribes is causing a weakening of these traditions.

Communication and Language

Most Native Americans speak English. Many maintain their traditional native languages as well. Native languages are taught in reservation schools (classes may be mandatory), in schools with a high number of Native American students, and in urban Indian centers and other urban organizations. Just as one tribe can have wide variation in its beliefs and customs, so can one tribe's language. There are three dialects within the Hopi Nation, for instance, and six in the Tohono O'odham.

When having a conversation, Native Americans tend to keep a wide space between themselves and others, especially on first meeting. Tribes differ in how much eye contact is acceptable. In some, avoiding looking a person in the eye is a sign of respect; in others, it signals disrespect and disinterest. If your patient is accustomed to having little eye contact, quickly scan the person's or family member's face every so often for signs of confusion. There is also no consensus on handshakes or embraces when greeting. In some tribal cultures, these are fine; in others, they are offensive. If you are uncertain whether the person and family shake hands, wait to see if they extend theirs. An ability to listen well is greatly valued. People who are serene and modest are highly appreciated. Talking is of less value, especially to elders. Assertiveness is to be avoided, because it may be interpreted as disrespect or aggression.

CASE EXAMPLE

As a bilagáana *(White) nurse giving care to Navajo people, I needed to be able to communicate more effectively. Even after attending classes, my Navajo language skills remain basic, although are still quite useful. The cultural lessons learned are priceless, though. For example, the beautiful Navajo word for "to pray" is sodiszin, which translates as "holy tongue." The Navajo people believe that language is a sacred gift from the Holy People. Language is to be used respectfully and with kindness and honor. Language should never harm, embarrass, abuse, or insult others in any way.* (Niela Redford)

When communicating with an Native American, always be fully present with them. That is, sit quietly and listen, and involve the person as well as the family. Solicit the elderly peoples' feelings and ideas about their condition and circumstances. Actively involve them in planning care.

Factors such as language fluency, literacy, and whether a statement is age appropriate are of great importance when conducting an assessment or educating clients and families. Consider speaking at a slower pace, especially with elderly people. They may be hard-of-hearing or have trouble following English. Answers to questions posed to elderly people may be provided through storytelling. When asking questions, the caregiver should demonstrate genuine concern.

The use of gentle humor is an effective way to establish rapport with the person and family. Humor should not be directed at anyone. Lillian Tom-Orme (2002), an expert on transcultural nursing, says, "When a client or family uses humor with nurses [or other caregivers], it is a good sign that trust has been established." Native American humor may take the form of teasing or friendly little jokes.

Address the individual as Mrs. or Mr. until rapport develops. The patient and family will often indicate that trust has been established by asking the caregiver what his or her first name is. From then on, the caregiver, patient, and family will likely be on a first-name basis. It is perfectly all right to ask the patient or family how to pronounce their names if their names are unusual.

Non–Native Americans may find what seem like long pauses in the conversation. Tribal elders may complain that English speakers "talk too fast" or are too direct. According to Lee Begay, Elder Services director for the Intertribal Council of Arizona:

> *Anglos tend to ask direct questions without establishing relations. Tribal elders usually will not respond and will stop listening if they are asked direct questions by a stranger. Establishing a rapport with a tribal elder is very important. It might take hours or even days. Overall, silence is valued, and long periods of silence between speakers are common. Interruption of the person who is speaking is considered extremely rude, especially if that person is an elder. Storytelling is common and is a way to convey thoughts and emotions, often through the use of metaphors. (Hendrix, 2001)*

Other cultural considerations should be taken into account when working with Native Americans. Emotional expressiveness may be controlled, except for humor. Body movements may be minimal. Touch is usually unacceptable, although friendly touching may be initiated by the Native American person once rapport is there. Always explain the purpose of touching someone. Ask permission first, especially if you need to touch the head and hair, which may be considered sacred. If the hair needs to be cut, be sure to explain why, save the hair, and give it to the family.

Some elders speak only their native tongue. Literacy levels and language abilities should always be assessed, especially if written forms or educational materials are used. When using interpreters, an adult of the same gender as the client is preferred. *Probability* statements such as, "There is a slight possibility that he will get better" or "I am quite certain this behavior will not change" do not translate grammatically in some Indian languages, and may be misinterpreted as fact or prediction. Even the greeting "How are you?" may cause the patient to feel they are less than well. Learn and use the greeting words of the people to convey respect and welcome.

Older Native Americans may need time to translate concepts into their language or thought and then back into English or Western thought before they answer. Over-the-phone translation services, such as Language Line Services, are available, but may not have translators who are proficient in Native American languages or in the particular language your client speaks. Some 200–210 Native American tongues are still spoken in the United States.

CASE EXAMPLE

A Tohono O'odham elder, admitted to a Phoenix hospital, smiled and took my hand in hers when I greeted her on Monday morning with, "Sa:pa i masma." She replied, "Oh, thank you! I have not heard any of my language since I got here. I was so lonesome. Now I feel safe." (Niela Redford)

Family Roles and Relationships

An elderly person's healthcare can be a challenge for the family. It is made complicated by the reverence for the old ones that people have. The following confession a grown child made to a doctor reflects the deep sadness families face as their elder fades into dementia:

> Doctor, I don't know what I should do about my mother. She gets mad a lot, and she is mean too. She's 85 years old and has always been very healthy. Now she isn't the same. She doesn't want to wash, and sometimes I have to make her clean herself. That isn't like her; she always taught us to keep ourselves clean. She used to like to go to town, and now she doesn't want to go places. She just wants to stay at home. She gets after the neighbors for nothing and accuses them of stealing things, and I know they don't do that. I guess she's just getting old, but I don't know why she's like that.

Before assessing a Native American home and family, one must have knowledge of tribal ways. It is unlikely, for instance, that someone who is an outsider or who has not established rapport with the patient, family, and perhaps even the community will be admitted into the home. This can include unfamiliar home health aides, public health nurses, community health representatives, or representatives from outside agencies (e.g., physical therapists, medical equipment deliverers, and Medicaid or Medicare case managers).

Once there is rapport, when making a home visit the healthcare provider should drive into the yard, park where they can be recognized, honk the horn a couple of times, then wait for someone to appear. This may be repeated once. If no one appears, the household does not wish to be visited at that time. A subsequent visit will be anticipated by the household, and should be scheduled with timely notification by letter or a community worker. It is recommended that on a first visit the non–Native American healthcare provider be accompanied by someone from the community.

CASE EXAMPLE

On the other hand, in certain Navajo communities, just honking the car horn is considered rude. Navajos are taught to invite people into their homes. For non–tribal members, it is best to have a Navajo individual with you when you are out visiting, so you will not get lost in the remote areas. In the case of non–family members visiting a Navajo for the first time at their home, someone will come out to greet you when you first arrive. They will want to know the purpose of your visiting. From that point, they will decide if they want to invite you in their home. (Lee Begay)

In a home assessment, the following factors should be considered: the absence or presence of electricity or a generator and what the available means are if the person needs to obtain help (e.g., nearby family or neighbors, telephone, walkie-talkies, radio communication). Other assessment factors should include likelihood of falls and burns, ability to obtain good nutrition, ability to maintain personal and household cleanliness, whether there is a potable water supply, adequate heating and cooling, adequate toilet facilities, the health of pets and livestock, and the quality of area for sleep and rest.

A family assessment should note the number and relationships of people in the home, their health and mobility, and the extent of their understanding of dementia. A cultural assessment should include information on diagnosis and treatment by traditional healers, use of traditional medicines and methods, and attitudes toward Western medicine providers, agencies, and facilities. It is also important to note any evidence of alcohol or drug use by the patient or others in the home, and any signs of elder exploitation or abuse.

The person's and their family's economic status greatly determines whether care plans will succeed. It can dictate whether the patient is able to acquire medical supplies or resources needed for continued care and wellness (e.g., running water, electricity, telephone, adequate space, healthful or specific diet). Clinic visits may not be kept because the person lacks money for gas. Recommendations for care with lower-income persons must be sensitive to these kinds of considerations.

CASE EXAMPLE

The monetary system is not as important as family values and support. Ke', or relationships, is very important to a Navajo. Many Navajo elders that we interviewed years ago thought of themselves as wealthy even though they were living below the poverty level. Navajos value kinship, livestock, personal health, and spiritual or traditional beliefs. (Lee Begay)

There is widespread variability from tribe to tribe on how acculturated tribal members are to mainstream America. Native Americans have a deep, strong cultural base, but their communities remain among the poorest places in America. Communities suffer from high unemployment and an inability to create new jobs because of the dearth of resources, shaky infrastructures, lack of capital, and remote locations. The poverty rate reported for Native Americans is more than twice (25.9% vs. 11.3%) that of non–Native Americans.

In addition to home safety, issues to consider include family care patterns, gender taboos, and feelings about outsider assistance in the home. Gender roles differ widely among tribes or nations; some are matrilineal whereas others are patrilineal.

Family is of utmost importance to the Native American. The Navajo say, "To be poor is to be without family or kin." Family consists of extended members, from all generations, who share commonality through the maternal and paternal grandmothers' family. Clan members are expected to provide care to an ill person by visiting the home, hospital, or long-term care facility. Most native people believe that presence or "being with" encourages that person to regain health and balance.

Medical decisions may depend on how the family is affected and, thus, the entire family may be included in making these important decisions. Gathering the family for decision making may take several days. The actual decision, if not made by the elders, will usually be made by a consensus.

In the past, Native Americans have suffered from the misuse of signed documents by non–Native Americans. This has resulted in a collective distrust of outsiders. Some persons may be unwilling to sign an informed consent, advance directives, or power of attorney forms, given this history of broken promises. A verbal agreement is perceived as being sufficient. When the person or family is reluctant to complete advance directives or medical power of attorney, the verbal agreement may be considered legally valid if there has first been a conference with the family, person, and a physician. The attorney for the community or healthcare facility can answer questions. With clear and thorough documentation in the patient's medical record, the decisions and agreements are generally followed. It is wise to have all those involved in the conference sign the documentation, if possible.

A reluctance to discuss topics related to death and dying is common among many tribal groups. The subject must be addressed with careful words and great sensitivity. Direct references to death are to be avoided. When healthcare professionals need to discuss these issues with Native Americans, one experienced in and knowledgeable of their ways should be present.

Nutrition

Food offers not only sustenance but is of great spiritual and social significance to the Native Americans. Food accompanies celebratory and ceremonial events, such as healing and religious events. Corn is a major part of the diet of many tribal groups. Corn products such as pollen and corn meal are important to traditional medicine and ceremonies.

Traditional foods and food preparation should be investigated and provided to persons with advanced dementia. Typical traditional foods among tribes include the following:

- Navajo—corn, beans, squash, mutton, antelope and deer meat, wild spinach and onions, melons, and other foods;
- O'odham—tepary beans, squash, melons, chilies, various wild foods (e.g., cholla buds, saguaro fruit, prickly pear pads, mesquite pods, and chia), and meat from wild animals (e.g., deer, javelina, rabbits);
- Apache—acorns, corn, agave, juniper berries and walnuts, beans and berries, and meat from deer, rabbits, and other wild animals;
- Northern Plains people—buffalo (believed to be a sacred gift from the Creator; it provides nutrition and is important in many practices and social events); and
- Chippewa (Anishinaabe, Ojibwa) and other northern people—wild rice has long been grown for nourishment, ceremonial use, as well as for profit.

Religion and Spirituality

Spiritual practices and religious beliefs will often influence a patient's decision about medical treatment. Because of their religious faith, patients may request diagnosis but not treatment. If a particular treatment is necessary, providers may find it helpful to talk with the patient's spiritual leader. Patients who seek mainstream medical care may also seek treatment from healers in their tribe. Rather than discouraging this, especially if the alternative treatment is not harmful, providers and their staff may want to incorporate traditional healing into the general treatment plan. The healthcare providers should know of traditional practitioners available for bedside healing and blessings.

Having an awareness of Native American traditional practices is important to the caregiver. Combining traditional beliefs with modern treatments not only provides culturally competent care but also contributes to survival of heritage. Medicine men and women are usually receptive to questions that are not intrusive and relish teaching caregivers about Native American spiritual practices. When a traditional ceremony is being performed at someone's bedside, it is wise for the caregiver to remain nearby to prevent interruptions (although native healers will understand that interruptions may be unavoidable in a critical care setting). The caregiver may offer assistance. Fresh water in a clean glass is used during the blessing and, afterward, will usually be drunk by the medicine person. Water is considered sacred and therefore is not wasted.

Most Native Americans share six spiritual concepts. First, a belief in unseen powers or what some people call the Great Mystery. Second, the knowledge that all things in the universe are dependent on each other. Third, a belief that personal worship reinforces the bond between the individual, the community, and the great powers. Worship is a personal commitment to the sources of life. Fourth, an understanding that sacred traditions and people knowledgeable in sacred traditions are responsible for teaching morals and ethics. Fifth, most communities and tribes have trained practitioners who have been given names such as medicine man or woman, priest, and so forth. These individuals also have titles given them by the people. They are responsible for specialized, sometimes secret knowledge that is kept stored in memory. They pass knowledge and sacred practices from generation to generation. The spiritual leaders have access to greater power than ordinary individuals do. They have special gifts, such as healing abilities. They provide healing and counseling and conduct ceremonies. Finally, there is a belief that humor is a necessary part of the sacred. Human beings are often weak—we are not gods—and our weakness leads us to do foolish things; therefore clowns and similar figures are needed to show us how we act and why.

Special hair adornments, a medicine bag, jewelry, or other regalia may have special spiritual meaning to a patient. It is best to clarify and understand this if these items have to be removed from the person for some reason. If possible, items of importance like this should remain with the person at all times.

Spirituality is central to people's existence and centers on harmony with nature. Self-awareness is considered necessary for harmony. All ceremonies and events start and close with prayer. Spiritualism brings families closer together and unites them with other Native Americans.

Death Rituals

Traditional belief systems comfort those receiving palliative care, as well as those caring for loved ones whose spirits are being lost to dementia. The long-practiced rituals surrounding this final stage of life and the processes of dying and death give structure for the work of caring and conclusion to the activities surrounding life's end. Death, burial, and grief customs may vary within a tribe, from village to village, and from family to family. In each tribe, death customs are practiced according to each family's beliefs.

Apache people treat the body with deep respect. Preparation of the body for burial traditionally includes reverent bathing, with washing and combing of the hair. Close relatives then dress the person in his or her good clothes and the body remains inside the family dwelling (*wickiup*) throughout the night. The old ways are still practiced by many today. Among the San Carlos and White Mountain Apache, funerals are conducted in a respectfully integrated manner. The priest performs a church service for a Catholic tribal member, incorporating the sacred elements of cedar and water. He accompanies the mourners to the burial grounds, says a prayer, consoles the bereaved, and returns to the church. The traditional burial ground rituals are then fulfilled. It is very important to the Apache that as many family members as possible be with the person at the time of his or her death.

The burial takes place in the morning, signifying a new beginning. During the night, relatives and friends gather at the deceased's home to comfort the family, to mourn, and to provide nourishment and help. Very early in the morning, some of the men may shoot guns, symbolizing departure from the earth. A meal may be served at midnight, as in the old times. Laughter is thought to send the deceased person happily on his or her journey. Nothing is taken from the burial site (i.e., flowers, mementos, gifts). The dead person is buried facing the east, with bread and clear water to nourish him or her as he or she travels to the Land of the Dead.

CASE EXAMPLE

At one recent Apache burial, the deceased woman's son placed her teacups, saucers, and spoons into her grave. He added her sewing kit saying, "Well, Mom, you won't be needing these here anymore." At another, my friend's family placed the new rug that had been purchased for his room beneath the coffin. A large duffle bag with his belongings was placed on top. (Niela Redford)

The dead person's name is never repeated again after the death rituals. The immediate family holds a dinner 1 year after the death. Those who helped during the grieving time are served a meal to show the family's appreciation. The departed one is honored.

Variations of the funeral rites exist among the tribes. The Maricopa, also known as the Pee Posh, share many customs with the Chemehuevi, Quechan, Mohave, and

Cocopah (Yuman) tribes. Traditional Maricopa families cremate their dead in a very sacred manner. The next of kin, often the mother or sister, decides the type of burial to be held. No children are allowed at a traditional ceremony. A member of the bereaved family, who is on a peer level with the burial specialist, must approach the specialist about preparations and carrying out the cremation. Strict protocols cover this negotiation, based on traditional beliefs. There are "cry houses" where the body is laid out for visitation. People come from afar and are fed by the women of the family.

Hopi people observe traditional and nontraditional spiritual practices. When a Hopi dies, the body is traditionally washed and then clothed in the garb of the special brotherhood or society to which the person belonged. When a hospital patient dies, the body is removed from the hospital as soon as possible. The idea of an autopsy violates Hopi beliefs, as it does with many other tribes. If the person dies close to home, the body is buried the same day or night. Immediate burial is important because the day after the death occurs is the first of 4 days during which the spirit leaves the grave and, it is said, goes to the bottom of the Grand Canyon. Food (e.g., pinto beans, piki bread, blue cornmeal pudding) is taken to the grave on the third day. The spirit departs early on the fourth.

The life of the Hopi is considered a journey from birth to death. Each stage—childhood, youth, adulthood, and old age—has its own accepted behaviors. Through death, the person is reborn into the underworld. The ceremony that follows the death of a Hopi is the simplest and shortest of all Hopi ceremonies. A loved one's death is handled with great reverence; reverence for life leads automatically to reverence for death.

Traditional spiritual practices remain very important to most of the Tohono O'odham. The people often integrate aspects of other religions, such as Catholic, Pentecostal, or Presbyterian. The deceased Tohono O'odham person is brought home from the funeral parlor for an all-night vigil in the home, in the village community center, or, if weather is suitable, outside beneath a ramada (*watto*). Individuals are often not embalmed because of a belief that the person will return to earth. The family, men or women, prepare the body according to ritual, cleansing and dressing it in clothes the person wore. Sometimes a suitcase is packed and buried with the body, as well as some of the deceased's favorite personal items (e.g., a man's horse blanket, a favorite hat, or a lady's sewing kit or favorite cup).

Most families hire a group to recite the rosary, say prayers, and sing throughout the night. Small signs are often posted across the Tohono O'odham nation to announce the wake and burial. The wake begins around sundown, continuing through the night until the burial at sunrise. During the wake, friends and family come to support the bereaved family and pay respect to the deceased. They take turns staying up during the wake so family members may rest.

The Tohono O'odham are among the groups who believe they will wander throughout eternity looking for any missing body parts. It is extremely important to ask the O'odham people and others about preserving body parts that have been amputated or removed (including bone fragments, fatty tissue, and hair) after surgery or injury for return to the individual or family. The tissue or organ will be buried at the place where the person eventually lies. O'odham people who do not know where their lost limb, tissue, or organ is may grieve for that unsaved part, dream about it, lose sleep, become depressed, lose their appetite, or even die.

The Navajo believe that when one dies, the spirit that represents the good in life goes to an afterworld. The journey takes 4 days and the person's spirit is guided to the afterworld by deceased relatives and friends. The afterworld is an underworld and is entered through the hole of emergence from which the first Navajo people came forth at the beginning of time. The afterworld is like life on earth and the inhabitants live the same way the living Navajos do, but it is a good life with happy times.

CASE EXAMPLE

Navajos generally do not talk about death. They know that death will come sometime in the cycle of life, but to talk about it now is believed to bring harm or sickness to one's self or family members. The majority of Navajos do not have a will or durable power of attorney. When an individual is near death, the family will want to extend their life for as long as possible. Doctors make the mistake of directing questions to male members of the family about life-support. Men do not make these decisions; it's usually the females. When a decision is made to let a person die, the majority of the family members will leave the facility and not stay around for the individual to die. Navajos currently use the mortuary to make all of the funeral arraignments. Burial must be done on the fourth day. (Lee Begay)

When a person dies, the good part of the person leaves with the spirit, whereas the evil part stays with the physical body. When a person dies, an evil spirit, or *ch'iindi*, is released with the dying breath. The ch'iindi is considered very dangerous and causes sickness and misfortune. The Navajo are very fearful of the ch'iindi and take every precaution to avoid contact. They take great caution to avoid the dead, graves, and anything connected with death. When a person dies in a hogan, the hogan is destroyed. Even today, families will bring their dying relatives to the hospital to prevent them from dying in the home. Many Navajos will avoid hospitals as they feel the buildings are filled with ch'iindis. One who has touched a dead body must undergo a ceremony known as the *Enemy Way* to purify and release the ch'iindi spirit.

Healthcare Practices and Practitioners

The Western social service network is not typically a part of Native American culture. The Indian Health Service serves many Native Americans and is the source of health care for many on and off the reservation. If you do provide care for someone who is Native American, a cultural assessment is an important first step.

> **CASE EXAMPLE**
>
> *The middle-aged daughter of a hospitalized elderly person suffering advancing dementia came to a Native American case manager's office in tears. She stood wringing her hands, and said, "I am so ashamed that my mother fell and got hurt. I just can't do this any more. I have teenagers in school, my husband and I work, and I am the only one in the family who can take care of our mother. I am so tired. I don't know what to do." The case manager (CM) quietly listened to this devoted, exhausted daughter as she continued to express her shame and sadness. Care alternatives for the mother were then discussed.*
>
> *The CM plays a crucial role in these situations. In this case, the CM collaborated with the Tribal CM, Social Worker, and Elder Services to assist the family. The most acceptable resolution for this family was the arrangement of periodic respite care in a nearby culturally competent care center. A weekday tribal caregiver was arranged through Elder Services. The daughter was relieved of her shame, the family remained intact, and the elderly person was well cared for.* (Niela Redford)

The case manager (CM) plays a crucial role in such situations. In the previous case example, the CM collaborated with the tribal CM, social worker, and elder services to assist the family. *Elder Services* is a term used within the Native American community. The most acceptable resolution for this family was the arrangement of periodic respite care in a nearby culturally competent care center. A weekday tribal companion or caregiver was arranged through Elder Services. The daughter was relieved of her shame, the family remained intact, and the elder was well cared for.

The family's knowledge and willingness to care for a dependent elder can be assessed with questions such as, "What will your family do when he [she] can no longer do for himself [herself]?" It may be necessary, because of mitigating circumstances, to place the person in an extended-care facility. This undesirable option can take the elder far from home, making regular family visits difficult. Food in the new place may not be culturally appropriate, the environment and furnishings will be unfamiliar, and the loneliness that can result can do harm to the spirit.

The person or family may be reluctant to disclose information and a health history. General distrust from historical events may prohibit consent and information sharing. This will be especially true if a caregiver approaches with any kind of blaming attitude, is critical of traditional healing, or dismisses explanations. When gathering social, family, and personal information, avoid negative or accusatory words or statements that emphasize problems or might be taken to indicate the person is responsible for his or her illness. Examples of questions that can be used to elicit the patient's perspective include the following: What do you think caused your problem? Why do you think it started when it did?

What do you call it? What do you think your sickness does to your body? How does it work?

Similarly, the activities of daily living (ADLs) should be assessed, using ADL and Instrumental ADL (IADL) scales and your own inquiries. For example, what kind of activities are they used doing? Did they ever use a telephone or balance a checkbook? Do they chop wood and carry water, or engage in activities such as leatherwork, beading, or weaving?

Native Americans are modest and value privacy and confidentiality highly. Before and during a physical exam, simple, gentle explanations should be given for why the body is being touched. Touching (by a stranger or family member) in some Indian cultures is inappropriate. Permission should be requested before the use of touch or before uncovering any part of a patient's body. The person may still refuse to disrobe. In some reservations, clothes are removed only if necessary. Requests should be accompanied by an explanation that is made in a quiet, calm, and pleasant manner. Loudness and brusqueness are associated with aggression.

If severe disease complications are apparent, such as requiring measures like surgery or in even more extreme circumstances, amputation, avoid using predictive statements such as, "Those toes are so dark and cold that they will have to be cut off if blood flow doesn't improve." If the toes do have to be amputated, the caregiver may be thought to have used witchcraft or put a curse on the person and be held responsible.

Depression is seldom the stated reason for an elder's clinic visit, although subjective and objective observations may reveal symptoms. The existence of depression is more likely to be expressed in cultural metaphors (e.g., "heavy heart," "lack of balance or harmony"). The family may be aware of diminishing memory and changes in behavior. These changes may be considered just as "part of life" until the patient's bodily functions and ability to get around show deterioration. Family and community often minimize memory loss and dementia, and may not present for treatment unless physical function is impaired.

Native Americans may underreport pain and report only that they are uncomfortable. Physical, mental, emotional, or spiritual distress may be expressed through storytelling. The caregiver is responsible for identifying signs and degrees of pain by observing facial expression or body language. He or she may notice a "pain face"—a frown, tight lips and jaw, tears, or look of fear or high anxiety. The eyes may be closed as the person attempts to escape the pain. The person may moan or pray. He or she may keep his or her body curled, or stretched tightly with toes curled. His or her hands may be tensely closed or may be pulling at the bed linen. People with advanced dementia will demonstrate pain in some way but usually cannot articulate it.

End-of-life preferences should be ascertained, but not until a relationship has been developed that includes some degree of trust. Healers, called *mahkai* (Tohono O'odham) and *hataalii* (Navajo) are highly regarded in Native American society. Western medical providers and caregivers may be placed in similar high esteem when they provide care that is respectful, kind, knowledgeable, and competent.

CASE EXAMPLE

Beverly Warne, a Lakota nurse, relates a childhood incident when she asked her grandmother about an uncle whose behavior she did not understand. He was fading into what was then called "being senile." The grandmother responded, "Do kashne [It's okay, don't worry]." She explained that to the Lakota, when this happens to people, it means the spirit is getting ready to go to the Great Mystery and the body is finishing up life's tasks. This example of deep reverence for the human being affected by dementia reflects a generally held belief in the value of human life, and a belief that change is simply part of life.

As in other groups, Native Americans often mistake Alzheimer's for general aging; it is referred to as "old timer's" disease. Although little is known about dementia's prevalence in the Native American community, Alzheimer's is thought to be relatively rare. Evidence suggests it is having a growing impact, however. According to figures from the Indian Health Service, the number of Native American deaths from AD increased some 300% recently. With high diabetes rates, as the Indian population ages, vascular-type dementias may be more common than in the Anglo population. For a proud culture made stronger by centuries of honoring its elders, these increases are significant.

◼ EUROPEAN AMERICANS

Overview and Heritage

Although it is almost impossible to characterize approximately 230 million people, a few general statements about European Americans (also known as Euro-Americans and, sometimes, White Americans) can be made. "Anglo-American" is a term sometimes used in the southwestern United States in place of European American. The European American population has sometimes been eclipsed or obscured by the erroneous notion that European Americans are more or less the U.S. population—and that there are few substantive differences among Americans. Within the U.S. population, those who have emigrated from European countries or whose forbears have emigrated from European countries comprise the majority (Leininger, 2002). Many European Americans have mixed European ancestries. The nations of origin include the eastern European nations, former Soviet bloc nations, and the former Soviet Union (Spector, 2004).

European Americans rarely understand that they also are an ethnic/cultural group. European American values are pervasive, and it is sometimes assumed that all who would come under the heading "European American" closely resemble one another. Actually, it was not until the 1980 census that questions on ancestry were asked (Spector, 2004). It was the first time that persons were asked to identify their race and/or ethnicity. The United States is a land of immigrants—except of course for Native Americans, who are indigenous to this land. History informs us of periods and events when discrimination, segregation, and racism by and large separated European Americans from other ethnic and cultural groups. There have been longstanding economic disparities, including health-related disparities, between European Americans and other U.S. subpopulations (National Center on Minority Health and Health Disparities, 2006). Ethnopharmacology, which (among other things) correlates health statistics and health patterns with specific ethnic groups, is in its infancy (Muñoz & Hilgenberg, 2005). Purportedly American world-views have more often than not been expressed and communicated from European American perspectives.

Related to demographics: the average life expectancy for European American males is 74.89 years, and for females, 80.67 years (Central Intelligence Agency [CIA], 2005b). U.S. government figures report that 81.7% of the population is White. Large cities in the United States, such as New York, Chicago, and Los Angeles, have in the past been predominantly European American, but this trend has been reversed. Arizona reported a 75.5% White population during the 2000 census, with Whites comprising 71.1% of the Phoenix population (U.S. Census Bureau, 2000b).

Many researchers have studied prevailing European American cultural attributes and values. Some of these attributes and values may be mistakenly represented as stand-ins for "American" attributes and values, and so: when identifying anything as purely American, caution is in order. European American attributes and values may include: individualism and self-reliance; independence and freedom; competition, assertiveness, and the value of achievements; materialism; dependence on technology; relative amounts of gender equality; youth and beauty; reliance on "scientific facts" and numbers; and generosity and helpfulness in crises (Leininger, 2002, p. 289).

European Americans are likely to value their individual autonomy and "getting ahead." They dislike restrictions on their freedoms, suppression of their values, and "being left behind." Material goods, possessions, and modern technologies tend to be highly valued. For European Americans, very often "time is money." European Americans value productivity and "doing." There is the claim that, among European Americans, decisions are made on the basis of hard facts—as exemplified by the maxim "prove it to me." Other values held in common may include a focus on the passage of time, control over time, self-promotion, and collaboration based on authority (Elliott, Adams, & Sockalingam, 1999b). European Americans are very often seen as being goal-directed and future oriented—often driven by financial gain.

Some European American ethnic groups may have become segregated according to generational segments. For example, Italian Americans may be divided among elderly persons residing in Italian enclaves, second generation persons living in urban neighborhoods, younger persons living in the suburbs, and new immigrants (Spector, 2004). In the past Italian immigrants have largely settled in New York and Boston, whereas immigrants from Poland very often first migrated to Texas and moved on from there. It is a reasonable expectation that newly arrived immigrants are going to settle where persons of similar background and ethnicity reside concurrently. This provides needed orientation, ongoing support, and guidance in a new country. Reasons for migration have been as varied as are the number of countries represented in America.

Communication and Language

English is the dominant language; however, different European American ethnic groups may hold on to their original language as their primary or secondary means of communication. The voice volumes of European American persons may be perceived by some as being loud (Elliot, Adams, & Sockalingam, 1999b). A loud voice may be misconstrued as reflecting anger and a person may be misunderstood (Purnell & Paulanka, 2008). For all groups, the specific context in which a statement is made plays an important role in communication. Many idioms that have made their way into American English and are heard often in conversational language may include atypical forms of speech, and may not even be translatable into other languages.

Some European American communication styles and "trademarks" may be perceived as denoting disrespect (Elliot, Adams, & Sockalingam, 1999a). European Americans may have a proclivity toward asking direct questions and expecting direct answers. Other European American communication "styles" may include a preference for written versus verbal communication, a penchant for speaking freely at meetings, and a directness of rhetorical style that might be described as "getting to the point." As a group, European Americans tend to be willing to share their thoughts and feelings among family, friends, and even strangers (Purnell & Paulanka, 2008). Support groups may be a preferred mechanism for family members to get needed information and guidance during difficult times. European Americans may be more willing to be part of support groups so that family members are less burdened.

European Americans tend to be noncontact persons, in comparison to persons of other groups, for whom hugs, embraces, and other gestures may be the norm. For European Americans, touch may be more acceptable within family circles or among close, personal friends. To some, European Americans may appear to be aloof and distant. Regional variations also exist, as, for example, European Americans who reside in the southern United States tend to be more accepting of contact and touch (Spector, 2004).

In general, European Americans prefer eye contact (Elliot, Adams, & Sockalingam, 1999b). Lack of eye contact may be perceived as indifference, as an effort to conceal something, or as just not being engaged. European Americans typically extend their hands for a handshake, and this serves as a welcoming gesture. Firm, long handshakes are the norm. Comfort zones related to personal space are alleged to be at around 18 inches (Purnell & Paulanka, 2003). Married women typically assume their husbands' last names and may hyphenate their maiden and married names. Variations exist within European American groups, so to be culturally sensitive, it is best to gather information on a specific group's preferred method of greeting, conversation style, and comfort zone related to personal space.

The sense of time (and a tendency to focus selectively on the past, present, or future) varies among European American groups. Overall, for European Americans, the future prevails over the present (Spector, 2004). German Americans may place more importance on the past, whereas other European Americans may be more future oriented. There is a general expectation of punctuality and the keeping of calendar commitments—although "better late than never" is an acceptable idiom.

Family Roles and Relationships

Social organization for European Americans includes the nuclear and extended family structures (Spector, 2004). The European American family unit may be varied, with many types of living arrangements, including married couple households, unmarried couple households, single parent households, or other domestic partner structures. Same-sex relationships are relatively more accepted in recent years.

Family patterns are mixed for many European American groups. For example, the patriarchal household is prevalent among Italian Americans (Spector, 2004). Other European American groups tend to be more egalitarian. Among European Americans, it is often acceptable for women to be career oriented, and child care, household work, and other kinds of routine work may be shared among both parents, or among parents and hired help. Children learn early on the value of independence (Leininger, 2002). The legal age of adulthood, 18 years of age, is often considered a time of emancipation from the family, and there is a push for persons coming of age to become self-reliant.

European Americans place a high value on the raising of children, and yet family members may or may not be expected to care for each other. The elderly may be viewed as less important. This is often owing to a cultural bias, not uncommon, whereby valued persons are those who are productive, self-sufficient, and independent. Youthfulness is valued, and "getting older" is typically not welcomed. European Americans typically do not defer to older persons in a group (Elliott et al., 1999a). Caring for an ill family member at home may be less important than achieving independence and success. Women are typically the caregivers. Families may be more likely to consider institutionalization for family members when the physical and emotional tasks of caregiving exceed their resources.

Nutrition

Food of course is a means of survival, yet the meaning of food and drink, common rituals related to food, and common food practices vary among European American cultures. Special holidays or events are connected to certain foods—such as turkey, stuffing, and corn for Thanksgiving, and hot dogs at a baseball game. For many groups, it is not permissible to eat some foods during specific religious holidays, such as the avoidance of meat on Fridays or during Lent among Catholics. Other groups may have certain practices related to cooking, such as the Jewish preparation of kosher foods. Members of older generations may seem to prefer "meat and potatoes" where members of younger generations may thrive on "fast food." Many specifically ethnic foods and dishes have been adapted or incorporated into meal planning for the general population. Italian-style pizza, Irish corned beef and cabbage, the Mexican burrito, and Chinese rice may all be staple items in European American kitchens.

Typical European American foods are: grains, including bread, pasta, oatmeal, and breakfast cereals, grits, and, to a lesser degree, rice. Common vegetables include broccoli, green beans, peas, corn, carrots, potatoes, lettuce, tomatoes, and squash. Common fruits include apples, bananas, berries, grapes, melons, peaches, pears, oranges, and other citrus products. Milk, yogurt, cheese, and ice cream are popular dairy products. Meats include cuts of beef, lamb, pork, and chicken. Eggs are typically scrambled, fried, or poached. Canned or fresh fish is eaten but may not have the same popularity as for other ethnic groups who rely on it for meals. However, regional differences may make fish more popular in locations near the ocean than in, say, Arizona. Dried beans are more likely to be found in mixed dishes, such as chili or soup, or used in preparing Mexican-style meals. Food can be prepared by frying, broiling, boiling, or roasting, or on a charcoal barbeque—a popular outdoor favorite.

It would be culturally astute to ask a family member of a person with dementia about that person's food preferences. Additionally, one should inquire about specific foods that he or she enjoys, including specialty dishes and treats.

Religion and Spirituality

The religions of European Americans are as diverse as their countries of origin. The Christian religions are dominant. A 2002 general estimate of all religious affiliation in the United States reveals the following: Protestant, 52%; Roman Catholic, 24%; Mormon, 2%; Jewish, 1%; Muslim, 1%; other, 10%; none 10% (CIA, 2005b). Many religious holidays are recognized and celebrated across the United States. It is best to ask family members of the personal religious affiliation of a person with dementia, and of any religious holidays that should be acknowledged or celebrated.

Death Rituals

An individual's personal religious beliefs may be exemplified during death rituals and traditions. Family traditions may also play a role. There are no universally prescribed practices or rituals. A 1- to 2-day waiting period prior to burial, during which there may be a wake or public viewing, is common. Placement of the deceased person's name in an obituary section of the newspaper is also common. Cremation and burial are acceptable practices, and the choice may center on individual preference, religious background, family tradition, and/or financial contingency. For example, cremation is not practiced by religious Jews, but is allowed for Lutherans (Spector, 2004).

There may be common ways of describing death that vary according to regional location and religious difference. For example, the term *passed away* may be a more common expression in New York, Dallas, and Los Angeles, and more prevalent among Catholics, Jews, Baptists, and followers of the Church of Christ (Spector, 2004). Death rites may vary among ethnic groups. Among German Americans, crying in private is sometimes expected. Irish Americans practice watching or "waking" the dead, the origin of which was to keep evil spirits away. Norwegian family members stay close to the dying person, as they believe that no one should die alone. A family member's death may be remembered by anniversary masses, memorial celebrations, or other events. In traditional Italian American families, women may wear black for extended periods to signify loss. Other mourning traditions may be relevant for other groups (Spector, 2004).

European Americans may be perceived by some as holding back during the grieving period. There is sometimes an ethic whereby family members are expected to be strong during difficult times — and therefore not show a lot of emotion when death has occurred or during the days that follow. To others, European Americans may appear to be indifferent or stoic, particularly relative to other cultural groups in which there is more of a proclivity toward celebrating the deceased person's life. Prolonging life via medical intervention is preferred among Seventh Day Adventists and Catholics; whereas a peaceful death is preferred among Mormons (Spector, 2004). Italian American Catholics prefer a closed casket. Lutheran Americans believe that the body dies when the person dies, with the soul going to heaven to enjoy everlasting life. Differences in mourning customs among European Americans are not restricted to religious-based differences, and so other kinds of differences may be important, and individual preferences should be ascertained.

Healthcare Practices and Practitioners

European Americans rely primarily on modern Western medicine. At the same time, more and more individuals are using complementary and alternative medicine and therapies, and even folk medicine. Some value self-education and self-responsibility vis-à-vis their health and healthcare, whereas others may rely totally on healthcare practitioners to manage their healthcare. Older adults may be more likely to follow a physician's directions without question, in contrast to younger persons who may be more likely to question and to require rationales and/or evidence that supports the physician's patient management decisions. Some individuals procrastinate and wait until their healthcare needs are urgent, while others adopt attitudes of self-empowerment and assume responsibility.

To some German Americans, health may consist more of freedom from illness, rather than a state of well-being. Polish Americans may define illness as something wrong with the body, mind, and spirit, whereas Italian Americans are likely to fully reveal their ailments to family members and expect immediate treatment (Spector, 2004). Overall, there are no standards of care for the management of health and illness, and individual values apply.

The prevalent illnesses and causes of death for European Americans of all ages are heart disease, cancer, cerebrovascular disease, respiratory disease, accidents, diabetes, influenza and pneumonia, and AD (Anderson & Smith, 2005). AD is the fifth leading cause of death for European American women older than 65 years, and seventh for men of the same age. Dementia may be perceived as part of the aging process—almost an expectation, and as inevitable as one grows older.

The Alzheimer's Association estimates that there are more than 5.2 million Americans with dementia. It is difficult to form an estimate of the number of European Americans specifically who have dementia. Dementia's impact is profound, regardless of ethnicity or race. Providing culturally sensitive and appropriate care for persons with dementia is the fundamental principle.

▓ MEXICAN AMERICANS

Susana Marquez and Bianca Martinez

Overview and Heritage

Hispanics or Latinos are Spanish-speaking ethnic groups in the United States that include cultures from Mexico, Central and South America, and some Caribbean countries. Although each has a unique culture, there are similar characteristics. Mexican Americans are included in this Hispanic or Latino category.

Although they are known as *La Raza*, Mexican Americans are not a race, but a mix of the Indians who originally inhabited the region now called *Mexico* and the Europeans who first began arriving there 500 years ago. The word *mestizo* is used to refer to a person of mixed blood. The union of the Spanish and Indian cultures provided the cultural foundation of modern-day Mexico. Mestizos have long suffered discrimination, first from the Spanish because they were not pureblood Spaniards, and later, in the United States, from Anglo-Americans. This discrimination that has prevailed throughout the centuries has shaped the worldview of many Mexican Americans.

The area that is now Arizona was regarded as New Spain until Mexico declared its independence from Spain in 1810. It then became part of the United States. The border that divides the United States and Mexico was open and people crossed without difficulty until the early 20th century, when restrictions were imposed. Mexican immigrants at first settled mostly in the Southwest and California and lived in barrios or neighborhoods where they continued speaking their language and following their cultural practices. More recently, migration has spread to all other states.

U.S. labor and immigration policies have shaped the destiny of Mexican Americans from the time of the Great Depression until today. People from Mexico (as well as Central America and some South American countries) come here in search of a better life. Most end up with low-paying and arduous jobs with few benefits and are ineligible for public assistance. Unlike Cubans who came here because of political oppression and were granted political asylum, many people from Mexico have entered without documentation. Undocumented people live in constant fear of being deported. This fear may not abate, even when legal status is obtained.

Because Mexican American is not a race but a mixture of races and nationalities, there is no one particular way that they look. Some have brown skin and predominantly Indian features, others European features and lighter skin; the majority fall somewhere in between. Generational and acculturation variables influence the extent to which much Mexican Americans adhere to old-world behaviors, such as venerating machismo and *personalismo* (emphasizing personal relationships), or speaking primarily Spanish. Someone who is third generation Mexican American is more likely to use English.

Communication and Language

Mexican Americans have been persistent in maintaining their traditions, language, and culture. Their communication style is indirect or circular. When stating a point, a speaker may present information in a roundabout manner to avoid conflict. Very direct communication can come across as cold or confrontational. Mexican Americans may perceive an English speaker as yelling, whereas an English speaker may perceive a Mexican American as shy or lacking self-confidence. On the other hand, when expressing emotion, a Mexican American can become loud and quite animated and to others, may appear out of control. Idioms or sayings, "*dichos*," are often used to clarify or emphasize a point. Spoken communication is preferred over written because it is more personal.

A caregiver will have better communication with a Mexican American person or his or her family if personalismo is fostered. Personalismo is a way of behaving that emphasizes personal concern. This can be initiated with a pleasant greeting, addressing the person by name, or engaging in small talk about the person's family and interests before proceeding on with the business at hand. Mexican Americans see the quality of the social interaction as more important than the length. This kind exchange is not considered too nosy or personal. On the contrary, it is expected and will go far toward establishing trust (*confianza*) and respect (*respeto*).

The culture places an emphasis on displaying a degree of respect that depends on another person's age, gender, social position, and level of authority. Even the language reflects this. Spanish has two forms of the pronoun *you*, familiar and formal. The familiar you, *tu*, is used with younger people and family members. The formal you, *usted*, is used as a form of respect when addressing someone in authority or with an older family member. Titles are important. When addressing an older person, *Don* or *Doña* may be used in front of the first name. *Señor* is for a man, *Señora* is for a woman who is or was married, and *Señorita* is for an unmarried woman regardless of her age.

When talking, Mexican Americans stand closer than Anglos do. If an Anglo keeps a wider distance, the Mexican American may perceive them as cold or unfriendly. These unconscious differences can create uncomfortable feelings as each person tries to adjust the space between them. Mexican Americans tend to use their hands freely to make a point and may reach out and touch the other person. In greetings, they usually ask about the welfare of the family (an example of personalismo). Greetings and farewells include reference to God: *Si Dios quiere* (God willing), *Vaya con Dios* (go with God). Hugs, *abrazos*, are a common way of greeting and saying good-bye to family and friends. They may be exchanged between members of the same gender. Handshakes are also acceptable.

In Latin American countries where socioeconomic levels range from very high to very low, a subordinate avoids making direct eye contact with people in authority as a gesture of respect. New immigrants to this country may continue using the practice for a while, but usually discard it as they become acculturated.

Time sense is more fluid for Mexican Americans. They tend to live in the present and be more flexible about time than many cultures are. They are less ruled by the clock. Appointment times are understood to be approximate and schedules are not strictly followed. Social gatherings are often expected to start later than was stated. Many Hispanics are averse to a hurried pace, especially given the expectations of personalismo.

Family Roles and Relationships

Roles are clearly defined in traditional families. The father is the decision maker and is responsible for the financial support of the family. Machismo is a cultural trait whereby men are expected to provide for and protect their families, but it can also mean the subjugation of women, along with heavy drinking and other behaviors to prove one's manliness. The wife and children are submissive. The woman's role is to raise the children and maintain the house, even if she works outside the home. Acculturation will often modify these roles.

The Mexican American family places great value on closeness and togetherness. Even if the family is dysfunctional, it maintains its closeness. Problems are kept within the house and outside intervention is avoided. It is considered the family's responsibility to take care of their elders. Assistance from adult children is expected and does not result in a parent's diminished feelings of self-worth. Grown children, especially daughters, visit the elders to provide care and assistance. The strong filial obligations contribute to the lower numbers of Mexican Americans in nursing homes and families who use hospice. There is usually a large network of people, related and not, who give support to each other. This can be seen at hospitals when the Mexican American patient receives a large number of visitors. Family obligations and the perception of family responsibility changes with the level of acculturation, but the expectation of family support does not.

In Latino cultures, older people are believed to have inner strength. At the same time, they consider themselves important members of the family and are not ashamed to ask for help. Elderly Latinos occupy a central position and are treated with respect (*respeto*), status, and authority. Often, the grandmother continues her role as maternal caregiver by babysitting the grandchildren. As families become more acculturated, though, elders may feel less respected as younger members adopt new lifestyles.

Nutrition

Food is central to many aspects of Mexican American culture. It symbolizes family, friendship, and hospitality and even religious beliefs. Families not only share meals, but also prepare special foods together, such as tamales. It is considered good hospitality to offer food to visitors. Food has a prominent role in social occasions. Special dishes mark the celebration of different holidays and special occasions—such as mole for weddings, pan de muerto for the Day of the Dead, and tamales for Christmas.

Providing a Mexican American with dementia familiar comfort foods adds to their enjoyment of life. Foods they likely grew up with include dishes made with corn (e.g., tortillas, enchiladas, tamales, champurrado), or thick corn-based drinks, and stews or sopas that are prepared with beans, chilies, and squash. Mexican Americans like spicy salsa on food. They use corn or flour tortillas as bread. Chocolate and sweet bread are favorite treats.

Food is often connected to religious celebrations. *Dia de los Muertos*, or Day of the Dead, is a Catholic/Aztec feast that is celebrated on November 2nd. The favorite foods and drinks of a deceased loved one are arranged on an altar, in the belief that the spirit of the loved one comes to visit and partakes of the food through the aroma. After a certain time, when it is thought that the spirit of the loved one has left, the family enjoys the food while remembering their deceased relative.

Traditional Mexican food is high in fat, which contributes to health problems. Obesity, cardiovascular disease, dental caries, and overnutrition or undernutrition are prevalent in the population. Approximately 10%–12% of the adults have diabetes, most of them, the non–insulin-dependent type. Mexicans in the United States eat more meat and saturated fats than Anglos do and use fewer low-fat dairy products. They are less likely to recognize when foods are high in fat. Hispanic women and children are more likely to be overweight or obese. Despite the obesity epidemic, segments of the population also suffer from malnutrition, especially among the socially isolated and poor. The high poverty rate contributes to poor nutrition.

Although a lot of material about health is available in Spanish, it is not always culturally relevant. For example, material encouraging exercise might show activities that Mexican Americans are not likely to participate in (e.g., step aerobics) and not likely to share activities they are likely to participate in (e.g., soccer). That, coupled with the complexity of the U.S. healthcare system and existing low levels of health literacy (i.e., understanding medical terms and techniques), can limit Mexican Americans' ability to benefit from the material.

Religion and Spirituality

Most Hispanics are Catholic. Mexican Americans believe that strength is gained through prayer and the support of the family and community. Prayer is used to petition God for favors and is a source of comfort and hope. A strong belief in destiny and predetermination exists. People will say, "It was his time" or "God had His plan and that is why it happened." These *dichos* denote the belief that God's punishment or will determines a person's health and life. Even people who are not churchgoers follow religious practices. It is common to have an altar to a venerated saint in a prominent place in the home, and to wear religious medals and carry rosaries. Mexican Americans with dementia who had grown up with these traditions will very likely find great comfort in having these articles at hand.

> CASE EXAMPLE
>
> *A 62-year-old single mother of a teenage son, who suffered from arthritis and diabetes and worked full-time seemed hesitant to seek placement for her mother. I became increasingly concerned about her situation, especially when her only vehicle broke down. She slowly opened up to the idea of placing her mother. She spoke to various family members who agreed that placement was in her mother's best interest. However, placement was not sought until she spoke to her priest, who reassured her placing a loved one was not a sin.* (Bianca Martinez, Mexican American social worker)

Death Rituals

When a person is considered close to death, a priest administers the sacraments of Anointing of the Sick, Reconciliation, and Holy Communion. Sometimes, however, the family is reluctant to call the priest because they do not want to scare the person. Usually, a mass is offered at funerals. The rosary novena is prayed at the deceased's home following the burial. A mass may also be held on the anniversary of a person's death. The grave is visited on All Souls' Day.

After the death of a loved one, a family may observe *luto* (traditional mourning). People wear black for a length of time that depends on their relationship to the deceased. Participating in any kind of entertainment or activity then is seen as disrespectful to the deceased.

Healthcare Practices and Practitioners

The notion of health is generally taken to mean being and looking clean, being able to rest and sleep well, feeling good and happy, and having the ability to perform one's expected role. A sense of well-being (*bienestar*) is thought to depend on emotional, physical, and social balance. Imbalance may produce illness. The wife or mother usually takes the lead in obtaining healthcare for a family member but may also discuss the person's condition and treatment with other family members. Advance directives may be a foreign concept to older Mexican American people because they rely on the family or physician to make those decisions for them. Less-acculturated older adults believe that people should not be told if they have a terminal illness; the younger generation thinks that the truth is better. Mexican Americans commonly use herbal and folk remedies, but as supplements to standard medical regimens. Many self-medicate with home remedies or over-the-counter drugs because of the high cost of prescription medicine and a lack of insurance coverage. Prayer, faith in God, and rituals are key elements in healthcare practices. A small percentage of traditional Mexican Americans consult faith healers (*curanderos*).

When treating the Mexican American, the healthcare practitioner needs to consider the cultural traits that have been described in this chapter—personalismo, the emphasis on respect, machismo, traditional family dynamics, the importance of religion, and Mexican time orientation—as well as to determine the level of acculturation and consider the population's history of discrimination. All these factors influence how the patient views the healthcare system. The person may mistrust the system because of past discrimination, may be fearful because of real or imagined immigration status issues, or may not speak English. A non-English speaker may be discouraged by an inappropriate translator, perhaps a young family member, from sharing pertinent information. If the healthcare practitioner rushes and does not take the time to develop rapport or personalismo, the person may feel uneasy about being examined or disclosing information. When consulting with the practitioner, the person may nod as if in agreement to save face but may not necessarily agree or comprehend and may be too shy to ask questions. Religious beliefs may dictate acceptable treatment. For instance, the Jehovah's Witnesses, which have a following among Latinos, do not countenance blood transfusions.

CASE EXAMPLE

Nasha was raised in a family who considered nudity sinful and immoral. Girls were taught to always be modest in their behavior and dress. She lived with that code of conduct until her death at 91. As the years had passed and Alzheimer's had taken its toll, she'd lost her ability to walk, speak, and take care of herself, but never her sense of modesty. When she was bathed or changed, her caregivers were always careful to respect her privacy by keeping her away from the eyes of others and covering her body as much as possible. Her dignity and modesty were never compromised. The caregivers were the same gender she was. (Susana Marquez, Mexican American social worker)

Pain and sickness may be seen as God's punishment for past sins. A person may decline pain medication to suffer and pay for their sins. Praying, tensing or relaxing, acceptance, and drinking teas are ways that Mexican Americans manage their pain.

Mental health disorders are downplayed or not addressed. Mental illness stays within the family and is not shared with outsiders, for it is regarded as shameful and humiliating. Limited knowledge about Alzheimer's or any cognitive impairment may be the reason why Mexican Americans view the disease as a mental illness or as part of the normal aging process. Some see Alzheimer's as God's will or punishment for past sins. Usually the family caregiver provides care with the belief that that they must "bear this cross." There is a high level of burden and stress among Hispanic caregivers. It is important for the family to maintain social appearances and respect; they may be reluctant to seek outside help.

Mexican decor, icons, symbols, and music are integral parts of the Mexican American life. People take great pride in the art, symbols, and music that reflect their heritage. They like warm colors: red, orange, yellow, and magenta. A caregiver who helps provide a Mexican American patient with the sensual experiences they are used to—who arranges for the presence of these colors in their room, or for them to listen to music that is familiar—will greatly enhance the level of comfort they feel. Mexican music may be preferred over music in English. Mexican Americans with dementia could feel more comfortable when they listen to the music they enjoy and are exposed to the familiar colors, designs, and textures of the culture.

■ GUIDELINES FOR INCORPORATING CULTURALLY APPROPRIATE CARE

The following is a list of guidelines that support the delivery of culturally appropriate and culturally sensitive dementia care, regardless of setting. Incorporating these guidelines into everyday healthcare practices is fundamental to providing quality dementia services to persons and their families.

1. *Consider each person as an individual as well as a product of his or her religion, ethnic background, language, and family system.* Each person is unique and has his or her own history. People's worldview is a composite of this history as well as the familial, community, and societal influences they have lived with. Their cultural perspectives are formulated and are incorporated into their own life stories. These result in people from the same culture having different perceptions on things like aging, views about caring for elderly family members, and issues related to cognitive impairment.

   Professional caregivers need to incorporate key aspects of a person's cultural background into everyday practices and into the care delivery system. Rachel Spector, a well-known expert in cultural diversity, recommends the following four questions to gain information about a person's ethnic background. They can be asked of the individual or of the family about the individual and will provide insight into family closeness, ties to friends, and customary nutrition, religion, and traditions.
   a. Do you mostly participate in social activities with members of your family?
   b. Do you mostly have friends from a similar cultural background as you?
   c. Do you mostly eat foods that are traditional in your family?
   d. Do you mostly participate in the religious traditions of your family?
   Questions that are answered "yes" can be explored further to learn more about a person's heritage. A heritage assessment will also be useful (see Appendix D).

   A person's life story can address individual preferences that incorporate cultural considerations. To ensure that cultural considerations are assessed and addressed, healthcare providers should clarify and discuss with family members the person's ethnicity, religion, spoken language, and cultural heritage. This information should be documented in the person's life story and be readily available for other caregivers to use.

2. *Acknowledge and support the family structure and caregiver roles.* The family structure is often central to a person's identity. Individual beliefs and values

are derived in part from the family. The term *family* encompasses any group of two or more people who are emotionally involved with each other. Family roles evolve with changes in age, generations, marital status, relocation, and economic status.

CASE EXAMPLE

Traditional Asian families are bound together by a shared understanding about family hierarchy, which dictates roles and responsibilities. The family is the center of all things, and all actions are dedicated to ensuring its health and dignity. (National Resource Center on Diversity)

The family is a significant part of one's culture. To ensure that cultural variations are addressed, healthcare providers should clarify and discuss with family members information related to their culture. To do this, elucidate and document a person's history as it relates to individual values and autonomy. Investigate relationships between family members, the ways they support each other, any alienation that exists, and other key factors. Identify the family structure and caregiver roles within the family. For example, the oldest adult child may have a greater role in family support or the only female adult child may be designated as the primary caregiver. Describe the available support system. This can include family, church, the community, and public or private associations. It may be an embarrassment for a Native American or Asian family to ask for help; therefore, resources may need to be explored. *Determine* the family views on long-term care or assistance in the home. Native Americans may consider it shameful for their elders to be placed in long-term care. Identify the decision maker(s) within the family. Decision making may be bound by traditional family values, specified roles, or other cultural determinants. Determine if the person(s) has legal authority to make important healthcare and financial decisions.

3. *Address language barriers and support positive approaches to communication.* Language is one of the fundamental determinants of culture. The healthcare provider must be aware of the dominant language and any dialects that exist when communicating to the person, even if the healthcare provider is not fluent in the person's native language. Words may have formal and informal meanings. Jargon, idioms, verbal intonations, and voice levels that are inappropriate may complicate communication.

   If the person and his or her family are not fluent in English, it may be necessary to use interpreters. Standards adopted by the Office of Minority Health in 2002 can provide guidance on this issue. The National Standards for Culturally and Linguistically Appropriate Services in Healthcare, or CLAS Standards, "address the needs of racial, ethnic, and linguistic population groups that experience unequal access to health service" (a synopsis is located in Appendix C of this chapter). Healthcare providers should refer to them when developing culturally and linguistically appropriate models of care.

To ensure that cultural variations are addressed, healthcare providers should consider the following when developing culturally sensitive dementia care. They should identify any need for interpreter services. The use of family members as interpreters is discouraged, as the opportunity to misread the transferred information may exist. Contact local resources, such as the Area Agency on Aging (e.g., the Asian Language Bank), for assistance. If something needs to be repeated, speak more clearly instead of loudly because a raised voice can be interpreted as yelling or intimidation. Paraphrase what the patient or family has told you in order to help avoid misunderstandings. Adopt a patient and calm manner. Use clinically appropriate tools that have been translated. Many pain assessment scales have been translated in a culturally sensitive manner into other languages. If possible, have other essential materials, such as advanced-dementia program services and tools, translated for use with individuals and families who are not proficient in English. Apply culturally competent review protocols and transcultural guidelines in the development and translation of materials for culturally and linguistically diverse populations.

4. *Recognize that fear of discrimination may impede care.* The National Resource Center on Diversity (2005) reports, "the history of racism and discrimination in the United States seriously impact the comfort level and sense of confidence that African Americans would like to feel in seeking care and assistance—thus many go without." Some Native Americans have fears related to exploitation. Anger may exist because of mistrust. On the other hand, the reputation that Asian Pacific Islanders have for being a "model community" may undermine help-seeking behaviors. The patient's previous feeling of discrimination and real or perceived disparities related to access of healthcare services in the past may adversely affect the patient's attitude toward those providing care.

   Care providers need to understand the linguistic, economic, and social barriers that individuals from different cultures face and that limit their access to needed healthcare and social services. To ensure that cultural variations are addressed, caregivers should clarify and discuss with family members whether the person has suffered from any past health disparities, what his or her health beliefs are, and how best to allay any lingering fears or anger that may have arisen during unfavorable past experiences.

5. *Support a person's preferences for traditional and mainstream care.* Families from different cultures consider and use alternatives to Western healthcare. In addition, different cultures may have different healing persons or special healers. The National Resource Center on Diversity (2005) notes, for instance, that "for many American Indians, the combination of traditional approaches to healing with mainstream services results in the most effective approach to end-of-life care." To ensure that cultural variations are addressed, healthcare providers should discuss with family members the persons' use and acceptance of traditional medical care practices, including herbal remedies, their use and acceptance of mainstream medical practices and practitioners, and their beliefs as they relate to medical interventions, healthcare decisions, and end-of-life care.

6. *Incorporate knowledge related to ethnopharmacology in practice.* Healthcare providers need to incorporate ethnopharmacologic research findings into the practice. Ethnopharmacology examines the relationship between ethnicity and drug response. It focuses on specific reactions people from different cultures might have with drug absorption, distribution, metabolism, and excretion. Most research has been done using only White males for the study subjects (although recently, that situation has changed some). The study results have then been applied to the entire population, when in fact, particular ethnic groups and White women can respond differently to some medications. Being aware that these differences exist is essential.

Healthcare professionals are urged to seek more information on how ethnicity can affect drug response and the corresponding safety risks for people with AD. To ensure that cultural variations are addressed, healthcare providers should discuss with family members the person's medication history, reactions to past and current medications, and the use of traditional and alternative therapies and medications. Information obtained regarding the safety and efficacy of medications should be shared with the person's primary care provider and incorporated into the care plan (see chapter 8 on appropriate use of medications in advanced dementia for more information).

7. *Respect and support religion and spirituality.* Religious diversity is as common as cultural diversity in the United States. The growth of religious diversity is, in and of itself, an important social phenomenon and has implications beyond religion. One's religious affiliation or spiritual beliefs may define or coexist with their cultural identity. All the same, it is important to remember that simply because a person is identified as a member of a particular ethnic group or religion does not necessarily mean that the person or the person's family share the same set of beliefs as other members of the ethnicity or religion do.

To ensure that religious and cultural variations are addressed, healthcare providers should discuss ethnic background and religious beliefs with family members. While respecting boundaries and confidentiality, ascertain the persons' religion and spiritual beliefs. Determine their preferences for worship. Ensure affirmation of their religion. Engage the persons' faith community as a critical support system for them and their family, if appropriate. Determine how religious icons, practices, beliefs, and hymns can be integrated into the persons' current experiences. Identify their perspective on suffering and how that may influence caregiving. Identify religious or spiritual preferences as they relate to end-of-life discussions and beliefs. Incorporate these findings into the life story and plan of care.

8. *Respect boundaries and issues related to personal space, touch, and body language.* Respect cultural preferences regarding how much physical distance should be kept between people engaged in conversation, casual touch, eye contact, and what constitutes a recommended volume of voice. Determine, for instance, if permission should be asked before touching someone. To ensure that cultural variations are addressed, healthcare providers should have a discussion with family members about a person's preferences with regard to personal space and touch. Determine if explanations may be needed in the use of touch while delivering care. Document this information in the care plan.

9. *Support cultural practices related to food and nutrition.* Food practices have fundamental values and meaning within a culture. To ensure that cultural variations are addressed, healthcare providers should discuss this area with family members. Explore what the persons' food preferences and prohibitions are, particularly any that are different from the facility's or institution's practices. Identify specific foods, preparation techniques, and rituals important to them, bearing in mind that these considerations may be related to their religious practices. Identify any food intolerances, nutritional deficiencies they have, or native food limitations that may cause problems for them. Use these findings when developing the life story and care plan.

10. *Address beliefs about pain, acknowledging differences among cultures.* Cultural beliefs about pain vary widely. In some cultures, pain is perceived as inevitable with aging. In others, it is regarded as the persons' "cross to bear." To ensure that cultural variations are addressed, healthcare providers should discuss with family members what their culture's conceptions about pain are. Determine the persons' medical history as it relates to pain. Assess any disabling, painful condition they may have. Ascertain how the persons treated any pain in the past, particularly if traditional remedies were used. Identify any cultural influences that could support or detract from adequate pain management. Identify how suffering is regarded. Determine the most appropriate, culturally sensitive strategies to minimize pain and suffering, accounting for individual and cultural variations. Incorporate any findings and the best pain management strategies into the care plan (consult chapter 7 for further details).

11. *Respect cultural variations related to death and dying.* Various cultures hold different beliefs about death and dying. Healthcare providers must be aware of their patients' beliefs. It is important to develop various communication strategies for dealing with end-of-life issues as they apply to various cultures. Caregivers working with people with AD must account for cultural variations when addressing death-and-dying needs. To do this, understand that a family's culture may influence ethical choices that might have to be made about artificial nutrition, life support, and whether to perform an autopsy. Respect individual choices for end-of-life care. Identify if oral transmission of decisions is common in their culture and make accommodations to ensure that end-of-life wishes are respected. Determine if placement in long-term care or facility-based hospice is acceptable. Provide education on death, dying, advance directives, and end-of-life care choices to family members, as appropriate. Review any advance directives. Secure information on the person's healthcare decisions. Incorporate these findings in the healthcare record and make notations in the care plan. Secure additional resources to support advance care planning.

12. *Use the interdisciplinary care team.* Culturally appropriate and sensitive care is best provided through an interdisciplinary approach. Caregiving staff who has been trained in assessment and interventions to meet cultural needs can offer tremendous support to the persons and their families.

    Professional caregivers can meet these needs by promoting collaborative efforts among the interdisciplinary team members. These efforts can include the development of cross-cultural training materials for caregivers and families, the integration of cultural assessment into care-planning documents, and the development of evaluation measures that account for cultural processes. Caregivers can identify specialty team members who may be best equipped to work with persons and families of diverse cultures. It may be important over time to expand the caregiving team to include others who may be helpful, such as traditional healers.

To ensure that cultural variations are addressed, healthcare providers should discuss with family members how cultural considerations for the person can be explored at interdisciplinary care planning meetings. Ensure that each member of the team is aware of cultural determinations and that these aspects of care are included in the care plan.

13. *Use available resources for learning more about culture.* For many caregivers, learning about different cultures is a new experience. For others, working with people from different cultures may be more commonplace. Regardless, contact with other cultures can be unsettling. Learning about culture starts with completing a cultural self-assessment, including reassessment of values, beliefs, and views. Learning more about different cultures will help alleviate uneasiness—awareness and knowledge will follow. More important, it will establish genuine links to persons with advanced dementia. Self-assessment is critical in identifying personal attitudes, bias, and/or prejudice. You can find a listing of current cultural self-assessment tools at www.nccccurricula.info/resources_mod2.html.

Healthcare facilities have both the responsibility to ensure culturally sensitive care for people with AD, and to support caregivers' efforts to attain necessary knowledge (see Exhibit 15.1). A list of cultural and dementia information available on the Internet appears in the appendixes at the end of this book.

EXHIBIT 15.1

Standards of Care for Providing Culturally Sensitive Care

A. The healthcare facility shall:
1. Form an action committee that examines and develops organization-wide, culturally sensitive dementia care programming.
2. Assess the organization's diversity and incorporate components of culturally sensitive care into the mission, philosophy, practices, policies and procedures, and the care delivery setting that address all dementia services.
3. Conduct a facility cultural assessment (for more information access http://www.alz.org/Resources/Diversity/downloads/GEN_ASSESS-CultCompSelfAssessProtocol.pdf) and identify interventions necessary to promote culturally sensitive care.
4. Build staff resources and capabilities to address cultural diversity at the organizational and unit level within the facility.

5. Convert necessary materials (e.g., AD care-program material, care-giver information, healthcare record documents) into other languages as needed and for the appropriate literacy levels (for more information access: http://www.alz.org/Resources/Diversity/downloads/GEN_TRANS-TransculturationGuidelines.pdf).

6. Build a cultural diversity intervention program that:
   a. Regularly conducts diversity assessments;
   b. Observes ongoing efforts to improve dementia care;
   c. Develops staff resources and capabilities through education and role modeling;
   d. Identifies voluntary change resources within the organization; and
   e. Increases responsiveness to concerns of diverse groups.

7. Institute mandatory orientation and ongoing education for caregivers related to cultural diversity that examine:
   a. Direct care issues and ADL;
   b. Family and caregiver roles and support;
   c. End-of-life care preparation and advance directives;
   d. Nutrition and food preferences;
   e. Religion or spirituality; and
   f. Expectations and understanding of dementia-specific care.

8. Ensure that language and communication needs of culturally diverse individuals are assessed and addressed.

9. Provide healthcare services tailored to a person's level of acculturation, avoiding stereotyping and exercising regard for individual preferences.

10. Develop a quality-monitoring program that incorporates continuous evaluation of the cultural diversity program standards.

B. Healthcare staff shall:

1. Conduct a cultural or heritage assessment with each person and document relevant findings in the life story and healthcare record.

2. Examine how cultural values and norms influence help-seeking and comfort-rendering responses for persons with advanced dementia and their families. Use these findings in developing and executing the care plan.

3. Examine the role that cultural values and norms play in helping to define and give meaning to Alzheimer's and dementia across various cultural groups. Use these findings in care delivery programs within the facility and for persons with advanced dementia and their families.

4. Examine the influence that cultural values have on caregivers' and recipients' physical and emotional health. Use these findings in care delivery programs within the facility and for persons with AD and their families.

5. Make culturally appropriate interventions to care for persons of differing cultures that include communication, nutrition and dietary practices, religion, family and social roles, and other practices that impact healthcare delivery (e.g., ceremonies, death rituals, etc.). Use these

Continued

Exhibit 15.1 *Continued*

findings in care delivery programs within the facility and for the persons with AD and their families.

6. Use information from ethnopharmacologic research to determine what drugs may elicit varied responses in persons from different ethnic groups. Use these findings in care delivery programs within the facility and for persons with AD and their families. Discuss these concerns, considerations, and findings with the facility pharmacist and medical director.

7. Monitor the persons with AD to determine therapeutic responses to medications as they relate to possible ethnic considerations.

8. Identify and document end-of-life decisions related to advance care planning and other considerations such as the nondisclosure of the terminal illness, the placement of the dying person or the body after death, and other culturally specific rituals and practices.

C. The person with advanced dementia shall expect:

1. Consideration of his or her background, family, personal history, and culture influences in determining what services are most appropriate.

2. Incorporation of his or her cultural background into the life story and care plan.

3. Respect for wishes and desires that may be culturally based, such as pain management practices, end-of-life care, and spiritual affiliations.

Note: These are general recommendations. The CLAS standards may supersede them.

REFERENCES

Alcantara, A. (1994). Gender roles, fertility, and the status of married Filipino men and women. *Philippine Sociological Review, 42*(1–4), 94–109.

Alzheimer's Association. (2005a). *10 steps to providing culturally sensitive dementia care.* Retrieved January 26, 2010, from http://www.alz.org/Resources/Diversity/downloads/GEN_EDU-10steps.pdf

Alzheimer's Association. (2005b). *Culturally sensitive dementia care.* Asian/Pacific Islander Cultures. Retrieved January 26, 2010, from http://www.alz.org/resources/diversity/downloads/asianoutreach_tipsandcitations.pdf

Alzheimer's Association. (2005c). *Providing culturally sensitive dementia care.* Retrieved January 26, 2010, from http://www.alz.org/Resources/Diversity/downloads/ABOUT_CulturallySensitive DementiaCare.pdf

Alzheimer's Association. (2006). *Research grants program announcement.* Retrieved January 26, 2010, from http://www.alz.org/Researchers?RGP/overview.asp

Alzheimer's Association. (n.d.) *African Americans and Alzheimer's disease: The silent epidemic.* Chicago: Author. Retrieved January 26, 2010, from http://www.alz.org/national/documents/report_africanamericanssilentepidemic.pdf

Alzheimer's Association, Desert Southwest Chapter & Delta Sigma Theta Sorority, Phoenix Metropolitan Alumnae Chapter. (n.d.). *Alzheimer's disease in the African-American community.* Phoenix, AZ: Authors.

Alzheimer's Association, Southeastern Pennsylvania Chapter. (n.d.). *Ten steps to start an African-American Support Group.*

Andersen, J. N. (1983). Health and illness in Pilipino immigrants. *Western Journal of Medicine, 139*(6), 811–819.

Anderson, R. N., & Smith, B. L. (2005). Deaths: Leading causes for 2002. *National Vital Statistics Reports, 53*(17), 1–90.

Anglo-America. (2010, April 22). In *Wikipedia, The Free Encyclopedia*. Retrieved April 2010, from http://en.wikipedia.org/w/index.php?title=Anglo-America&oldid=357551296

Applewhite, S. L. (1995). Curanderismo: Demystifying the health beliefs and practices of elderly Mexican Americans. *Health and Social Work, 20*(4), 247–53.

Arizona Commission of Indian Affairs. (n.d.). *Arizona tribal income and poverty statistics, 1999.* Retrieved from http://www.indianaffairs.state.az.us/

Beal, T. (2004, September 19). The way I heard the story. *Arizona Daily Star.*

Beck, P., Walters, A., & Francisco, N. (2001). *The sacred ways of knowledge, sources of life.* Tsaile, AZ: Navajo Community College Press.

Blackhall, L., Murphy, S., Frank, G., Michel, V., & Azen, S. (1995). Ethnicity and attitudes toward patient autonomy. *The Journal of the American Medical Association, 274*(10), 820–825.

Brandt, E. A. (n.d.). *Encyclopedia of North American Indians, Apache, Western.* Retrieved January 26, 2010, from http://college.hmco.com/history/readerscomp/Naind/html/na_002100_apachewester.htm

Braun, K. L., & Browne, C. V. (1998a). Cultural values and caregiving patterns among Asian and Pacific Islander Americans. In D. Redburn & R. McNamara (Eds.), *Social gerontology* (pp. 155–182). New York: Greenwood Press.

Braun, K. L., & Browne, C. V. (1998b). Perceptions of dementia, caregiving, and help seeking among Asian and Pacific Islander Americans. *Health & Social Work, 23*(4), 262–274.

Braun, K. L., Takamura, J. C., & Forman, S. M., Sasaki, P. A., & Meininger, L. (1995). Developing and testing outreach materials on Alzheimer's disease for Asian and Pacific Islander Americans. *Gerontologist, 35*(1), 122–126.

Calhoun, M. A. (1985). The Vietnamese woman: Health/illness attitudes and behaviors. *Healthcare for Women, 6*(1–3), 61–72.

Campinha-Bacote, J. (1998). African American. In L. D. Purnell & B. J. Paulanka, (Eds.), *Transcultural healthcare. A culturally competent approach* (pp. 53–73). Philadelphia: F. A. Davis.

Central Intelligence Agency. (2004). *The world factbook – Vietnam.* Retrieved January 26, 2010, from http://www.cia.gov/library/publications/the-world-factbook/index.html

Central Intelligence Agency. (2005a). *The world factbook – Korea North and South.* Retrieved January 26, 2010, from https://www.cia.gov/library/publications/the-world-factbook/index.html

Central Intelligence Agency. (2005b). *The world factbook – United States.* Retrieved January 26, 2010, from https://www.cia.gov/library/publications/the-world-factbook/index.html

Central Intelligence Agency. (2006). *The world factbook – Japan.* Retrieved January 10, 2006, from https://www.cia.gov/library/publications/the-world-factbook/index.html

Chee, Y. K., & Levkoff, S. E. (2001). Culture and dementia: Accounts by family caregivers and health professionals for dementia-affected elders in South Korea. *Journal of Cross-Cultural Gerontology,16*(2), 111–125.

Chen, H., Foo, S. H., & Ury, W. (2002). Recognizing dementia. *Western Journal of Medicine, 176*(4), 267–270.

Chinese Americans and Dementia. (2006). Retrieved January 26, 2010, from http://www.ethnicelders-care.net/ethnicity&dementiachinese.htm

CHISPA E-learning Environment: Caring for Hispanic Patients Interactively. *E-pocket book for caring for Hispanic patients.* Retrieved January 26, 2010, from http://itdc.lbcc.edu/chispa/#

Chong, N. (2002). *The Latino patient: A cultural guide for health care providers.* Yarmouth, MA: Intercultural Press.

Church, T. (1987). Personality research in a non-Western culture: The Philippines. *Psychological Bulletin, 102*(2), 272–292.

Condon, J. C. (1997). *Good neighbors: Communicating with the Mexicans.* Yarmouth, MA: Intercultural Press.

Corbett, J. M. (2000). *Religion in America.* Upper Saddle River, NJ: Prentice Hall.

Dahozy, C. (2004). Cultural practices and beliefs of birth and death of Southwest Native American Tribes. *The IHS Primary Care Provider, 29*(3), 49–52.

D'Avanzo, C. E. (1992). Bridging the cultural gap with Southeast Asians. *American Journal of Maternal Child Nursing, 17*(4), 204–208.

Delta Sigma Theta Sorority, Phoenix Metropolitan Alumnae Chapter, & Alzheimer's Association, Desert Southwest Chapter. (2005a.) *The impact of age-related memory loss in the African-American community: What do we know and what can we do?* [Conference materials].

Delta Sigma Theta Sorority, Phoenix Metropolitan Alumnae Chapter, & Alzheimer's Association, Desert Southwest Chapter. (2005b.) *Standing in the gap.* [Conference materials].

DiPasquale-Davis, J., Hopkins, S. J. (1997). Health behaviors of an elderly Filipino group. *Public Health Nursing, 14*(2), 118–122.

Dolan, R. E. (1993). *Philippines: A country study.* Washington DC: Federal Research Division, Library of Congress.

Elliott, C., Adams, R. J., & Sockalingam, S. (1999a). *Awesome library: Multi-cultural toolkit.* Retrieved January 26, 2010, from http://www.awesomelibrary.org /multiculturaltoolkit-introduction.html

Elliott, C., Adams, R. J., & Sockalingam, S. (1999b). *Normative communication styles and values.* Retrieved January 18, 2006, from http://www.awesomelibrary.org/multiculturaltoolkit-introduction.html

Finke, B. (2000). The elder with dementia or confusion. *The IHS Primary Care Provider, 25*(5), 86–87.

Folstein, M. F., Bassett, S. S., Anthony, J. C., Romaniski, A. J., & Nestadt, G. R. (1991). Dementia: Case ascertainment in a community survey. *Journal of Gerontology, 46*(4), 132–138.

Fox, P. G. (1991). Stress related to family change among Vietnamese refugees. *Journal of Community Health Nursing, 8*(1), 45–46.

Froehlich, T. E., Bogardus, S. T., & Inouye, S. K. (2001). Dementia and race: Are there differences between African Americans and Caucasians. *Journal of the American Geriatric Society, 49*(4), 477–484.

Geographia. (n.d.). *Vietnam.* Retrieved January 2010, from http://www.geographia.com/vietnam/

Gerdner, L. A., Cha, D., Yang, D., & Tripp-Reimer, T. (2007). The circle of life: End-of-life care and death rituals for Hmong-American elders. *Journal of Gerontological Nursing, 33*(5), 20–29.

Gerdner, L. A., Xiong, S. V., & Cha D. (2006). Chronic confusion and memory impairment in Hmong elders: Honoring differing cultural beliefs in America. *Journal of Gerontological Nursing, 32*(3), 23–31.

Giese, P. (1997). *US Federally Non-Recognized Tribes, State by State.* Retrieved January 26, 2010, from http://www.kstrom.net/isk/maps/tribesnonrec.html

Gold, S. J. (1992). Mental health and illness in Vietnamese refugees. *Western Journal of Medicine, 157*(3), 290–294.

Goldrick, M., Giordano, J., & Pearce, J. (1996). *Ethnicity & family therapy.* New York: The Guildford Press.

Goldstein, M. Z., & Griswold, K. (1988). Cultural sensitivity and aging. *Psychiatric Services, 49*(6), 769–991.

Grebler, L., Moore, J. W., & Guzman, R. C., & Berlant, J. L. (1970). *The Mexican American people: The nation's second largest minority.* New York: The Free Press.

Grober, P. (2002). *Geo-demographics of aging in Arizona: State of knowledge.* Retrieved January 26, 2010, from http://www.slhi.org/publications/studies_research/pdfs/CoA_Geo-demographics_of_Aging.pdf

Guzmán, B. (2001). *The Hispanic population, census 2000 brief.* Retrieved January 26, 2010, from http://www.census.gov/prod/2001pubs/c2kbr01-3.pdf

Halporn, R. (1992). Introduction. In C. L. Chen, W. C. Lowe, D. Ryan, A. H. Kutscher, R. Halporn, & H. Wang (Eds.), *Chinese Americans in loss and separation* (pp. v–xii). New York: Foundation of Thanatology.

Hendrix, L. R. (2001). *Ethnogeriatrics curriculum module: Health and health care for American Indian/Alaska Native elders.* Retrieved April 1, 2006, from http://www.stanford.edu/group/ethnoger/

Henkel, G. (2004). Cultural humility. *Caring for the Ages, 5*(12), 50–55. Retrieved January 26, 2010, from http://www.amda.com/publications/caring/december2004 /culturalhumility.cfm

Henry J. Kaiser Family Foundation. (2005). *Arizona population figures.* Retrieved July 11, 2005, from http://www.statehealthfacts.org

Hickey, G. C. (1994). *Village in Vietnam.* New Haven, CT: Yale University Press.

Hinton, L. (2002). Improving care for ethnic minority elderly and their family caregivers across the spectrum of dementia severity. *Alzheimer Disease and Associated Disorders, 16,* (Suppl. 2), S50–55.

Hoffman, L. (n.d.). *The psychology of color, the fine art of creativity.* Retrieved January 5, 2005, from http://creativeartist.com/decArts/psycheColour.asp

Holmes, E. R., & Holmes, L. D. (1995). *Other cultures, elder years.* Thousand Oaks, CA: Sage Publications.

Hoobler, T., & Dorothy, H., & Takei, G. (1996). *The Japanese American family album.* New York: Oxford University Press, Inc.

The Hopi Tribe. (2006). *Welcome to the Hopi Tribe*. Retrieved May 7, 2010, from http://www
.libertyparkusafd.org/lp/Native%20Americans/North%20American%20Tribes/The%20
Hopi%20Tribe.htm

Indian Health Service. (2005). *Diabetes. Heritage and Health & IHS Profile, 2005*. Retrieved
January 3, 2006, from http://info.ihs.gov

Indian Health Service. (2002). Health and Heritage Brochure. *Indian Health Service: An Agency
Profile; 2002*. Retrieved April 17, 2006, from http://info.ihs.gov/IHSProfile.pdf

Japanese Americans and Dementia. (2005). Retrieved November 21, 2005, from http://www
.ethnicelderscare.net/ethnicity&dementiaasia.htm

Jervis, L. L., & Manson, S. M. (2002). American Indians/Alaska Natives and dementia. *Alzheimer's
Disease and Associated Disorders, 16*(Suppl. 2), S89–S95.

Joaquin, A., Jr. (April 17, 2000). *Waila: Tradition*. Pulse of the Planet Program 2121. Jim Metzner
Productions & National Geographic Society©.

Jones, B. (2003). *Executive summary: American Indians and Alaska Natives: A demographic perspective,
population resource*. Washington, DC: Author.

Kaiser Foundation Health Plan, Inc. (2003). *Culturally competent care toolkit*. Created by the
National Diversity Department, Institute for Culturally Competent Care.

Kim, K. C., Kim, S., & Hurh, W. M. (1991). Filial piety and intergenerational relationship in Korean
immigrant families. *International Journal of Aging & Human Development, 33*(3), 233–245.

Kim, K. H., Shin, H. R., & Nakama, H. (1994). Health consciousness in relation to education in Korea—
focusing on seven preventable health risk factors. *Asia-Pacific Journal of Pubic Health, 7*(1), 3–9.

Kim, K. K., Yu, E. S., Liu, W. T., Kim, J., & Kohrs, M. B. (1993). Nutritional status of Chinese-, Korean-,
and Japanese-American elderly. *Journal of the American Dietetic Association, 93*(12), 1416–1422.

Korea National Statistical Office. (2005). *Population. Society*. Retrieved February 14, 2006, from
http://www.nso.go.kr

La France, M., & Mayo, C. (1978). Cultural cues. In *Moving bodies: Nonverbal communication in
social relationships* (pp. 171–189). Monterey, CA: Brooks/Cole.

Le, C. N. (2005). A Modern Day Exodus. *Asian-Nation: The Landscape of Asian America*. Retrieved
January 27, 2010, from http://www.asian-nation.org/exodus.shtml

Lee, I., & Ramsey, S. (2000). *The Korean language*. New York: New York Press.

Lee, J. K. (1998). Religious factors historically affecting pre-modern Korean elite/higher education.
The SNU Journal of Education Research, 8, 31–63.

Lee, E. (1997). *Working with Asian Americans. A guide for clinicians*. New York: Guilford Press.

Leininger, M. (2002). Anglo-American (United States) culture care values, beliefs, and lifeways.
In M. Leininger & M. R. McFarland (Eds.). *Transcultural nursing: Concept, theories, research,
practice* (3rd ed., pp. 287–299). New York: McGraw-Hill.

Liu, C. (1991). From san gu liu po to 'caring scholar': The Chinese nurse in perspective. *International
Journal of Nursing Studies, 28*(4), 315–324.

Lipson, J. G., Dibble, S. L., & Minarik, P. A. (1996). *Culture and nursing care: A pocket guide*. San
Francisco: University of California San Francisco Nursing Press.

Lomatewama, R. (1998, November 4). *Hopi culture*. Lecture presented at Northern Arizona
Museum, Flagstaff, AZ: Author.

Lopez, D., Reader, T., & Buseck, P. (2002). *Community attitudes toward traditional Tohono O'odham
foods*. Tohono O'odham Community Action & Tohono O'odham Community College. Retrieved
January 27, 2010, from http://www.tocaonline.org/Oodham_Foods/Oodham_Foods.html

Lourie, E. J., & Attico, N. B. (2000). Elder health care: A challenge for the provider and the family.
The IHS Primary Care Provider, 25(5), 82–84.

Lum, O. (1995). Health status of Asians and Pacific Islanders. *Clinics in Geriatric Medicine, 11*(1), 53–67.

Lynch, F. (1973). Social acceptance considered. In F. Lynch & A. de Guzman II (Eds.), *Four readings
on Philippine Values* (4th ed.). IPC Papers No. 2, (pp. 1–68). Quezon City, Philippines: Ateneo
de Manila University Press.

Matocha, L. K. (1998). Chinese Americans. In L. D. Purnell & B. J. Paulanka, *Transcultural health
care – A culturally competent approach* (pp. 163–188). Philadelphia: F. A. Davis Company.

Matsuoka, J. K. (1990). Differential acculturation among Vietnamese refugees: Implications for
social work practice. *Social Work, 35*, 341–345.

Matsuoka, J. K. (1991). Vietnamese Americans. In N. Mokuau (Ed.), *Handbook of social services for
Asian and Pacific Islanders* (pp. 117–130). New York: Greenwood Press.

Mayers, M. K. (1980). *A look at Filipino lifestyle*. Dallas, TX: The Illinois Museum of Anthropology.

McBride, M. (1994). *Health and health care of Filipino American elders*. Stanford: CA: Stanford Geriatric Education Center, Stanford University School of Medicine.

McNeill, J. A., Sherwood, G., Palos, G., & Starck, P. (2002). *Supporting pain management across the lifespan measuring pain management outcomes in Spanish speakers*. Nursing for Target Populations, University of Texas-Houston, HSC, School of Nursing, Houston, TX, and Pain Research Group, UT M. D. Anderson Cancer Center, Houston, TX, USA.

Melnick, R. (2002). *The coming of age. Four scenarios of Arizona's future*. Phoenix, AZ: St. Luke's Health Initiatives.

Miranda, B., McBride, M., & Spangler, Z. (1998). Filipino-Americans. In L. Purnell & B. Paulanka (Eds.), *Transcultural health care: A culturally competent approach* (pp. 245–272). Philadelphia: F. A. Davis Company.

Morano, C. L., & King, M. D. (n.d.) *African American caregiver training program. Caregiver resource manual*. Baltimore, MD: University of Maryland.

Morgan, M. G. (2002). African Americans and culture care. In M. Leininger & M. R. McFarland (Eds.), *Transcultural Nursing. Concepts, theories, research & practice* (3rd ed.). New York: McGraw-Hill.

Muñoz, C., & Hilgenberg, C. (2005). Ethnopharmacology. *American Journal of Nursing, 105*(8), 40–48.

National Center on Minority Health and Health Disparities. (2006). *Strategic research plan to reduce and ultimately eliminate health disparities. Volume 1. Fiscal years 2002–2006*. Retrieved January 27, 2010, from http://ncmhd.nih.gov/our_programs/strategic /pubs /VolumeI_031003EDrev.pdf

National Resource Center on Diversity. (2005). *Talking in circles. Cultural perspectives in end-of-life care*. Washington, DC: Author.

Native Seeds/SEARCH (n.d.) Retrieved January 27, 2010, from http://www.nativeseeds.org

Navajo Nation Museum. (n.d.). *Traditional Navajo Food Pyramid*. Retrieved February 10, 2006, from http://reta.nmsu.edu/sacred/lesson/pdfs/food_pyramid.pdf

New World Order. (1994). A new TB threat. *Asiaweek: Hong Kong*.

Niiya, B. (1993). *Encyclopedia of Japanese American history. An A-to-Z reference from 1868 to the present*. New York: Facts On File, Inc.

North Carolina Institute of Medicine. *NC Latino health 2003*. Durham, NC: Author. Retrieved January 27, 2010, from http://www.nciom.org/projects/latino /latinopub/C3.pdf

Northern California Cancer Center. (1993a). *Average annual age-adjusted incidence rates for selected sites, 1986–1990, for men in the San Francisco Bay Area* (unpublished paper). Union City, CA: Author.

Northern California Cancer Center. (1993b). *Average annual age-adjusted incidence rates for selected sites, 1986–1990, for women in the San Francisco Bay Area* (unpublished paper). Union City, CA: Author.

Nowak T. T. (2003). People of Vietnamese heritage. In L. D. Purnell and B. J. Paulanka (Eds.), *Transcultural health care: A culturally competent approach* (pp. 327–343). Philadephia: F. A. Davis Co.

Office of Minority Health. (2001). *National standards for culturally and linguistically appropriate services in health care. Final report*. Retrieved January 27, 2010, from http://www.omhrc.gov/assets/pdf/checked/finalreport.pdf

Office of Minority Health. (2000). Assuring cultural competence in health care: Recommendations for national standards and outcomes-focused research agenda. *Federal Register, 65*(247), 80865–80879.

Organisation for Economic Co-operation and Development. (n.d.). *Statistics*. Retrieved February 14, 2006, from http://www.oecd.org

Paz, J. J. (1993). Support of Hispanic elderly. In H. McAdoo (Ed.), *Family ethnicity*. Newbury Park, CA: Sage.

Pfeifer, M. E. (2001). U.S. Census 2000: An overview of national and regional trends in Vietnamese residential distribution. In *US Census 2000*. Retrieved January 27, 2010, from http://hmong-studies.com/ PfeiferReviewofVietnameseStudies2001.pdf

Hsueh, K., Phillips, L., Bursac, K., & Guo, G. (2005). Prevalence of Alzheimer's disease in Arizona: Future projections and implications. *Arizona Geriatrics Society, 10*(2), 19–24.

Pineda, E. (1989). *The family code of the Philippines: Annotated*. Quezon City, Philippines: Central Law Book Publishing Co., Inc.

Program for Multicultural Health – Japanese. Retrieved January 27, 2010, from http://www.med .umich.edu/multicultural/ccp/japanese.htm

Purnell, L. D., & Paulanka, B. J. (2008). The Purnell Model of Cultural Competence. In L. D. Purnell & B. J. Paulanka (Eds.), *Transcultural health care. A culturally competent approach* (3rd ed., pp. 8–39). Philadelphia: F. A. Davis.

Rallying Points. (2002). African American aging and health care relevant to care and caring near and at the end of life. *National Resource Center on Diversity in End-of-Life Care: Diversity Notes.*

Redford, N. (2005). *Cultural considerations in caring, educational series for caregivers, Maricopa Integrated Health System.* Phoenix, AZ: Author.

Rhode Island Office of Minority Health. *Latino/Hispanic culture health.* Retrieved January 27, 2010, from http://www.health.ri.gov/chic/minority/lat_cul.php

Rutledge, P. J. (1992). *The Vietnamese experience in America.* Bloomington, IN: Indiana University Press.

San Francisco Department of Public Health. (1992). *AIDS Surveillance report: AIDS cases between 1981–1992.* San Francisco: Author.

Sabogal, F., Marin, G., Otero-Sabogal, R., VanOss-Marin, B., & Perez-Stable, E. J. (1987). Hispanic familism and acculturation: What changes and what don't? *Hispanic Journal of Behavioral Sciences, 9*(4), 397–412.

Servin, M. P. (1974). *An awakened minority: The Mexican-Americans.* (2nd ed.). Beverly Hills, CA: Glencoe Press.

Sharts-Hopko, N. C. (2003). People of Japanese heritage. In L. D. Purnell & B. J. Paulanka, (Eds.), *Transcultural health care—A culturally competent approach* (pp. 218–233). Philadelphia: F. A. Davis Company.

Sheikh, A. A., & Sheikh, K. S. (1989). *Healing East and West: Ancient wisdom and modern psychology.* New York: John Wiley & Sons, Inc.

Spector, R. (2004). *Cultural diversity in health and illness.* (6th ed.). Upper Saddle River, NJ: Pearson Prentice Hall.

Stauffer, R. Y. (1991). Vietnamese Americans. In J. N. Giger & R. E. Davidhizar (Eds.), *Transcultural nursing, assessment and intervention* (pp. 402–434). St. Louis: Mosby Year Book.

Still, O., & Hodgins, D. (2003). Navaho Indians. In L. D. Purnell & B. J. Paulanka (Eds.), *Transcultural healthcare. A culturally competent approach* (pp. 279–283). Philadelphia: F. A. Davis.

Suh, Sharon A. (2004), *Being Buddhist in a Christian World: Gender and Community in a Korean American Temple,* (pp. 3–5). Seattle: University of Washington Press.

Talamantes, M. A., Gomez, G., & Braun, K. L. (2000). Advance directives and end-of-life care: The Hispanic perspective. In K. L Braun, J. H. Pietsch, & P. L. Blanchette (Eds.), *Cultural Issues in end of life decision making* (pp. 83–100), Thousand Oaks: CA: Sage Publication.

Talamantes, M. A., Lawler, W. R., & Espino, D. V. (1995). Hispanic American elders: Caregiving norms surrounding dying and the use of hospice services. *Hospice Journal, 10*(2), 35–49.

Tanabe, M. K. G. (n.d.). *Health and health care of Japanese-American elders.* Retrieved January 27, 2010 from http://www.stanford.edu/group/ethnoger/japanese.html

The American Heritage® Dictionary of the English Language. (2000). (4th ed.). Houghton Mifflin Company.

Tom-Orme, L. (2002). Transcultural nursing and health care among Native American peoples. In M. Leininger & M. R. McFarland (Eds) *Transcultural nursing: Concepts, theories, research & practice* (pp. 429–440). (3rd ed.). New York: McGraw-Hill.

Tom, L. A. S. H. (2006). Health and health care for Chinese-American elders. *Stanford Ethnogeriatric Curriculum Module.* Retrieved January 27, 2010, from http://www.stanford.edu/group/ethnoger/chinese.html

Tuskegee Syphilis Experiment. (2005). Retrieved January 27, 2010, from http://www.infoplease.com/ipa/A0762136.html

University of Washington Medical Center. (2007, April). Communicating with your American Indian/Alaskan Native patient. *Culture Clues™.* Retrieved January 27, 2010, from http://depts.washington.edu/pfes/PDFs/AmericanIndianCultureClue.pdf

U.S. Census Bureau. (1990). *Census 90.* U.S. Department of Commerce and Statistics Administration.

U.S. Census Bureau. (2000a). *Introduction to census 2000 data.* U.S. Department of Commerce Economics and Statistics Administration.

U.S. Census Bureau. (2000b). *Census 2000, Fact sheet: Arizona.* Retrieved January 27, 2010, from http://factfinder.census.gov/home/saff/main.html?_lang=en

U.S. Department of Agriculture. *MyPyramid.gov* Retrieved January 27, 2010, from http://www.mypyramid.gov/pyramid/index.html

U.S. Department of Health and Human Services. (n.d.). Healthy people 2010, *19 nutrition & over-weight-disparities.* Retrieved January 27, 2010, from http://www.healthypeople.gov/Document/HTML/Volume2/19Nutrition.htm

Valle, R. (1998). *Caring across cultures: Working with dementing illness and ethnically diverse populations.* Bristol, PA: Taylor & Francis.

Villa, R. F. (1991). La fe de la mujer. In M. Sotomayor (Ed.) *Empowering Hispanic families: A critical issue for the 90s* (pp.43–58). Milwaukee, WI: Family Services America.

Voss, M. (1996, March 12). *Cross-cultural manners* (p. 2T). *Des Moines Register,* 2T.

Wentz, R. E. (1998). *The culture of religious pluralism.* Boulder, CO: Westview Press.

White, B. (2004). Culturally competent care. In S. Lewis, M. Heitkemper & S. Dirksen, (Eds.), *Medical-surgical nursing: Assessment & management of clinical problems* (6th ed.). St. Louis, MO: Mosby Year Book, Inc.

Yee, B. (2005). *Health and health care of Southeast Asian American elders: Vietnamese, Cambodia, Hmong and Laotian elders.* Retrieved January 27, 2010, from http://www.stanford.edu/group/ethnoger/index.html

Yeo, G., Hikoyeda, N., McBride, M., Chin, S., Edmonds, M., & Hendrix, L. (1999). *Cohort analysis as a tool in ethnogeriatrics: Historical profiles of elders from eight ethnic populations in the United States.* Palo Alto, CA: Stanford Geriatric Education Center.

Yeo, G., & Lieberman, M. (1993). *Cases in the California ADDTC data bank by ethnicity* (unpublished data).

Yin, Y. W., & Hu, L. T. (1994). Public outpatient mental health services: Use and outcome among Asian Americans. *American Journal of Orthopsychiatry, 64,* 448–455.

Youn, G., Knight, B. G., Jeong, H. S., & Benton, D. (1999). Differences in familism values and care-giving outcomes among Korean, Korean American, and white American dementia caregivers. *Psychology and Aging, 14*(3), 355–364.

Young-mee, C. (2000). *Integrated Korean: Beginning 1.* Hawaii: Hawaii Press. In S. Young & A. Moon (Eds.). (1998). *Korean American women: From tradition to modern feminism.* Westport, CT: Praeger Publishers.

Zemke, R., Raines, C., & Filipczak, B. (1999). *Generations at work: Managing the clash of veterans, boomers, xers, and nexters in your workplace.* AMACOM: A Division of American Management Association.

Zhan, L. (2003). *Asian Americans: Vulnerable populations,model interventions, and clarifying agendas.* Sudbury, MA: Jones and Bartlett Publishers.

Zoucha, R., & Purnell, L. (2003). People of Mexican heritage. In L. D. Purnell & B. J. Paulanka, (Eds.). *Transcultural health care: A culturally competent approach* (pp. 264–278). Philadelphia: F.A. Davis Company.

HEALTHCARE DECISIONS FOR PERSONS WITH ADVANCED DEMENTIA

Paul Harrington, Jill Preston, Dawn Savattone, and Barbara Volk-Craft

▉ INTRODUCTION

The following chapter offers a look at the legal principles guiding the healthcare decisions that must be made either for or by people with advanced dementia. It provides practical tips to assist the caregiver in clarifying and honoring those choices. The first part describes common decisions that arise and suggests principles for how to make them. The second part describes protocols for advanced decision making when someone with dementia retains the ability to express his or her wishes, and guidelines for applying substitute judgment standards when a person has lost the decision-making capacity.

▉ AREAS OF POTENTIAL DECISION MAKING

Common healthcare decisions that face people with advanced dementia include the choice to pursue, withhold, or withdraw the following.

Cardiopulmonary resuscitation (CPR) involves efforts to maintain heart and breathing functions, usually in the event of cardiac arrest. CPR can also include the use of respirators or ventilators when a person has problems breathing. These efforts may or may not succeed in restarting the heart and breathing, and may be painful and even cause bodily injury. If successful, life may be extended on life-supporting devices, but the potential exists for reduced quality of life. If the person or a surrogate decision maker chooses not to pursue resuscitation, the person's physician will be asked to complete and sign a do-not-resuscitate (DNR) order, which is placed in the medical record. A DNR order is limited to resuscitation and does not preclude other interventions and long-term care services.

Feeding tubes become a consideration in advanced dementia as eating and swallowing difficulties occur and lead to weight loss. Most studies provide little evidence that feeding tubes extend life or prevent infections, and some have shown higher levels of aspiration pneumonia, diarrhea, and the use of physical restraints. Conscientious feeding programs and an approach focused on palliative care are alternatives to tube feeding.

Although *intravenous (IV) hydration* may provide temporary fluid replacement, it cannot maintain nutrition and probably decreases comfort. In the absence of nutrition and hydration, the body develops endorphins, which are morphine-like substances that blunt nerve endings. Increasingly, evidence suggests that this form of dying is comfortable and can be enhanced by supplemental pain management.

Pneumonia, often a result of problems with swallowing food, and urinary tract infections are common in persons with advanced dementia. *Antibiotics* may or may not improve these conditions. Aggressive treatment may be determined by a person's advance care planning, cultural background, and clinical features of the dementia episode. If a person decides against the use of antibiotics, medications and other pain management approaches often can effectively manage discomfort.

Hospitalization is an important consideration because changes in the environment can be stressful and disruptive for a person with dementia, even in the early stages. Hospitals are particularly challenging environments because they typically lack the calmness, familiarity, and predictability that people with Alzheimer's need. Alternatives to hospitalization, such as the delivery of services in a long-term care facility, physician's office, or an outpatient surgery center, along with do-not-hospitalize (DNH) orders should be considered.

Hospice services provide support to the person and his or her surrogate during the terminal stages of dementia. Using a palliative care approach, hospice programs focus on providing services to keep the person comfortable to maintain dignity and quality of life during the dying process. Hospice care is provided in a person's home, assisted-living homes and centers, nursing homes, and palliative care units. An interdisciplinary team including nurses, physicians, social workers, pastoral and bereavement counselors, and volunteers address the physical, emotional, and spiritual needs of the person and his or her surrogate.

Research participation usually involves clinical trials in which participants either receive a drug under investigation or a placebo. A placebo is an inactive substance that is used in medical research. In most studies, neither researchers nor participants know who is getting the actual drug. Clinical trials vary considerably on inclusion criteria (criteria required for participation) and exclusion criteria (conditions that exclude involvement).

Brain autopsy remains the only way to confirm that a person had Alzheimer's or another type of dementia. Because brain autopsy requires special arrangements, the decision to perform one should be made well in advance of the person's death.

▦ PRINCIPLES TO GUIDE HEALTHCARE DECISIONS

Advance directives specify person's wishes related to healthcare should he or she be unable to execute these decisions on his or her own. The next section identifies more clearly the principles and considerations used in making these decisions.

Self-Determination

Understanding the principles of making healthcare decisions starts with the concept of self-determination. Self-determination refers to an individual's right to choose one's own path in life (see Exhibit 16.1). Healthcare decisions are very personal expressions of this. Self-determination is an important legal and ethical principle that influences how and by whom healthcare decisions are made.

EXHIBIT 16.1

An Example of Self-Determination

Let us explore an example of self-determination. Suppose you decide to buy a car. Certain basic requirements must be met before you could. You must be an adult to enter into the purchase contract, and you must have the money to pay for the car. Similarly, an individual must be an adult to make healthcare decisions for himself or herself, and must be able to think about and communicate those choices to others. Once those basic requirements are met, you could make an independent decision.

You might not know very much about the safety of the cars that are available, and you might refer to a consumer guide that compares safety records. Similarly, an individual might not know very much about the healthcare choices facing him or her, and might listen to a physician's or other specialist's advice. Although expert advice may help you weigh your options and the opinions of family, friends, and other loved ones may be important, the principle of self-determination declares that you will make the decision for yourself.

An adult who has the ability to understand, think, make choices, and communicate those choices is responsible to make his or her own healthcare decisions. Those decisions must be honored by all others, including family, physicians, and institutions. It is only when the individual is not able to make or communicate decisions that another person is permitted to make decisions on another's behalf.

Express Wishes

An adult who has the ability to understand, think, and make healthcare choices can express healthcare wishes directly. If an individual has written down healthcare choices and then lost the ability to communicate, then others, including family, physicians, and healthcare institutions, must honor those express (written) wishes. A person's right to self-determination does not end when that person is no longer able to communicate. Express wishes will continue to direct treatment.

Substitute Judgment

When a person is not able to understand, make choices, or communicate, that individual is not able to participate in self-determined healthcare decision making. The loss of these abilities may be temporary or permanent, but during this time someone else must make decisions for the individual. The person who steps in is called a *surrogate decision maker*. The process of making the decisions is called *substitute judgment*.

Surrogate decision makers must try to imagine what the incapacitated person would have wanted and to substitute the imagined feelings and choices of the person they are representing for their own. The surrogate must consider the expert advice and the opinions of others who know about the situation, then ask, "In these circumstances, what would that person want?"

Best Interest

If the individual's express wishes are not known, and the surrogate decision maker is unable to imagine what the individual would want, then the decision is made in the best interest of the person (see Exhibit 16.2). The best interest standard is used rarely. Usually surrogate decision makers, such as family or friends are able to imagine what their loved one would want in the circumstances. Best interest is most often used when no one knows the individual well, or when the individual has no close relatives or friends to make decisions on his or her behalf.

EXHIBIT 16.2

A Case Study of Self-Determination, Express Wishes, Substitute Judgment, and Best Interest

Mr. M is a healthy and active retiree, who is living with his wife in a pleasant senior community. Mr. M completed an advance directive, appointing his wife as his healthcare power of attorney and describing his wishes in a living will. In his living will, Mr. M wrote that he would not want to be kept alive following an accident or injury if there was no hope of his recovery to an independent level again. Several years after he completed the advance directives, Mr. M suffered a stroke and was rushed to the hospital. The doctors tell Mrs. M that immediate surgery is needed to relieve the swelling on Mr. M's brain. The doctors believe that if the surgery goes as planned, Mr. M has a good chance of a successful recovery. A decision to accept or refuse surgery must be made. What principles of healthcare decision making should be used?

1. *Self-Determination.* Mr. M is too ill to participate in the decision himself. He is not able to understand, think, make choices, or communicate. Mr. M

is not capable at this time of a self-determined decision regarding the potential surgery; therefore, Mr. M's previously expressed wishes must be consulted.

2. *Express Wishes.* Mr. M had previously expressed his wishes in a living will. Mr. M's living will gives directions that he should not be kept alive following an accident or injury if there is no hope of his recovery to an independent level again. Did Mr. M express his wishes clearly about this current situation? No, he is not in a situation of no hope of recovery. Mr. M's physicians report that he has a good chance of a successful recovery. His wishes about his current situation, when the doctors think he has a good chance for a successful recovery, were not expressed in the living will. Mr. M's express wishes do not address the question of the proposed surgery; therefore, a surrogate decision maker must be asked to consider the question using substituted judgment.

3. *Substitute Judgment.* Mrs. M was appointed as her husband's healthcare power of attorney and has the responsibility of being his surrogate decision maker. Without Mr. M's express wishes, Mrs. M. must imagine what Mr. M. would want for himself in this circumstance. Mrs. M must ask herself, "If Mr. M could communicate right now, would he agree to the surgery?" Mrs. M's decision to accept or refuse the surgery must be made based on her ability to imagine her husband's wishes for himself.

4. *Best Interest.* Because Mrs. M will likely be able to make a decision on behalf of Mr. M using substitute judgment, the best interest standard is not needed. However, if Mrs. M was so overwhelmed by the situation that she could not make a decision, or if she refused to make a decision on behalf of her husband, then the physicians caring for Mr. M would be required to decide whether to perform the urgent surgery. The physicians do not know Mr. M and therefore would not be able to use the substitute judgment standard to imagine what he would desire in this circumstance. If the physicians were required to decide, they would need to use the best interest standard. What would be in Mr. M's best interest in this situation?

▨ CONSIDERATIONS FOR MAKING HEALTHCARE DECISIONS

Unfortunately, relatively few people with dementia complete an advance directive and even if one does exist, the document may not address all possible treatment decisions or contain adequate language to clearly provide guidance with decision making. As a result, family or surrogates may encounter circumstances when, because the express wishes are unknown or unclear, a decision must be made through the process of substitute judgment.

To make a decision based on substitute judgment, the family or surrogate decision maker should consider what the person would have wanted, as well as the benefits and burdens of the particular treatment. The following are some questions that may help:

- What would the person have wanted if able to make the decision on his or her own?
- Did the person ever make any comments about healthcare decisions or end-of-life care in response to situations addressed in the media?
- What cultural, religious, or spiritual values may have influenced the person's decisions about medical treatments or attitudes about quality of life and death?
- Did the person ever make or participate in healthcare decisions for a relative? If so, do factors in that decision relate to his or her personal beliefs?
- Are there financial factors related to the healthcare decision that would have influenced the person's decisions?
- Did the person ever mention how much discomfort he or she would be willing to endure?

In terms of questions specific to a particular treatment, consider the following:

- How will the treatment benefit the person?
- What can be expected in terms of functional improvement (or decline)?
- How will the treatment affect the person's level of comfort?
- Can the treatment be provided for a limited time to see if it is helpful?
- How (and when) will I know the treatment is helpful?
- If the treatment is started, can it (and how will it) be withdrawn at a later time?
- What are the alternatives?
- What are the risks and burdens (including discomfort) of the treatment?
- Are there ways to minimize these risks and burdens?
- How can comfort be maximized during the treatment?
- Will the treatment require a move from the person's current care setting?
- What are the financial implications of the treatment?

In addition to asking the questions about benefits and burdens to the person's physician and members of the treatment team, it can be helpful for the family or surrogate to discuss treatment options with other family members and supports, including friends and clergy. If additional guidance is needed, consultation with a local healthcare organization's ethics committee can prove invaluable.

Helpful Hints for Providers

When faced with a situation of healthcare decision making, it is sometimes automatic to move right to the final answer. Do not skip to the end. Train yourself to move down the list; from top to bottom, to be sure you have considered each standard for decision making (see Exhibit 16.3). Can the person make a decision now (self-determination)? Did the person write a decision down when he was able to do so (express wishes)? What would the person want in these circumstances if he or she were able to communicate (substitute judgment)? What would be in the person's best interest (best interest)?

EXHIBIT 16.3

A Case Study of Considerations for Making Healthcare Decisions

Mr. A is an 85-year-old man diagnosed with Alzheimer's disease. Although currently unable to make healthcare decisions, he had appointed his wife as his healthcare power of attorney and completed a living will 3 years ago when he was first diagnosed. A healthcare power of attorney is a document that designates an agent who can make decisions about care. A living will gives instruction about future choices to the healthcare power of attorney.

Over the past year, Mr. A has experienced increasing difficulty with swallowing food. He has aspirated while eating and developed pneumonia several times. Until now, the facility's medical director treated these infections with oral antibiotics. Recently, the facility hired a new medical director who spoke with Mrs. A about whether or not to continue treating these infections. Mrs. A referred to the living will, but unfortunately, it only addressed decisions about CPR and feeding tubes. In this case, Mrs. A is faced with having to make a substitute judgment. By reviewing the first set of questions listed earlier, she was able to gain clarity about the decision that Mr. A would have likely made had he been able to express his wishes about antibiotics.

In addition to asking the questions to the person's physician and members of the treatment team about benefits and burdens, it can be helpful for the family or surrogate to discuss treatment options with other family members and supports, including friends and clergy. If the need for additional guidance is needed, consultation with a local healthcare organization's ethics committee can prove to be an invaluable resource.

Remember, a person speaks first for himself or herself, and then a written document such as a living will speaks for the person. A surrogate decision maker only speaks for a person if the person cannot, and there exists no express wishes that answer the question to be considered. A surrogate decision maker, including a healthcare power of attorney, cannot override the previously-expressed wishes (living will) of a person.

■ WHEN A PERSON IS ABLE TO PARTICIPATE IN DECISION MAKING: EXPRESS WISHES

A person with advanced dementia will virtually never retain the capacity needed to fully participate in healthcare decisions. With early diagnosis, good planning, and wise professional guidance, individuals can help their families prepare for the inevitable loss of decision-making abilities. This section will review the opportunities to plan ahead for an individual with dementia who is able to participate in decision making.

Principles for Participation in Decision Making

Individuals have the legal and ethical right to participate in self-determined healthcare decisions. Each person should have the opportunity to understand the options, the benefits and risks of each option, and what experts recommend. After a review of this information, each person should have the opportunity to make his or her own choice about healthcare treatment, including the choice to accept or refuse specific medical interventions.

Tasks for the Person With Dementia and the Family or Surrogate

If an individual is able to participate in healthcare decisions, now is the time to discuss those preferences with family members and get those preferences written down. Individuals can document future healthcare preferences in advance directives. The advance directive will preserve their express wishes to guide healthcare choices that in the future will need to be made on their behalf. The following steps should be considered:

1. *Appoint a healthcare power of attorney (including mental healthcare power of attorney).* Only an individual can appoint a healthcare power of attorney (also known as a medical power of attorney) to make healthcare treatment choices on his or her behalf during times of incapacity, including mental incapacity. A healthcare power of attorney should be readily available in an emergency, but the person appointed does not need to live in the same town or the same state. A person selected to serve as a healthcare power of attorney should agree to act on the individual's behalf. It is very important that the individual and the selected healthcare power of attorney have a detailed conversation about what healthcare the individual would want and would not want in the future.
2. *Complete a living will.* A living will gives instructions about future choices to the healthcare power of attorney, family members, physicians, and institutions. A living will must be completed while a person retains the ability to make decisions. There are many possible forms that can be used and a living will may even be handwritten. The living will is a very personal document. Each person's living will may look very different.
3. *Seek professional assistance with financial preplanning.* An individual with dementia will require an increasing level of personal and professional care as the disease progresses. The required care will have significant financial consequences to the individual and his family. Professional assistance from a financial planner and eldercare attorney with financial planning, particularly while the person retains decision-making ability, is recommended.
4. *Communicate values, choices, preferences, and decisions to the surrogate.* If persons with dementia are able to communicate, efforts should be made for them to share their values, choices, preferences, and healthcare decisions with family members and friends. It is often difficult for loved ones to hear a person discuss these issues. Family members may have concerns or disagreements about the choices. By discussing the issues while the person is still capable of decision

making, they will have time to convey their feelings and talk about their differences. An individual's expressed choices for his or her own healthcare treatment must be honored by surrogate decision makers, family and friends, and all healthcare providers, even if members of the family do not agree with the choices. These conversations will ease the family's burden in the future and ensure that the individual's wishes are honored.

5. *Copy and distribute advance directives.* Advance directives are of little use if no one has a copy or knows what they say. Advance directives should be distributed widely. Make several copies of each advance directive document and the living will. Give copies to the medical or mental healthcare power of attorney, other family members and close friends, and the person's physician for the office file. Give one to any healthcare facility where the person may seek care, including the hospital, nursing home, assisted-living home, or hospice.

Tasks for Healthcare Providers and Caregivers

If a person with dementia possesses the ability to participate in healthcare decisions when he or she enters first encounters with a healthcare provider or facility, processes should be in place to systematically solicit and document key healthcare choices of that individual at the earliest possible opportunity (see Exhibit 16.4). The opportunity for an individual with advanced dementia to participate in detailed advance care planning will be lost with the passage of time and the advancement of the disease. The more detailed a description of preferences the healthcare provider is able to obtain from an individual who's still able to express them, the better able the caregivers will be to honor the preference.

1. *Review advance directives.* The healthcare provider or caregiver should review the individual's advance directives and assist the person and family with advance care planning discussions and advance directive completion. An opportunity to discuss common care choices that the individual will face should be arranged, and if the individual agrees, the discussions should include interested family members, loved ones, and friends. A person with dementia may choose to update previously-executed advance directives, adding healthcare treatment preferences specific to the needs that accompany dementia.

2. *Collect, copy, and file all advance directive documents.* The healthcare provider or institution should have a systematic process to collect, copy, and file each person's advance directives. The advance directives may not have been included in the transfer papers a referring hospital sent, or family members may have neglected to provide a copy. For instances like these, the healthcare provider or caregiver should develop a follow-up process that ensures the advance directives are located and a copy is filed in the medical record.

3. *Keep advance directives available.* Individuals with dementia may undergo significant changes and require emergency medical intervention at any time. While a person is in an institution's or facility's care, his or her advance directives

should be readily available for review. If the person is transferred to a hospital or acute care setting for treatment, copies must accompany them. If a copy machine is not accessible at all times, several extra copies should be made in advance and stored in the medical record for emergency transfers.

4. *Reassess advance directives with condition change.* As a person with dementia's condition changes, his or her preferences for healthcare treatment may change. If the person retains the ability to make decisions, the healthcare provider or caregiver should arrange for them to review and update the advance directives and previous treatment choices. If the individual agrees, these discussions should include family members, loved ones, and friends. Even if the individual elects to continue as before, the caregiver should document the discussion in the medical record and assure the person that he or she has the option to review the choices again at any time.

5. *Offer educational opportunities.* Caregivers, healthcare providers, individuals, and their families should have an opportunity to learn more about advance care planning and advance directives. Education can be provided on-site at facilities, or through resources in the community. An educated caregiver will be better able to understand and honor individuals' advance directives. An individual who is more informed will be more effective in communicating healthcare preferences. A family that is more knowledgeable will be better able to represent their loved one's wishes for care when that individual loses his or her capacity to participate in treatment decisions.

EXHIBIT 16.4

A Case Study of the Ability to Express Wishes

Mr. P is admitted to a care facility following a 5-day hospital stay for dehydration and pneumonia. Mr. P is 86 years old, a retired plumber, and lives at home alone. Mr. P has been having memory problems and no longer drives. His daughter lives nearby and assists him with grocery shopping, meal preparation, and housecleaning. On admission, Mr. P is quite weak, unable to walk without assistance, and falls asleep easily. He appears to understand what is going on around him and speaks in a soft voice. Mr. P has a diagnosis of pneumonia and dementia.

Tasks for Mr. P and his family or surrogate include:

■ Providing the care facility with a copy of all advance directive forms (if completed).
■ Discussing Mr. P's condition and future care needs and complete advance directives.
■ Naming a healthcare power of attorney and complete a living will (if not completed).
■ Consulting with a financial planning professional.

Tasks for the healthcare provider or caregiver include:

▦ Arranging a meeting with Mr. P and his family to review advance directives.
▦ Collecting and copying advance directives, and storing copies in the medical record for easy access.
▦ Providing Mr. P.'s daughter with copies of advance directives for filing and future use at other healthcare institutions.
▦ Reassuring Mr. P and his daughter that advance care planning will be reviewed as his condition improves or otherwise changes.
▦ Coordinating the education of staff, individuals, and their families on advance directives.

▦ WHEN A PERSON IS NOT ABLE TO PARTICIPATE IN DECISION MAKING: SUBSTITUTE DECISION MAKING

When an individual with dementia is no longer able to understand or communicate, the responsibility for healthcare decisions is transferred to a substitute decision maker or surrogate. This section reviews the role of the surrogate decision maker and discusses how a person's wishes can be honored after he or she can no longer participate in decision making.

Principles for Substitute Decision Making

When an individual loses the ability to understand or communicate, that person does not lose the right to have his or her healthcare choices acknowledged. Substitute decision makers and healthcare providers are required by legal and ethical principles to determine and respect that person's wishes (see Exhibit 16.5). Choices that were written down before the loss of decision-making capacity must be reviewed and must guide the healthcare choices made on his or her behalf. The surrogate must use the substitute judgment standard in making healthcare decisions: "What would this person want?" If the person did not adequately express his or her wishes and if the surrogate's knowledge of the person's values is not deep enough to make a decision, the surrogate must make decisions to the best of his or her belief.

EXHIBIT 16.5

A Case Study of Substitute Decision Making

Mrs. T is admitted to a long-term care facility following a 4-day hospital stay for infected leg ulcers. Her husband died 3 years ago and she has a daughter living out of state who handles her financial affairs. Prior to her hospitalization,

Continued

Exhibit 16.5 *Continued*

Mrs. T was living with her older sister in a small home, and her sister reports that Mrs. T has become more confused and has been unable to manage her personal care over the past few months. Mrs. T is admitted to the care facility for continued treatment of her leg ulcers and with a diagnosis of dementia. The facility staff determines that Mrs. T is not able to understand or communicate her healthcare choices because of her advanced dementia.

Tasks for Mrs. T's family or surrogate include:

- Locating Mrs. T's healthcare power of attorney and living will documents (she has a copy in her dresser drawer and her daughter has a copy).
- Bringing copies to the facility and keeping extra copies at home.
- Reviewing Mrs. T's living will in relationship to her current condition— does she express any wishes about long-term care, hospice care, or end-of-life care, or does she make other statements that can guide current choices?
- Having Mrs. T's daughter review her responsibilities, as healthcare power of attorney, with the facility staff including providing emergency contact phone numbers.
- Discussing common healthcare decisions that Mrs. T will face with facility staff and medical professionals caring for her. These conversations can be conducted in person or by phone, because Mrs. T's daughter is out-of-state.
- Thinking about these common healthcare decisions and discussing as a family what Mrs. T would want done in those circumstances. These family discussions can occur over a period of time and be held over the phone.
- Having Mrs. T's daughter, as healthcare power of attorney, make decisions now about future medical care needs and communicate those choices to the facility staff. Mrs. T's daughter can write these choices down and mail them to the facility, or they can be written down by the staff during a phone conversation with Mrs. T's daughter.
- Advocating for what Mrs. T would want for herself by being available to answer staff questions about care and treatment, and by always making treatment choices based on consideration of what Mrs. T would want in a particular circumstance.

Tasks for healthcare provider and caregiver include:

- Reviewing Mrs. T's advance directives, and keeping several copies readily available for review and facility staff use.
- Contacting Mrs. T's daughter and determining her ability or willingness to serve as Mrs. T's medical power of attorney.
- Obtaining and documenting emergency contact phone numbers for Mrs. T's daughter and ensuring that the numbers are available to all facility staff at all times.

> ▦ Arranging a time to talk to Mrs. T's daughter in detail about her mother's current condition, what Mrs. T has stated in her advance directives, and common healthcare decisions that Mrs. T may face as her dementia progresses, offering to have the medical professionals providing care to Mrs. T speak with the daughter if needed.
> ▦ Encouraging Mrs. T's daughter to think about common healthcare choices that Mrs. T may face, and asking herself, "What would she want in those circumstances?"
> ▦ Documenting in advance of a medical emergency healthcare treatment choices that Mrs. T's daughter makes on her mother's behalf being sure that all decisions are readily available for facility staff review at all times.

Many states have specific statutes that delineate the responsibilities of a surrogate. You should consult with your local state government to find out what statutes are currently in place. Below is an example from the Arizona Revised Statutes of how surrogate responsibilities can be delineated.

SURROGATE RESPONSIBILITIES

Arizona Revised Statutes
Title 36 Public Health and Safety
Chapter 32 Living Wills and Health Care Directives
36-3203 Surrogate; authority; responsibilities; immunity

The surrogate shall make health care decisions for the patient in accordance with the patient's wishes as expressed in the healthcare directive.

If the healthcare directive does not provide sufficient information to know what the patient would want in a particular circumstance, the surrogate shall base these decisions on the surrogate's knowledge of the patient's values if those are known or can be determined to the surrogate's satisfaction.

If neither the healthcare directive nor the surrogate's knowledge of the patient's values provides a sufficient basis for making a healthcare decision, the surrogate shall decide based on the surrogate's good faith belief as to what is in the patient's best interest.

Tasks for the Person With Dementia and the Family or Surrogate

1. *Locate, copy, and review any previously written advance directive.* The family and close friends of the person with dementia should locate any previously-written advance directive. There may be copies already in their possession, or in the individual's personal effects, a safety deposit box, or in a lawyer's or financial

planner's file. Provide those documents to the care facility staff and ask them to make copies; always store an extra copy in a safe and accessible place. The surrogate decision maker, as well other interested family members and friends, should take the time to carefully read the advance directives. These papers will provide some insight and guidance into what the person who wrote them would want in the future.

2. *Review surrogate decision maker's role.* A surrogate decision maker has agreed to a serious responsibility. The surrogate decision maker, whether appointed through a healthcare power of attorney or having taken on the role because of the close relationship with the incapacitated person, is responsible to act on that individual's behalf. The surrogate decision maker must repeatedly ask, "What would this person want?" The surrogate decision makers should use any advance directives and previously expressed wishes to help answer that question as if they were in the person's shoes.

3. *Understand and plan for common healthcare decisions.* Dementia is a disease that progresses along a predictable course. The timing of the progression may vary, but the decisions that will be faced about medical treatment are predictable. The surrogate decision maker responsible for medical treatment choices should understand and plan for the predictable healthcare choices that will develop. The surrogate decision maker should seek guidance and education from the professional medical staff. Ask: "What can I expect in the next few weeks? Or months?" The surrogate should consider the decisions to be faced, future options for care and treatment, and what the person with dementia would want in future circumstances. The surrogate should write down the decisions arrived at and share them with the caregiver at the facility (e.g., "If nasal congestion or cough develops, this is what I would like done. If my loved one is unable to swallow, this is what I would like done."). By planning ahead, the surrogate can take the time to understand the options; ask questions about the benefits or treatment risks; take previously expressed wishes into consideration; make careful, thoughtful decisions; and avoid last-minute, emotional, and high-stress decisions.

4. *Advocate for what the person with dementia would want.* A surrogate decision maker is often someone who has been close to the person with dementia, either a family member or friend. Regardless of the intimacy or length of the relationship, the surrogate decision maker must take the time to recall and consider the person with dementia's values, thoughts, and previous conversations. Did the person previously say something that suggested what his or her feelings might be about end-of-life care? "I would do that all over again if I needed to" about an earlier treatment, perhaps, or, "I would never want that kind of treatment again no matter what."

Tasks for the Healthcare Provider or Caregiver

Once a person with dementia has lost decision-making capacity, the healthcare provider or caregiver must ensure that the person's previously expressed wishes guide healthcare treatment choices. Those previously expressed wishes are often documented in an advance directive such as a living will. In addition to the guidance offered by the previously completed advance directives, the healthcare provider will look to a surrogate decision maker to act on behalf of a person incapacitated by dementia. The surrogate decision maker's role is to stand in for the incapacitated person and to answer the question, "What would this person want in these circumstances?"

1. *Collect, copy, and file all advance directive documents.* The incapacitated person's previously expressed wishes are the most important consideration in respecting that person's self-determination and personal treatment choices. The healthcare provider or caregiver should have a systematic process to collect, copy, and file each person's advance directives. The healthcare provider should ensure that these advance directives are always accessible to facility caregivers.
2. *Identify the legal surrogate decision maker.* In addition to the guidance offered in the previously completed advance directives, the healthcare provider or caregiver will identify a surrogate decision maker who is legally able to act on behalf of a person incapacitated by dementia. The surrogate decision maker's identity might be easily determined, as in a case where there is an existing healthcare power of attorney, or it may be less clear. If the incapacitated person does not have a guardian, and did not appoint a healthcare power of attorney when able to do so, the surrogate decision maker(s) must be determined by review of the state statute (law) that lists the order of surrogates responsible for making healthcare decisions. Each state has a different statute for determining surrogate decision makers. Once the surrogate decision maker has been identified, the caregivers must have easy access to his or her phone number. The surrogate's inclusion in healthcare choices is essential, both legally and ethically. Below is an example from the Arizona Revised Statutes of how surrogate decision makers are determined.

SURROGATE DECISION MAKERS

Arizona Revised Statutes
Title 36 Public Health and Safety
Chapter 32 Living Wills and Health Care Directives
36-3231 Surrogate decision makers; priorities; limitations

If an adult patient is unable to make or communicate treatment decisions, the patient's agent (designated by healthcare power of attorney) or court-appointed guardian shall act as the patient's surrogate.

If neither of these situations apply, the following individual(s) in the indicated order of priority, who are available and willing to serve as the surrogate, who then have the authority to make healthcare decisions for the patient and who shall follow the patient's wishes if they are known:

1. The patient's spouse (unless legally separated).
2. An adult child of the patient (if more than one adult child, then consent of a majority of the adult children who are reasonably available for consultation).

Continued

SURROGATE DECISION MAKERS *Continued*

3. A parent of the patient.
4. If the patient is unmarried, the patient's domestic partner if no other person has assumed any financial responsibility for the patient.
5. A brother or sister of the patient.
6. A close friend of the patient.

If no surrogate listed can be located, the patient's attending physician may make healthcare treatment decisions for the patient after the physician consults with and obtains the recommendations of an institutional ethics committee.

If this is not possible, the physician may make these decisions after consulting with a second physician who concurs with the physician's decision.

3. *Assist the surrogate decision maker with advance decision making.* Healthcare providers should review the individual's advance directives and assist the surrogate decision maker in reviewing common healthcare decisions in advance of emergency need. By doing this prior to an emergency, the surrogate decision maker has the time to understand the options and avoids having to make last-minute, emotional, and high-stress decisions. The surrogate's healthcare decisions made in advance of a medical emergency must be clearly documented and readily available to caregivers.

WHEN CAPACITY IS LIMITED OR UNCLEAR: INCAPACITY

Advance care planning includes the identification of an agent to act on one's behalf in the event of incapacity. What happens if no one has been appointed and decisions need to be made? A care provider will then need to determine whether the person with advanced dementia has the capacity to elect someone. The question becomes, "Is the person able to understand and tell us what he wants?" Determining capacity for persons with advanced dementia often proves to be a challenge for the family and for healthcare professionals.

Principles for Determining Capacity

What is capacity? In the legal context, the definition varies according to the scope of decision that is to be made. Essentially, capacity means that a person understands the nature and effect of his or her act. To appoint an agent to make medical decisions, a person must understand that he or she is naming someone to make those decisions for him or her. The individual must also understand that an agent will determine healthcare decisions for him or her when unable to personally make them. If the person understands those things, then he or she has the capacity to create a healthcare power of attorney. A diagnosis of dementia alone does not necessarily mean that the person lacks capacity. For instance, a person with dementia may be more confused in the evenings and, therefore, unable to make certain decisions at that time. However, the same person may be clear enough another time of the day to execute a particular document—to reasonably understand the nature and effect of executing that document.

Decisional capacity, or in healthcare terms an *informed consent*, means that the person can understand his or her health condition. This means that the person can consider the benefits, burdens, and risks of care options, can weigh the treatment consequences against his or her preferences and values, can reach a decision that is consistent over time, and can communicate that decision to others.

Determining capacity generally entails ethical considerations. Those considerations are often based on varying circumstances and add complexity to the process. For example, does the person want to designate an agent or are family members trying to force the issue? Are family members trying to ignore the capacity issues? Would any of the family members have reason to be concerned if an investigation were conducted into the matter? A combination of factors must be evaluated to determine a person's capacity. As each person's situation is different, the areas needing to be evaluated also differ. Looking at the person's total situation, medical, personal, financial, and psychosocial, is imperative.

If the person with advanced dementia is regularly unable to make responsible personal decisions, then the person probably does not have the capacity to create a healthcare power of attorney or other legal documents. In that event, a statutory surrogate or a court-appointed guardian would need to make the necessary decisions on the person's behalf.

Completing the Documents

Planning is the key to avoiding these types of dilemmas. Preferably, a healthcare power of attorney will be prepared before capacity is lost. However, if capacity is unclear, consider the following:

- Does the person understand, even if only for the moment, that he or she is agreeing to appoint another person to make health decisions for him or her?
- Are there family dynamics that exist that would raise concerns about someone's motives for "pushing" the creation of a healthcare power of attorney?
- Are there any family members avoiding the capacity issue?
- Has a physician been involved in determining capacity?

If a person is not able to execute a power of attorney, the healthcare professional will need to defer to the statutory surrogate or a court-appointed guardian. Many factors affect capacity. The timing of the approach, the manner in which the person is approached, and changing environmental circumstances can all have an effect on capacity. Table 16.1 offers advice for the family or surrogates, as well as advice for facility administration or staff that will assist in the success of naming an agent (see Exhibit 16.6).

TABLE 16.1

Helpful Hints to Facilitate the Preparation of a Power of Attorney Document

Helpful Hints for Family	Helpful Hints for Facility Administration and Staff
▦ Remember that time and patience are very important. A person might not be able to make a decision when it is convenient for you. In this case, re-approach the person during a different time of day, or during a less stressful time. The issue of capacity is determined the moment in which the documents are being executed, not later that evening.	▦ Document efforts, limitations, and why proceeding with the surrogate laws is needed.
▦ Establishing trust with the person will prove helpful in this process.	▦ Do not be afraid to repeatedly try to find that moment of capacity for the person.
▦ Many factors can contribute to capacity. Increased stress—mind, body, environmental—can make a person's dementia worse. Medical problems, such as a urinary tract infection or a cold, can aggravate the situation. If there are other factors affecting the person's capacity, resolve these issues and try again.	▦ Keep documentation of the healthcare power of attorney attempts in the medical record, as well as the decision to use the statutory surrogate laws, or the need to find someone to act as a surrogate.
	▦ Have a procedure in place for the cases when a person has no capacity, no healthcare power of attorney, and no surrogate, or the surrogate is not willing or able to carry out his or her responsibilities.

EXHIBIT 16.6

A Case Study of Healthcare Power of Attorney

Mr. S is in a nursing facility dementia unit. He has lost the ability to care for himself, although he can still communicate issues he is having to each of his daughters. On some days, he recognizes both of them. The daughters could act as surrogates but, because of a conflict with each other, they are not comfortable acting without some legal authority. Both daughters want their father to be taken care of; however, they have different ideas of what the care would include. If the surrogacy laws are to be applied, the daughters must reach a consensus on what the course of treatment should be. If the father could name one daughter as the agent under a healthcare power of attorney, the issue of responsibility would be resolved. If the facility staff approaches Mr. S during a time that he can communicate his preferences, is able to name one of the daughters as his agent, and is willing to sign the documents, then the directive would be valid and would avoid any misunderstanding between daughters. This does not mean that this process is easily done, rather that it is worth the effort to try. In the next chapter, we will examine situations like this more closely.

REFERENCES

Allen, R. S., DeLaine, S. R., Chaplin, W. F., Marson, D. C., Bourgeois, M. S., Dijkstra, D., et al. (2003). Advance care planning in nursing homes: Correlates of capacity and possession of advance directives. *The Gerontologist, 43*(3), 309–317.

American Geriatrics Society Ethics Committee. (1998). *Making treatment decisions for incapacitated elderly patients without advance directives* (monograph). American Geriatrics Society Position Statement. Retrieved January 25, 2010, from http://www.americangeriatrics.org/products/ positionpapers/treatdecPF.shtml

Chen, J. H., Lamberg, J. L., Chen, Y. C., Kiely, D. K., Page, J. H., Person, C. J., et al. (2006). Occurrence and treatment of suspected pneumonia in long-term care residents dying with advanced dementia. *Journal of the American Geriatrics Society, 54*(2), 290–295.

Cohen-Mansfield, J. (2002). Development of a framework to encourage addressing advance directives when resources are limited. *Journal of Aging & Health, 14*(1), 24–41.

Fabiszewski, K. J., Volicer, B., & Volicer, L. (1990). Effect of antibiotic treatment on outcome of fevers in institutionalized Alzheimer patients. *The Journal of the American Medical Association, 263*(23), 3168–3172.

Finucane, T. E., Christmas, C., & Travis, K. (1999). Tube feeding in patients with advanced dementia: A review of the evidence. *The Journal of the American Medical Association, 282*(14), 1365–1370.

Frisoni, G. B., Franzoni, S., Bellelli, G., Morris, J., & Warden, V. (1998). Overcoming eating difficulties in the severely demented. In L. Volicer & A. Hurley (Eds.), *Hospice care for patients with advanced progressive dementia* (pp. 48–67). New York: Springer.

General Powers and Duties of Guardian, ARS 14-5312 (A) and (8)(9), (n.d.).

Golleher v. Horton, 148 ARS 14-5506 (App. 1985).

Hirschman, K. B., Joyce, C. M., James, B. D., Xie, S. X., & Karlawish, J. H. T. (2005). Do Alzheimer's disease patients want to participate in a treatment decision, and would their caregivers let them? *The Gerontologist, 45*(3), 381–388.

Hurley, A. C., Volicer, B., Mahoney, M. A., & Volicer, L. (1993). Palliative fever management in Alzheimer patients: Quality plus fiscal responsibility. *Advances in Nursing Science, 16*(1), 21–32.

Karlawish, J. H., Casarett, D. J., James, B. D., Xie, S. X., & Kim, S. Y. (2005). The ability of persons with Alzheimer disease (AD) to make a decision about taking an AD treatment. *Neurology, 64*(9), 1514–1519.

Karp, N., & Wood, E. (2003). *Incapacitated and alone: Health care decision-making for the unbefriended elderly.* Washington, DC: American Bar Association.

Kayser-Jones, J. (1996). Mealtime in nursing homes: The importance of individualized care. *Journal of Gerontological Nursing, 22*(3), 26–31.

Kim, S. Y., Kim, H. M., Langa K. M., Karlawish, J. H., Knopman, D. S., & Appelbaum, P. S. (2009). Surrogate consent for dementia research: A national survey. *Neurology, 72*(2), 149–155.

Koppelman, E. R. (2002). Dementia and dignity: Towards a new method of surrogate decision making. *Journal of Medicine and Philosophy, 27*, 65–85.

Lamberg, J. L., Person, C. J., Kiely, D. K., & Mitchell, S. L. (2005). Decisions to hospitalize nursing home residents dying with advanced dementia. *Journal of the American Geriatrics Society, 53*(8), 1396–1401.

Leland, J. (2001). Advance directives and establishing goals of care. *Primary Care, 28*(2), 349–363.

Living Wills and Health Care Directives, ARS 36-3231 (1992).

Long, C. O. (2009). Palliative care for advanced dementia. *Journal of Gerontological Nursing, 35*(11), 19–24.

Luchins, D. J., Hanrahan, P., & Murphy, K. (1997). Criteria for enrolling dementia patients in hospice. *Journal of the American Geriatric Society, 45*(9), 1054–1059.

Mahoney, E. K., Volicer, L., & Hurley, A. C. (2000). Food refusal. In E. K. Mahoney, L. Volicer, & A. C. Hurley (Eds.), *Management of challenging behaviors in dementia* (pp. 155–170). Baltimore, MD: Health Professionals Press, Inc.

McCann, R. M., Hall, W. J., & Groth-Juncker, A. (1994). Comfort care for terminally ill patients: The appropriate use of nutrition and hydration. *The Journal of the American Medical Association, 272*(16), 1263–1266.

Morrison, R. S., Chichin, E., Carter, J., Burack, O., Lantz, M., & Meier, D. E. (2005). The effect of a social work intervention to enhance advance care planning in the nursing home. *Journal of the American Geriatric Society, 53*(2), 290–294.

Powers of attorney; best interest; intimidation; deception; definitions ARS 14-5506 (F)(2) (n.d.).

Protection of Person Under Disability, Definitions, ARS 14-5101 (n.d.).

Rhodes, R., & Holzman, I. R. (2004). The not unreasonable standard for assessment of surrogates and surrogate decisions. *Theory of Medical Bioethics, 25*(4), 367–385.

Sachs, G., Shega, J. W., & Cox-Hayley, D. (2004). Barriers to excellent end-of-life care for patients with dementia. *Journal of General Internal Medicine, 19*(10), 1057–1063.

Seal, M. K. (2004). *Arizona consumers guide to guardianship and conservatorship*. Mesa, AZ: JacksonWhite Law Firm, P.C.

Small, N., Downs, M., & Froggartt, K. (2006). Improving end-of-life care for people with dementia — the benefits of combining UK approaches to palliative care and dementia care. In M. L. M. Bere & G. M. M. Jones (Eds.), *Care-giving in dementia — research and applications*, (Vol. 4, pp. 365–392), London, & New York: Routledge & Sons.

Smith, S. J. (1998). Providing palliative care for the terminal Alzheimer's patient. In L. Volicer & A. Hurley (Eds.), *Hospice care for patients with advanced progressive dementia* (pp. 247–256). New York: Springer.

Volicer, L. (2008). End-of-life care for people with dementia in long-term care settings. *Alzheimer's Care Today, 9*(2), 84–102.

Volicer, L., Brandeis, G. H., & Hurley, A. C. (1998). Infections in advanced dementia. In L. Volicer & A. Hurley (Eds.), *Hospice care for patients with advanced progressive dementia* (pp. 29–47). New York: Springer.

Volicer, L., Rheaume, Y., Riley, M. E., Karner, J., & Glennon, M. (1990). Discontinuation of tube feeding in patients with dementia of the Alzheimer type. *American Journal of Alzheimer's Care and Related Disorders and Research, 5*, 22–25.

Volicer, L., Seltzer, B., Rheaume, Y., Karner, J., Glennon, M., Riley, M. E., et al. (1989). Eating difficulties in patients with probable dementia of the Alzheimer type. *Journal of Geriatric Psychiatry and Neurology, 2*(4), 188–195.

Warden, V. J. (1989). Waste not, want not. *Geriatric Nursing, 10*, 210–211.

White, R. A., Macdonald, E. K., & Seal, M. K. (2004). *Alzheimer's and the law*. Mesa, AZ: JacksonWhite Law Firm, PC.

Winzelberg, G. S., Hanson, L. C., & Tulsky, J. A. (2005). Beyond autonomy: Diversifying end-of-life decision-making approaches to serve patients and families. *Journal of the American Geriatric Society, 53*(6), 1046–1050.

17

THE CONTINUUM OF GRIEF

Kathryn B. Lindstrom, Rosemarie Bosch, Ruth M. Cohen,
Paul Fredericks, Geri R. Hall, Paul Harrington,
Deborah Hollawell, Kathy Kramer-Howe, Pat Priniski,
Jennifer Westlund, David Wilsterman, and Hank Zaremba

▓ INTRODUCTION

When people think about the term *grief*, they generally make the assumption that grief only occurs in the wake of a loved one's death. However, this is not true for the family members and significant others of people with dementia. For them, grief runs through the entire experience. It arrives long before the physical end.

Caregivers of persons with dementia go through anticipatory grief. This is likely to occur at significant moments during the process, including during the diagnostic disclosure, when symptoms progress from one level to another, and in the late stages of the disease.

When people have a loved one who is seriously ill with something other than dementia, it generally takes them about 18 months to deal with caregiving strain and prepare themselves for the death of a loved one. However, the course of dementia can run several years or longer. "A caregiver's grief may wax and wane, while they recycle again and again through the grief experience," social workers Ponder and Pomeroy (1996) write. Families who have someone ill with dementia may have more time to prepare for the death, but this does not necessarily help them arrive at an acceptance of the death.

The term *ambiguous loss* describes the situation for dementia caregivers. Their experience of loss is incomplete and uncertain. The people they care for are physically present but, increasingly, psychologically absent. As the individual's psychological decline increases, a caregiver's feelings of ambiguity typically builds. Family members become more uncertain about whether to think of the person as absent or present. As this continues, the likelihood of their experiencing symptoms of depression increases. A kind of social loss occurs as well, as friends and social groups behave as if the person is already gone. These experiences of psychosocial losses significantly complicate the grieving process, as spouses lose their mate and children lose their parent long before any physical death. One article eloquently summarized these losses: "As deterioration robs the family of dignity, intellect and personhood, feelings of loss and powerlessness ensue, an empty space begins to develop, and the caregiver is forced to let go of a relationship inch by inch" (Jones & Martinson, 1992).

As the demented person undergoes profound and disturbing changes in behavior, it is normal for loved ones to experience various thoughts, feelings, physical sensations, and behaviors. These reactions to anticipatory grieving, however, are frequently overlooked or mislabeled as depression or stress by health professionals. But in overlooking the role grief is playing in their lives, people involved in caring for a person with dementia can find their own ability to heal and cope disrupted. They inadvertently cut themselves off from a wider range of available interventions. Grief support is available from various sources. During the terminal stages of the disease, hospice services can be particularly helpful.

EXPERIENCE OF SPOUSE CAREGIVERS

In considering family members' predeath grief experience, spouses of persons with dementia have a very different experience than adult children. A caregiver's experience of loss is also influenced by the severity of dementia, whether it is mild, moderate, or severe.

For spousal care, partners of persons who have mild (or early-stage) dementia, grief intensity is usually low, although sadness may be in evidence. Their experience of loss is focused more on the person with dementia, their diminishing abilities and the changes they are undergoing in shared activities and the relationship. As the dementia progresses and the individual moves into the moderate stages of dementia, grief intensity steadily increases. The focus of loss remains on the person and shared activities or relationship, but caregiver-related sacrifices start to become distressing as the person needs increasing help with daily living activities. Emotional reactions include feelings of compassion, frustration, and sadness. The caregiver may redefine the relationship as increasing responsibilities are assumed. By the time the person reaches the advanced stages of dementia, grief intensity is at its peak. The focus of loss shifts to changes caregivers personally feel—for example, that they feel less like part of a couple now and more like an individual. Reactions may include sadness, uncertainty, loneliness, and general emptiness.

EXPERIENCE OF ADULT CHILDREN CAREGIVERS

Adult children experience different loss patterns. When the parent is in the mild or early stages of dementia, adult children also tend to have low grief intensity, but the sense of loss is focused more on their own personal sacrifices now. As the dementia progresses into the moderate stages and the parent loses more obvious capacity, grief intensity dramatically jumps and often corresponds with the adult child having to assume a decision-making role over his or her parent. Although the focus of loss remains on personal sacrifices, emotional reactions typically intensify into feelings of anger, guilt, and resentment.

With advanced dementia, grief intensity remains high, but the focus of loss may shift from sacrifice to loss of the relationship with the parent. Emotional reactions shift, from anger and frustration to a pervasive sense of sadness, regret, and resignation.

▨ EXPERIENCE OF FAMILY CAREGIVERS AFFECTED BY EARLY-ONSET DEMENTIA

A particular kind of dementia, early onset, requires special consideration. Because early onset, or dementia that occurs before the age of 65, is far less common than later onset, there has been little documentation of what the grief experience is like for family members because it comprises less than 5% of dementia cases. This much is clear, however, that the spouses and children are considerably younger and, therefore, face much different life issues than those with loved ones affected by more typical late-onset dementia. Spouses in the first group are more likely to be engaged in work and raising families. Their children may not yet have reached adulthood. One study found that caregivers of younger persons had significantly higher levels of burden; that, in fact, the burdens were inversely related to the affected person's age.

These caregivers face unique challenges in several areas—obtaining a diagnosis, financial worries, loss of employment, and family conflict. Of the population studied, 75% report that their children experienced psychological or emotional problems related to their parents' dementia. Many report experiencing social isolation and dissatisfaction with available services.

▨ PREDEATH GRIEF ASSESSMENT AND INTERVENTIONS

Predeath Grief Assessment

During the course of dementia, caregivers may experience grief in several ways: through feelings of personal sacrifice, in the sadness they experience about the effects of the disease, in the depression that comes from uncertainty about the progression and unexpected events, and in their feelings of isolation. The Marwit-Meuser Caregiver Grief Inventory (MM-CGI) provides a useful means of assessing the intensity and patterns of this grief (see Exhibit 17.1). The 50-item inventory provides a total score for grief intensity level, comprised of the scores on three subscales: personal sacrifice burden, heartfelt sadness and longing, and worry and felt isolation. An 18-item version of the MM-CGI is also available that yields the same total score and is much quicker and easier to administer. The MM-CGI can provide insights to caregivers on their experiences and may help direct them to more effective ways of coping during the caregiving journey.

EXHIBIT 17.1

Marwit-Meuser Caregiver Grief Inventory—Short Form

Instructions: This inventory is designed to measure the grief experience of family caregivers of persons living with a progressive dementia, such as Alzheimer's disease. Read each statement to the right carefully, then decide how much you agree or disagree. Circle the number 1–5 that reflects your response (1 = Strongly Disagree, 5 = Strongly Agree).

		ANSWER KEY 1 = Strongly Disagree // 2 = Disagree // 3 = Somewhat Agree // 4 = Agree // 5 = Strongly Agree		
1		I've had to give up a great deal to be a caregiver.	1 2 3 4 5	A
2		I feel I am losing my freedom.	1 2 3 4 5	A
3		I have nobody to communicate with.	1 2 3 4 5	C
4		I have this empty, sick feeling knowing that my loved one is "gone."	1 2 3 4 5	B
5		I spend a lot of time worrying about the bad things to come.	1 2 3 4 5	C
6		Dementia is like a double loss . . . I've lost the closeness with my loved one and connectedness with my family.	1 2 3 4 5	C
7		My friends simply don't understand what I'm going through.	1 2 3 4 5	C
8		I long for what was, what we had and shared in the past.	1 2 3 4 5	B
9		I could deal with other serious disabilities better than with this.	1 2 3 4 5	B
10		I will be tied up with this for who knows how long.	1 2 3 4 5	A
11		It hurts to put her/him to bed at night and realize that she/he is "gone."	1 2 3 4 5	B
12		I feel very sad about what this disease has done.	1 2 3 4 5	B
13		I lay awake most nights worrying about what's happening and how I'll manage tomorrow.	1 2 3 4 5	C
14		The people closest to me do not understand what I'm going through.	1 2 3 4 5	C
15		I've lost other people close to me, but the losses I'm experiencing now are much more troubling.	1 2 3 4 5	B
16		Independence is what I've lost . . . I don't have the freedom to go and do what I want.	1 2 3 4 5	A

| 17 | I wish I had an hour or two to myself each day to pursue personal interests. | 1 2 3 4 5 | A |
| 18 | I'm stuck in this caregiving world and there's nothing I can do about it. | 1 2 3 4 5 | A |

Source: Reprinted by permission from Meuser, Marwit, & Sanders, 2004, pp. 169–195.

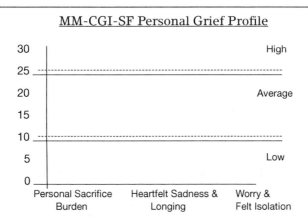

MM-CGI-SF Personal Grief Profile

What do these scores mean?

Scores in the top area are one standard deviation (SD) higher than average based on responses of other family caregivers ($n = 292$). High scores may indicate a need for formal intervention or support assistance to enhance coping. Low scores (one SD below the mean) may indicate denial or a downplaying of distress. Low scores may also indicate positive adaptation if the individual is not showing other signs of suppressed grief or psychological disturbance. Average scores in the center indicate common reactions. These are general guides for discussion and support only—more research is needed on specific interpretation issues.

Author Note: This scale may be copied and freely used for clinical or supportive purposes. Those wishing to use the scale for research are asked to e-mail for permission meusert@abraxas.wustl.edu (5/04).

Interventions for Predeath Grief

Few studies have been published about intervening with caregiver grief. Those studies that have been reported suggest that grief increases as the dementia's severity increases, and that family caregivers of persons with advanced dementia experience the highest levels of grief. Several themes emerge in the literature concerning the grief experience, including a yearning for the past, regret and guilt, isolation, restricted freedom, life stressors, and coping strategies. Coping strategies

TABLE 17.1

The Marwit-Meuser Caregiver Grief Inventory Subscales

Subscale	Focus and Examples	Targeted Interventions
Personal sacrifice burden	Addresses what the caregiver must give up to function in the caregiving role. Examples: ▪ "Independence is what I've lost . . . I don't have the freedom to go and do what I want." ▪ "I wish I had an hour or two to myself each day to pursue personal interests."	Provide practical services to ease the caregiver's physical burdens of care. Interventions include the involvement of family and friends to assist in care, formal respite services including adult day health care, and consideration of more comprehensive long-term care services, including placement outside the home, in some instances.
Heartfelt sadness and longing	Refers to the personal sadness and separation pain traditionally understood as grief in Western culture. Examples: ▪ "I feel very sad about what this disease has done." ▪ "I long for what was, what we had and shared in the past."	Use interventions aimed at helping the caregiver remain emotionally connected to the person while adjusting to their changing relationship. When the person loses verbal abilities, instruction on nonverbal ways of connecting through music, massage, aromatherapy, and other modes of sensory stimulation may be comforting to the person and healing for the caregiver. Self-expression through writing in a journal and keeping memory books may also help. Support groups provide a venue to share feelings.
Worry and felt isolation	Represents a more pervasive, depressive sense of uncertainty and withdrawal and/or isolation from others. Examples: ▪ "I lie awake most nights worrying about what's happening and how I'll manage tomorrow." ▪ "The people closest to me do not understand what I am going through."	Caregivers may benefit from help by identifying specific worries and developing practical plans to address these concerns. Issues related to isolation can be lessened through encouraging social connections. Social connections may include either formal supports such as Internet, telephone, and in-person groups or informal support of greater involvement of family and friends as well as connections with social and recreational activities.

used by high-grief caregivers include spiritual faith, social supports, and pets. It was suggested that these caregivers may benefit from supportive interventions that are based on reducing feelings of isolation, lack of freedom, and increased guilt and regret, while also addressing feelings of loss. Interventions that facilitate building a supportive network were also said to be helpful. In this regard, family caregivers need to feel appreciated and validated for their roles in caregiving and for continuing the connections with the persons for whom they care. Support groups or any form of emotional support that offers open discussion and nonjudgmental listening seems to help caregivers cope with anticipatory grief. It is not unreasonable to pursue grief counseling or psychotherapy at this phase. Various psychosocial interventions are articulated in the MM-CGI.

Although caregiving burdens would seem to lessen dramatically when a loved one enters a care facility, one study found that depression and anxiety levels remain just as high based on the added element of guilt that the caregiver feels for placing his or her loved one in a facility. Symptoms were particularly noticeable among spousal caregivers, those who were visiting the individual more frequently, and those who were less satisfied with the help they were receiving from others. Clinical services were found to be helpful for family caregivers; specific interventions include having a trained staff member guide the family through placement and mediation for anxiety and depression following placement. In addition, it helped when family and friends were recruited to support caregivers. It is crucial that caregivers with loved ones living in facilities receive adequate assessment of their needs as well as effective interventions that offer support. Table 17.1 presents explanations of the subscales and targeted interventions for the management of caregiver grief.

■ POSTDEATH GRIEF AND BEREAVEMENT

Postdeath Grief Experience

The grief experience that follows a death is often called *bereavement*. The word shares a root with the word *to rob*. Someone or something has been taken or stolen against our wishes. *Grief* and *mourning* more exactly describe the array of responses one has to this loss: the cognitive, emotional, physical, social, and spiritual reactions. People process their grief in different ways, including being numb. Someone can be bereaved without feeling intense emotions. People may grieve the loss of opportunity that has occurred, their hopes and dreams, the ideals or values connected with the person, and even the myths of how the world was supposed to be, in which bereaved persons indulged prior to their loved one's illness.

Time alone does not heal all wounds. Understanding of the loss, acceptance, and expressive action are also necessary. Grieving occurs in stages. One model identifies the following phases:

1. Accepting the reality of the loss
2. Working through the pain of grief
3. Adjusting to and creating an environment in which the deceased is missing
4. Relocating the deceased emotionally and/or spiritually and moving forward in life

Factors Affecting Family Adjustment in Bereavement

This section explores how dementia impacts families who are bereaved, what kind of support is most needed, and how some common expectations or assumptions about grief do not fit the reality.

Families of persons who die after a long progression through dementia have had many experiences of loss, grief, and caregiver burden before the death. The caregiving experience and the context in which the death occurred will have been significant influences. One study found that family caregivers who were able to keep their relative at home showed greater resilience in bereavement. Their depressive symptoms declined within 3 months of the death, and declined further within a year. Most of them said that they felt relieved by the death. Only a minority needed or wanted bereavement support services. In contrast, families in the study whose loved ones died in care facilities did not show the same relief from depression. The relief from caregiver burden that may come with placement is not necessarily balanced with relief from lingering depression in bereavement.

These findings raise important questions about what kind of impact placement has on the bereavement experience. In caregiver focus groups, the decision to institutionalize a loved one consistently emerged as one of the most difficult they faced. Even when the facility-based experience was positive, people frequently continued to feel that they had failed to care for a loved one in the way they might have hoped. There was often trauma associated with the decision to place a loved one in a care facility, accompanied by severe exhaustion, depletion of resources, financial constraints, and extreme immediate behavioral changes in the loved one, or family pressure. It should be quickly noted, however, that each family situation is unique.

A caregiver support group offered in the placement setting could help family caregivers work through difficult feelings. Being able to express themselves and find support with people who listen nonjudgmentally might prepare families for an easier bereavement later on.

How do families adjust to life going forward? One of the few research projects focusing specifically on dementia bereavement identified several common patterns. In one, when primary caregivers had intensely cried and grieved during the time of care, they often found that afterward, there were few tears left to shed. They were ready to move on with life. Their loved one had not been recognizable to them for some time and they had not been able to have a meaningful goodbye at life's end. The need to feel sorrowful grief in large part was met before the death. Most of these family members felt good about the caregiving they had provided.

Other caregivers said they were ready to let go, but expressed feelings of ambivalence and deep sorrow about the final loss. They remembered how their loved ones had lost all their former dignity and personhood and seemed to let go of living. They talked about how they prayed for death to relieve the extended twilight and their own heartbreak. During bereavement, these people felt some shame or guilt about this. It is important for people in this situation to normalize these reactions and resolve any conflicting reactions so they can begin to move forward.

Most families found that it was natural to feel relief at the time of death, but that the relief was often relief mixed with other feelings. When the loved one had been placed in a care setting, guilt, regret, and even anger often surfaced. Some people judged the facility as having failed them in their hopes for, and expectations of, good caregiving. They judged themselves as having let their loved ones down. They looked back at times of anger, frustration, helplessness, and physical decline with feelings of "if only," "should have," and "why." It might be helpful for families in this situation to review the course of the disease and the fact that a decline in eating and drinking, as well as an increased vulnerability to infection, often accompanies the end stage. A realistic review of the caregiving experience, focusing on all that was done and on the limits of control, can help them work through difficult thoughts and feelings. When guilt and anger can be converted into regret for having placed the loved one in a care setting, then mourning can begin.

Instrumental and Intuitive Grieving Patterns

In this culture, we typically think of grief and bereavement as a time of depression and sadness that is best processed by expressing feelings, crying, and attending support and therapy groups. In reality, the grieving experience is very individual. It is influenced by many factors, including one's relationship to the person who died, the circumstances surrounding the death, social and personal variables, and the personality of the bereaved. Many people, especially men, experience grief primarily in cognitive and behavioral ways. That pattern of grief is called *instrumental grieving*. When grief is experienced and expressed in a predominantly emotional way, it is described as *intuitive grieving*.

Instrumental grievers do experience the psychic energy that is generated by loss, but they channel this into thinking about aspects of the loss, solving problems, fulfilling obligations, and taking actions to memorialize the person who died. Most people experience a combination of these grieving patterns, but one usually dominates. These patterns are commonly thought of as male (instrumental) and female (intuitive). However, women who are mostly instrumental in their approach to grieving and men who are mostly intuitive may find very little social, family, and even subjective support for their reactions. They may be relieved to learn that their way of grieving is not abnormal or inadequate.

Providers of grief support can greatly help families by identifying and affirming each individual's unique pattern. Family members often fail to understand and accept each other's grieving pattern. Education can help resolve conflicts and boost mutual support. Various approaches to bereavement might be suggested, so each person can find what is most comforting to him or her. Planting a tree or funding a scholarship in a loved one's honor will appeal to instrumental grievers. Support groups and memory books are more helpful to intuitive grievers.

Finding New Roles and Moving Forward

Bereavement support can offer practical help to caregivers who report feeling lost and without a role in life following a loved one's death. Many have been out of social circulation and the job market for years, and must reestablish a social identity and find employment. They may have lost significant sources of support if they were too engaged in caretaking to continue spiritual practices. Caregivers who found comfort in Alzheimer's support groups now begin to lose connections with other members of the group. Others who have visited their loved ones in care facilities for several years may lose the relationships they had developed with staff, other residents, and their families. Encouraging people to list their support sources and to identify what kinds of support they derive from different people or places can be the beginning of reconnecting. They may have neglected their health and need encouragement to see their physicians and to pay attention to their personal well-being. Depleted caregivers often require months to restore their strength and reserves. They may find that they need to defer the hard work of mourning during this time. For others, bereavement becomes a time to rediscover meaning in life. It is important for those persons providing grief support to know what spiritual and psychological resources are available in the community and to be able to assess, give referrals, and provide coaching in rebuilding a meaningful life.

Bereavement Support for Professional Caregivers

Professional caregivers often develop long-term relationships with the individuals for whom they care and with their families. Their role entails the sort of nurturing, patience, and physical care that a parent gives a child. This kind of work can foster deep feelings of responsibility and protectiveness. As the individual's health declines, caregivers too may grieve the loss of the person they knew and the way things used to be.

When a person dies, the loss is felt on several levels. In a short time span, the caregiver has lost the person for whom he or she had been caring, contact with the family, and sometimes his or her employment. As a caregiver, he or she may have functioned as a trusted surrogate family member. As this role ends, a caregiver may feel unacknowledged and disenfranchised. If a caregiver works in a placement setting, he or she may lose contact with family members who stop visiting.

Caregivers' agencies, coworkers, and employers need to acknowledge their grief. Caregivers deserve validation and appreciation for all the care they provided, a chance to release themselves from any feelings of responsibility for the individual's decline or physical death, and the opportunity to attend a memorial service or funeral. Institutional rituals can help: quarterly bereavement meetings, a place for sharing photographs and mementos, and a meaningful interval being allowed to elapse before the person's bed is filled or the caregiver takes on a new assignment. Bereavement assistance from a religious community can also help.

■ REFERENCES

Boss, P. (1999). *Ambiguous loss: Learning to live with unresolved grief.* Cambridge, MA: Harvard University Press.

Boss, P., Caron, W., Horbal, J., & Mortimer, J. (1990). Predictors of depression in caregivers of dementia patients: Boundary ambiguity and mastery. *Family Process, 29*(3), 245–254.

Frank, J. B. (2008). Evidence for grief as the major barrier faced by Alzheimer caregivers: A qualitative analysis. *American Journal of Alzheimer's Disorders and Other Dementias, 22*(6), 516–27.

Freyne, A., Kidd, N., Coen, R., & Lawlor, B. A. (1999). Burden in carers of dementia patients: Higher levels in carers of younger sufferers. *International Journal of Geriatric Psychiatry, 14*(9), 784–788.

Holley, C. K., & Mast, B. T. (2009). The impact of anticipatory grief on caregiver burden in dementia caregivers. *Gerontologist, 49*(3), 388–396.

Jones, P. S., & Martinson, I. M. (1992). The experience of bereavement in caregivers of family members with Alzheimer's disease. *Image: Journal of Nursing Scholarship, 24*(3), 172–176.

Kiely, D. K., Prigerson, H., & Mitchell, S. L. (2008, August). Health care proxy grief symptoms before the death of nursing home residents with advanced dementia. *American Journal of Geriatric Psychiatry, 16*(8), 664–673.

Kovach, C. R., Wilson, S. A., & Noonan, P. E. (1996). Effects of hospice interventions on behaviors, discomfort, and physical complications of end-stage dementia in nursing home residents. *American Journal of Alzheimer's Disease, 11*(4), 7–10.

Lucero, M. (2004). Enhancing the visits of loved ones of people in late-stage dementia. *Alzheimer's Care Quarterly, 5*(2), 173–177.

Luscombe, G., Brodaty, H., & Freeth, S. (1998). Younger people with dementia: Diagnostic issues, effects on carers and use of services. *International Journal of Geriatric Psychiatry, 13*(5), 323–330.

Mack, K., & Thompson, L. (2004). *A decade of informal caregiving: Are today's informal caregivers different than informal caregivers a decade ago?* Washington, DC: Center on an Aging Society. Retrieved January 25, 2010, from http://ihcrp.georgetown.edu/agingsociety/pubhtml/caregiver1/caregiver1.html

Martin, T., & Doka, K. (2000). *Men don't cry . . . women do: Transcending gender stereotypes of grief.* Philadelphia: Brunner/Mazel Publishers, Inc.

Marwit, S. J., & Meuser, T. M. (2002). Development and initial validation of an inventory to measure grief in caregivers of persons with Alzheimer's disease. *The Gerontologist, 42*(6), 51–65.

Marwit, S. J., & Meuser, T. M. (2005). Development of a short form inventory to assess grief in caregivers of dementia patients. *Death Studies, 29*(3), 191–205.

Meuser, T. M., & Marwit, S. J. (2001). A comprehensive, stage-sensitive model of grief in dementia caregiving. *The Gerontologist, 41*(5), 658–670.

Meuser, T. M., Marwit, S. J., & Sanders, S. (2004). Assessing grief in family caregivers. In K. J. Doka (Ed.), *Living with grief: Alzheimer's disease* (pp. 169–195). Washington, DC: Hospice Foundation of America.

National Family Caregiver Association. (2005). *Common bonds of caregiving.* Retrieved January 23, 2010, from http://www.thefamilycaregiver.org/who_are_family_caregivers/common_bonds_of_caregiving.cfm

Ott, C. H., Sanders, S., & Kelber, S. T. (2007). Grief and personal growth experience of spouses and adult-child caregivers of individuals with Alzheimer's disease and related dementias. *The Gerontologist, 47*(6), 798–809.

Ponder, R. J., & Pomeroy, E. C. (1996). The grief of caregivers: How pervasive is it? *Journal of Gerontological Social Work, 27*, 3–21.

Rabow, M. W., Hauser, J. M., & Adams, J. (2004). Supporting family caregivers at the end of life: "They don't know what they don't know." *The Journal of the American Medical Association, 291*(4), 483–491.

Rando, T. A. (2000). Anticipatory mourning: A review and critique of the literature. In T. A. Rando (Ed.), *Clinical dimensions of anticipatory mourning: Theory and practice in working with the dying, their loved ones, and their caregivers* (pp. 17–50). Champaign, IL: Research Press.

Sanders, S., Marwit, S. J., Meuser, T. M., & Harrington, P. (2007). Caregiver grief in end-state dementia: Using the Marwit and Meuser Caregiver Grief Inventory for assessment and intervention in social work practice. *Social Work Health Care, 46*(1), 47–65.

Sanders, S., Ott, C. H., Kelber, S. T., & Noonan, P. (2008). The experience of high levels of grief in care-givers of persons with Alzheimer's disease and related dementia. *Death Studies, 32*(6), 495–523.

Schulz, R., & Beach, S. (1999). Caregiving as a risk factor for mortality: The Caregiver Health Effects Study. *Journal of the American Medical Association, 282*(23), 2215–2219.

Schulz, R., Belle, S. H., Czaja, S. J., McGinnis, K. A., Stevens, A., & Zhang, S. (2004). Long-term care placement of dementia patients and caregiver health and well-being. *The Journal of the American Medical Association, 292*(8), 961–967.

Schulz, R., Mendelsohn, A. B., Haley, W. E., Mahoney, D., Allen, R. S., Zhang, S., et al. (2003). End-of-life care and the effects of bereavement on family caregivers of persons with dementia. *The New England Journal of Medicine, 349*(20), 1936–1942.

Wasow, M., & Coons, D. (1987). Widows and widowers of Alzheimer's victims: Their survival after spouses' death. *Journal of Independent Social Work, 2*(2), 21–23.

Worden, J. W. (2008). *Grief counseling and grief therapy: A handbook for the mental health practitioner* (4th ed.). New York: Springer Publishing.

Zhang, B., Mitchell, S. L., Bambauer, K. Z., Jones, R., & Prigerson, H. G. (2008). Depressive symptom trajectories and associated risks among bereaved Alzheimer disease caregivers. *American Journal of Geriatric Psychiatry, 16*(2), 145–155.

ESTABLISHING HEALTHCARE-RELATED LEGAL OPTIONS FOR THE VULNERABLE PATIENT

Paul Harrington, Jill Preston, Dawn Savattone, and
Barbara Volk-Craft

▥ INTRODUCTION

When people with dementia have lost capacity and have no one with legal authority to make healthcare decisions for them, the facility must explore other options. These individuals are vulnerable, as they have no one to speak on their behalf. This group of individuals has been called the *unbefriended elderly* by the American Bar Association. It is estimated that 3%–4% of all nursing home residents fall into this category. Each healthcare provider must determine how to handle these types of situations. What can be done to assist these persons, ethically, and with ease, so that the facility and staff can provide appropriate care, and so that the rights of the individual are not compromised? There are two options to evaluate:

1. Using the legal system to appoint a guardian.
2. Finding alternatives to guardianship.

▥ GUARDIANSHIP AND CONSERVATORSHIP

A guardian is a court-appointed individual who makes personal, placement, and medical decisions for someone who is incapacitated. The incapacitated person is called the *ward*. A guardian has powers similar to those of a parent for a child, although the guardian is not required to provide financial support. A guardian makes decisions about the ward's living arrangements and medical care.

Conservatorship is a legal concept in the United States, whereby an entity or organization is subjected to the legal control of an external entity or organization, known as a *conservator*. Conservatorship is established either by court order (with regard to individuals) or via a statutory or regulatory authority (with regard to organizations). Many jurisdictions use the term *guardianship* to refer to the same legal principle (in California, conservatorships are for adults and guardianships are for children). A person under conservatorship is a *conservatee* or a protected person, whereas a person under guardianship is a *ward*. In most states, a court visitor or some other investigatory person or agency must review the case's facts and submit a report, usually required to be in writing, to the court before the court makes a decision on the request to establish a conservatorship or guardianship. Court visitors are often required to be experts in some appropriate field, such as social work or law. The court may appoint an attorney to represent the proposed conservatee or ward. If the proposed conservatee or ward is unable to have an attorney–client relationship because of some impairment, the court may appoint a *guardian-ad-litem* (who is often also an attorney). A guardian-ad-litem does not take instruction from the client, but rather tells the court what the guardian-ad-litem thinks is in the best interests of the proposed conservatee or ward, whether or not that is what the proposed conservatee or ward wants.

The legal guardianship process can be lengthy and costly. Once the court is petitioned for the appointment of a guardian, the court then schedules a hearing on the incapacity of the proposed ward. An attorney is appointed to represent the proposed ward. A court investigator is assigned to interview family members and friends and to make a report to the court. A physician's report regarding capacity issues is also necessary. At the hearing, the judge or commissioner hears testimony, considers the physician's report, and decides whether to appoint a guardian.

Generally, it takes about 6–8 weeks for a guardianship hearing to be held. If the situation is an emergency, a petition for the temporary appointment of a guardian can be filed. A hearing on the temporary appointment can be held within approximately 3–10 working days.

The guardianship and conservatorship process can be complicated. Guardianship is protection for the ward. Conservatorship is protection for the ward's finances. It is recommended that family members consult with an experienced attorney to evaluate their situation. The family should bring important legal documents, such as powers of attorney, trusts, and wills to the appointment for the attorney to review. The family should also bring documents identifying their loved one's financial assets. It is important that all legal and financial documents be provided for the attorney to review, so to facilitate the evaluation of the ward's information and provide appropriate guidance on steps to be taken. If a guardianship or conservatorship is necessary, the attorney can prepare the documents and initiate court proceedings.

The healthcare facility should identify which individuals are without an agent or surrogate before healthcare needs arise. Who are the unbefriended elderly in your facility? There still may be time to find a willing surrogate or name an agent. Waiting too long to begin this process may limit options. There may be other ways to handle healthcare decisions without a costly guardianship or conservatorship action. If guardianship is needed, the facility should have a list of qualified elder law attorneys available to use for referrals (see Exhibit 18.1).

EXHIBIT 18.1

A Case Study on Guardianship

Mrs. L has advanced dementia and is in a skilled nursing center. She is married and has no children and no family in the area. She no longer has the capacity to make medical or financial decisions. Her husband had been acting as her agent under her healthcare power of attorney, but unexpectedly, Mr. L had a heart attack and died. Mrs. L had not named a secondary agent. Who is going to act on her behalf? Because there are no family members or close friends to act in her best interest, and because there now is no one to handle her financial affairs for her, the facility must call on other resources available to them to petition the court to get a guardian and conservator appointed. This process could have been avoided if a secondary agent had been named prior to Mrs. L's loss of capacity.

Alternatives to Guardianship

Having an agent named in a healthcare power of attorney is really the best way to avoid the issue of guardianship. The use of an identified statutory surrogate is the next alternative. The mechanism by which to identify this surrogate varies from state to state. Having a plan in place to identify those who do not have an agent assigned and no known surrogate offers the potential of finding a voice for the person before a need occurs.

Names of possible surrogates, who were identified while the person was hospitalized, are often omitted from healthcare records that follow patients from one facility to another, because in some states surrogate decision-making powers are limited to each treatment decision. Key contacts and other valuable information are often lost forever.

A surrogate identification worksheet, such as the one shown in Exhibit 18.2, can be used as a tool to assist professionals in recognizing family members, friends, and

EXHIBIT 18.2

Sample of a Surrogate Identification Worksheet [a]

PATIENT'S NAME: _____ DOB: _____

Directions: This form is used to specify the type of surrogate who will make healthcare decisions for the above patient when s/he is unable to do so. The person responsible for locating a surrogate decision maker shall contact the following individual(s) in the indicated order of priority below who

[a] This identification of a surrogate worksheet is modeled from the one used in from Arizona. This is used as an example only. These worksheets will differ from state to state.

Continued

Exhibit 18.2 *Continued*

are available and willing to serve as a surrogate. Documentation of contacts/results may be noted on this form and/or in the patient's chart.

SELECT ONE:

APPOINTED SURROGATE(S): A person authorized to make healthcare decisions on behalf of the patient.

____ Guardian appointed for the express purpose of making healthcare treatment decisions (place copy in medical record).

____ Agent under healthcare power of attorney (place copy in medical record).

IF NEITHER IS AVAILABLE, make reasonable efforts to contact and verify that the person(s) is unwilling or unable to serve as surrogate decision maker before moving to the next in priority:

____ 1. The patient's spouse (unless the patient and spouse are legally separated).

____ 2. An adult child of the patient (if the patient has more than one adult child, the health provider shall seek the consent of a majority of adult children who are reasonably available for consultation) – list all children serving as surrogates below.

____ 3. A parent of the patient.

____ 4. If the patient is unmarried, the patient's domestic partner (if no other person has assumed any financial responsibility for the patient.

____ 5. A brother or sister of patient.

____ 6. A close friend of patient (an adult who has exhibited special care and concern for the patient, who is familiar with the patient's healthcare views and desires and who is willing and able to become involved in the patient's healthcare and to act in the patient's best interest).

IF NONE OF THE ABOVE CAN BE LOCATED:

____ Attending physician
   a. after the physician consults with and obtains the recommendations of an institutional ethics committee OR IF THIS IS NOT POSSIBLE
   b. after consulting with a second physician who concurs with the physician's decision

NOTES:

_____

_____

IDENTIFIED SURROGATE(S) – please include name, relationship to patient, address, and phone number(s) for each identified surrogate:

_____

_____

_____

PERSON COMPLETING FORM: _____ DATE: _____

TITLE: _____

HEALTH PROVIDER/FACILITY: _____

others close to the patient who are available to make healthcare decisions when needed. This worksheet should become a permanent part of the patient's records. Patients with dementia are often victims of either too much or too little treatment when a surrogate cannot be identified quickly, and valuable surrogate information can help keep them from becoming vulnerable within the system.

The facility's creation of a healthcare directive procedure is crucial to the success of naming an agent or surrogate. A qualified staff member can be assigned to coordinate the alternative to guardianship effort and keep tasks well defined. Often these issues are difficult for families to discuss. It is vital to provide a welcoming and professional environment for discussion.

The following example of a facility plan can be used to help identify decision makers (see Exhibit 18.3):

1. Identify a specific person in the facility to be in charge of this effort and act as an investigator of surrogates.
2. Identify the unbefriended elder before possible issues arise.
3. Review the person's abilities to execute a healthcare power of attorney.
4. Document expressed wishes.
5. Take proper steps to find a surrogate. Evaluate surrogacy possibilities and document on the Surrogate Identification Worksheet.
6. If no surrogate can be found, look at alternative options. Include outside resources to assist with plan.
7. Evaluate the financial options for legal guardianship process.
8. Call the local Area Agency on Aging (AAA) for further assistance.

EXHIBIT 18.3

A Case Study of Identifying Decision Makers

Consider the case study described earlier involving Mr. and Mrs. L. Now, instead of imagining them without children, let us assume that they have a grown child, a daughter, living out of state. The daughter, in this instance, was not listed as a secondary agent under the power of attorney. The facility used the Surrogate Identification Worksheet to investigate whether she wanted to be involved and asked her to act as surrogate. After the facility investigation, she consented to act as medical surrogate, but she did not want to be involved in financial matters. As there is now a surrogate for medical decisions, but not financial, this eliminated the need for the appointment of a guardian. Mrs. L's financial affairs still need to be managed. The daughter needs to hire an elder law attorney to petition the court for a conservator, thereby getting all surrogate decision makers in place.

It is a detailed process to determine who might be an appropriate agent, whether a healthcare power of attorney, statutory surrogate, or guardian. The process is never the same but the need for inquiry and investigation of appropriate surrogates remains. The burden for completing this process lies within the healthcare community. Although it is widely agreed that respect for autonomous decision making is a fundamental ethical principle that should consistently guide healthcare delivery, there is much to be done to make this a reality (see Exhibit 18.4).

EXHIBIT 18.4

Guidelines for Establishing Healthcare Facility Policy for Healthcare Decision Making

A. The healthcare facility shall:
  1. Establish a policy and procedure to solicit and document advance directives from individuals with dementia in a timely manner if they are able to participate in decision making. The policy and procedure will include:
    a. Designation of a person(s) or position(s) in the facility to be responsible for advance care planning activities;
    b. Identification of an acceptable time frame for staff to meet with person or family and assist the person with dementia to complete a new advance directive if needed; and
    c. Documentation of requirements that clearly communicate the process of advance care planning, what has been done, and what remains to be done.

2. Establish a policy and procedure to obtain and file previously executed advance directives (advance directives that were completed by an individual prior to admission to the long-term care facility) from an individual with dementia or family. The policy and procedure will include:
   a. Designation of a person(s) or position(s) in the facility to be responsible for follow-up efforts to obtain previously-executed advance directives;
   b. Identification of an acceptable time frame for staff to obtain and file previously executed advance directives;
   c. Identification of steps the staff will take if these previously-executed advance directives are not readily available, including notification of facility administrator for assistance; and
   d. Documentation of requirements that clearly communicate what steps have been taken to obtain these previously-executed advance directives, what staff members have been involved in the efforts, and what the outcome of the efforts is.
3. Establish a policy and procedure to identify the legal surrogate decision maker(s) for each individual with dementia who lacks decision-making capacity. The policy and procedure will include:
   a. Designation of a person(s) or position(s) in the facility to be responsible to identify the legal surrogate(s) who will make healthcare decisions on behalf of an individual with dementia who lacks decision-making capacity;
   b. Identification of an acceptable time frame for staff to identify and document the identity of the surrogate decision maker(s);
   c. Identification of a time frame to review advance directive documents (e.g., care-planning sessions) that may require changes or updating to meet the person with advanced dementia's needs;
   d. Ensuring that the identity of the legal surrogate decision maker(s) is readily available and accessible to care staff around the clock; and
   e. Outlining a follow-up process if a surrogate decision maker is not readily identified, including notification of the facility administrator.
4. Designate experienced person(s) or position(s) that will have the responsibility to meet with the person with dementia and surrogate decision makers to:
   a. Discuss the progression of dementia;
   b. Review the common healthcare decisions that a person with dementia will face over the course of the disease;
   c. Explain options for medical treatment, including risks and benefits;
   d. Facilitate the completion of advance directives documents (if the person with dementia has decision-making ability) or advance surrogate decision-making documents (if the person with dementia lacks decision-making capacity); and
   e. Review advance-care planning documents and treatment choices when the person with dementia experiences a significant change in condition.

Continued

Exhibit 18.4 *Continued*

   5. Provide (either directly or through community resources) educational opportunities for individuals, their families, and facility staff to learn about advance directives, the role of a surrogate decision maker, and other issues related to advance care planning.

B. Healthcare staff shall:
   1. Consistently obtain previously executed advance-directive documents from the person with dementia or his or her family.
   2. Place all advance-directive documents and advance surrogate decision-making documents in a readily accessible and confidential file (e.g., medical record or chart).
   3. Ensure that copies of all advance directive documents and advance surrogate decision-making documents are available at all times and that a copy of these documents accompanies the person with dementia any time that person leaves the facility premises for medical care.
   4. Meet with the person with dementia and surrogate decision makers to:
      a. Discuss the progression of dementia;
      b. Review the common healthcare decisions that a person with dementia will face over the course of the disease;
      c. Explain options for medical treatment, including risks and benefits;
      d. Facilitate the completion of advance directives documents (if the person with dementia has decision-making ability) or advance surrogate decision-making documents (if the person with dementia lacks decision-making capacity); and
      e. Review advance care planning documents and treatment choices with the person with dementia and/or family or surrogate whenever the person with dementia experiences a significant change in condition.

C. Persons with advanced dementia shall expect:
   1. Previously-executed advance directives are obtained, reviewed, filed, and remain readily accessible in their medical record to ensure that their expressed wishes are respected and honored.
   2. A designated and experienced facility staff person(s) to meet with them and/or their legal surrogate decision maker(s) to communicate the progression of dementia, common healthcare decisions encountered over the course of the disease, methods to maintain dignity and comfort, and medical treatment options, including risks and benefits.
   3. A facility staff person(s) to provide information about educational opportunities for persons, their families, and their legal surrogate decision maker(s) to learn about advance directives, the role of a surrogate decision maker, and other issues related to advance care planning.
   4. Depending on decisional capacity, a designated facility staff person(s) to attempt to either facilitate the completion of new advance directives or identify legal surrogate decision makers(s) in a timely manner (for persons who have not executed advance directives).

5. Healthcare and/or legal resources to be contacted if concerns arise related to healthcare decisions or advance directive issues.
6. Copies of all advance directive documents and surrogate advance decision-making documents to accompany them any time they leave the facility premises for medical care.
7. A designated, experienced staff person(s) to review advance care planning documents and treatment choices with them and/or their surrogate decision maker(s) whenever a significant change in condition occurs.

REFERENCES

Allen, R. S., DeLaine, S. R., Chaplin, W. F., Marson, D. C., Bourgeois, M. S., Dijkstra, K., et al. (2003). Advance care planning in nursing homes: Correlates of capacity and possession of advance directives. *The Gerontologist, 43*(3), 309–317.

American Geriatrics Society Ethics Committee. (1998). *Making treatment decisions for incapacitated elderly patients without advance directives* (monograph). American Geriatrics Society Position Statement. Retrieved March 27, 2005, from http://www.americangeriatrics.org/products/positionpapers/treatdecPF.shtml

Chen, J., Lamberg, J. L., Chen, Y., Kiely, D. K., Page, J. H. Person, C. J., et al. (2006). Occurrence and treatment of suspected pneumonia in long-term care residents dying with advanced dementia. *Journal of the American Geriatrics Society, 54*(2), 290–295.

Cohen-Mansfield, J. (2002). Development of a framework to encourage addressing advance directives when resources are limited. *Journal of Aging & Health, 14*, 24–41.

Fabiszewski, K. J., Volicer, B. J., & Volicer, L. (1990). Effect of antibiotic treatment on outcome of fevers in institutionalized Alzheimer patients. *Journal of the American Medical Association, 263*(23), 3168–3172.

Finucane, T. E., Christmas, C., & Travis, K. (1999). Tube feeding in patients with advanced dementia: A review of the evidence. *Journal of the American Medical Association, 282*(14), 1365–1370.

Frissoni, G. B., Franzoni, S., Bellelli, G., Morris, J., & Warden, V. (1998). Overcoming eating difficulties in the severely demented. In L. Volicer & A. Hurley (Eds.), *Hospice care for patients with advanced progressive dementia* (pp. 48–67). New York: Springer.

General Powers and Duties of Guardian, ARS 14-5312 (A) and (8)(9), (n.d.).

Golleher v. Horton, 148 ARS 14-5506 (App. 1985).

Hirschman, K. B., Joyce, C. M., James, B. D., Xie, S. X., & Karlawish, J. H. (2005). Do Alzheimer's disease patients want to participate in a treatment decision, and would their caregivers let them? *The Gerontologist, 45*(3), 381–388.

Hurley, A. C., Volicer, B. J., Mahoney, M. A., & Volicer, L. (1993). Palliative fever management in Alzheimer patients. quality plus fiscal responsibility. *Advances in Nursing Science, 16*, 21–32.

Kayser-Jones, J. (1996). Mealtime in nursing homes: The importance of individualized care. *Journal of Gerontological Nursing, 22*(3), 26–31.

Karlawish, J. H. T., Casarett, D. J., James, B. D., Xie, S. X., & Kim, S. Y. (2005). The ability of persons with Alzheimer disease (AD) to make a decision about taking an AD treatment. *Neurology, 64*(9), 1514–1519.

Karp, N., & Wood, E. (2003). *Incapacitated and alone: Health care decision-making for the unbefriended elderly.* Washington, DC: American Bar Association Commission on Law and Aging.

Koppelman, E. R. (2002). Dementia and dignity: Towards a new method of surrogate decision making. *Journal of Medicine and Philosophy, 27*, 65–85.

Lamberg, J. L., Person, C. J., Kiely, D. K., & Mitchell, S. L. (2005). Decisions to hospitalize nursing home residents dying with advanced dementia. *Journal of the American Geriatrics Society, 53*(8), 1396–1401.

Leland, J. (2001). Advance directives and establishing goals of care. *Primary Care, 28*(2), 349–363.

Living Wills and Health Care Directives, ARS 36-3231 (1992).

Luchins, D. J., Hanrahan, P., & Murphy, K. (1997). Criteria for enrolling dementia patients in hospice. *Journal of the American Geriatric Society, 45*(9), 1054–1059.

Mahoney, E. K., Volicer, L., & Hurley, A. C. (2000). Food refusal. In E. K. Mahoney, L. Volicer, & A. C. Hurley (Eds.), *Management of challenging behaviors in dementia* (pp. 155–170). Baltimore, MD: Health Professionals Press, Inc.

McCann, R. M., Hall, W. J., & Groth-Juncker, A. (1994). Comfort care for terminally ill patients: The appropriate use of nutrition and hydration. *The Journal of the American Medical Association, 272*(16), 1263–1266.

Morrison, R. S., Chichin, E., Carter, J., Burack, O., Lantz, M., & Meier, D. E. (2005). The effect of a social work intervention to enhance advance care planning in the nursing home. *Journal of the American Geriatric Society, 53*(2), 290–294.

Powers of attorney; best interest; intimidation; deception; definitions ARS 14-5506 (F)(2) (n.d.).

Protection of Person Under Disability, Definitions, ARS 14-5101 (n.d.).

Rhodes, R., & Holzman, I. R. (2004). The not unreasonable standard for assessment of surrogates and surrogate decisions. *Theory of Medical Bioethics, 25*(4), 367–385.

Seal, M. K. (2004). Arizona consumers guide to guardianship and conservatorship. Mesa, AZ: JacksonWhite Law Firm, P.C.

Smith, S. J. (1998). Providing palliative care for the terminal Alzheimer's patient. In L. Volicer, & A. Hurley (Eds.), *Hospice care for patients with advanced progressive dementia* (pp. 247–256). New York: Springer.

Volicer, L., Brandeis, G. H., & Hurley, A. C. (1998). Infections in advanced dementia. In L. Volicer & A. Hurley (Eds.), *Hospice care for patients with advanced progressive dementia* (pp. 29–47). New York: Springer.

Volicer, L., Rheaume, Y., Riley, M. E., Karner, J., & Glennon, M. (1990). Discontinuation of tube feeding in patients with dementia of the Alzheimer's type. *American Journal of Alzheimer's Care and Related Disorders and Research, 5*, 22–25.

Volicer, L., Seltzer, B., Rheaume, Y., Karner, J., Glennon, M., Riley, M. E., et al. (1989). Eating difficulties in patients with probable dementia of the Alzheimer's type. *Journal of Geriatric Psychiatry and Neurology, 2*(4), 188–195.

Warden, V. J. (1989). Waste not, want not. *Geriatric Nursing, 10*, 210–211.

White, R. A., Macdonald, E. K., & Seal, M. K. (2004). *Alzheimer's and the law.* Mesa, AZ: Jackson-White Law Firm, PC.

Winzelberg, G. S., Hanson, L. C., & Tulsky, J. A. (2005). Beyond autonomy: Diversifying end-of-life decision-making approaches to serve patients and families. *Journal of the American Geriatric Society, 53*(6), 1046–1050.

GLOSSARY

Activities of daily living (ADLs): Activities regularly performed by a person throughout the course of a normal day. These include walking, eating, dressing, grooming, toileting, and bathing.

Advance care planning: Care planning that identifies choices for end-of-life care. It includes written plans for future healthcare, particularly for the time when the person is unable to make his or her own decisions.

Advance directives: Documents that allow an individual to make decisions about future healthcare and to designate who will be authorized to make decisions on his or her behalf. These documents take effect when the person becomes mentally or physically unable to make or communicate wishes. Examples include a living will, healthcare or mental healthcare power of attorney, and prehospital medical care directives.

Artificially administered: Providing food or fluid through a medically invasive procedure. Examples include a tube inserted through the nose, a tube inserted into the stomach or intestine, or an intravenous needle.

Assisted-living facility: A residential care institution, including adult foster care, that provides or contracts to provide continuing supervisory care services, personal care services, or directed care services.

Bathing without a battle: Phrase used to describe bathing practices that minimize the distress experienced by persons with advanced dementia; also called towel or bed baths. Relates to interventions that promote a positive bathing experience and are often performed in bed using warm sheets and towels and a no-rinse soap. The experience may seem more like a gentle massage than a bath.

Best interest: A surrogate decision maker's good faith belief as to what is best for the incapacitated individual, applied in cases when the individual's expressed wishes are not known and the surrogate does not have enough information to imagine what the individual would want. Most often used when no one knows the individual well, or when the individual has no close relatives or friends to make decisions on his or her behalf.

Capacity: The ability to comprehend, make, and communicate a decision.

Caregiver: An adult who provides functionally impaired adults with supervision and assistance in the instrumental activities of daily living (caregiving).

Comfort care: Treatment and care given to protect and enhance a person's quality of life without artificially prolonging life. Pain management is emphasized.

Comfort food: In terms of dementia, any food that a person will accept, eat, and tolerate.

Consent: An agreement of one person to accept the actions of another on his or her behalf. A consent is voluntary given by one who still has the capacity to choose and who is fully informed of the implications of that choice.

Conservator: Person appointed by the court in a legal proceeding to act as the legal representative of a person who is mentally or physically incapable of managing his or her own finances.

Competency: Legal term for capacity.

Culturally appropriate care: Refers to an awareness of one's own existence, sensations, thoughts, and environment without letting it have an undue influence on those from other backgrounds. The ability of an individual, organization, or practitioner to recognize the cultural beliefs (in the context of cultural competence [see *culturally competent care*]), attitudes, and health practices of diverse populations and to apply that knowledge in every intervention at the systems level or at the individual level, to produce a positive health outcome.

Culturally competent care: Caregivers displaying *cultural competence* demonstrate knowledge and understanding of the patient's culture, acceptance and respect of cultural differences, and accordingly adapt to be congruent with the person's culture. Cultural competence refers to attention to the total context of care.

Culturally sensitive care: Culturally sensitive care refers to some basic knowledge of culture care with respect and attention to traditions and knowledge of the culture.

Culture: Culture is a system of shared symbols, serving as guides for interactions with others.

Delirium: State of temporary but acute confusion that is manifested suddenly. There are many possible causes. This state is considered to be life threatening and requires immediate medical intervention.

Dementia friendly: Any program or service interventions that provide comfort and palliative care for people with advanced dementia or other forms of dementia.

Directed care services: Programs and services provided to people who are incapable of recognizing danger, summoning assistance, expressing needs, or making basic care decisions.

Documentation: Written, supportive evidence, as in a person's medical record or healthcare facilities records.

Durable power of attorney: Written designation of an adult, called an agent, to make financial decisions on the author's behalf during periods of incapacity. The appointed agent does not have the authority to make healthcare decisions unless specifically stated in the document.

Express wishes: Decisions regarding healthcare treatment(s) that a person makes verbally or in writing.

Environment: This refers to the physical aspects of a milieu where a person with advanced dementia resides. Includes the dimensions and arrangement of the living space, all objects or items within that living space, lighting, temperature, and noise.

Extrinsic factors: Anything relating to the physical environment that is external to a person's body.

Family: A group of two or more individuals related by ties of blood, legal status, or affection to the individual and who consider themselves a family unit.

Grooming: The activities and care related to an individual's personal hygiene and outward appearance.

Guardian: Person appointed by the court to make personal, placement, and medical decisions for someone who is incapacitated.

Guidelines: Relevant principles that apply to defining or delivering care to persons with advanced dementia. The guidelines form the basis of the standards.

Healthcare decisions: Also known as healthcare directives or advance directives; these documents stipulate a person's choices for future medical care needs.

Healthcare facility or institution: An institution, building, or agency (nonprofit or otherwise) that provides medical, nursing, health screening, and other health-related service; supervisory-, personal-, and directed-care services; and includes home health agencies and hospice service agencies.

Healthcare power of attorney: Document designating an adult, called an agent, who can make healthcare decisions on the author's behalf during periods of incapacity. A healthcare power of attorney is considered durable if the appointment of the agent is not limited by time or circumstance. Sometimes referred to as a medical power of attorney.

Healthcare staff: Paid employees who perform direct or indirect services for a person in a healthcare facility or agency.

Home: A person's place of residence.

Home healthcare agency: A healthcare facility or institution that provides skilled nursing and other therapeutic services to those persons residing in homes or homelike settings.

Hospice: A healthcare facility, institution, program, or entity that provides end-of-life care for those in the later or final stages of life.

Incapacity: The inability to comprehend, make, or communicate personal decisions. Incapacity can be mental or physical and may be temporary or permanent.

Incontinence: Loss of bladder and/or bowel control.

Interdisciplinary team: Members who provide a wide diversity of clinical services and who typically collaborate to review, evaluate, and update the care plan for people with advanced dementia. May include members of the person's family, the primary care physician, a hospice or palliative care physician, registered nurses, caregivers or certified nursing assistants, social workers, a spiritual counselor, a bereavement counselor, an activity professional, trained volunteers, and therapists.

Intrinsic factors: Relates to a person's internal body system.

Life story: Also known as a *life history* or *biosketch*; a summation of a person's background and past that identifies the important people, milestones, pleasures, and life experiences.

Living will: A document that makes known a person's wishes regarding healthcare treatment. It is intended to guide or control treatment decisions that can be made on a person's behalf and is typically used in conjunction with a person's healthcare power of attorney.

Meaningful connections: Substantive interactions between the caregiver and the person with advanced dementia that result in positive reactions from the person during an activity.

Medication: Refers to an administered or self-administered prescription or nonprescription drug, administered to or self-administered by a person to maintain health or to prevent or treat an illness or disease.

Mental healthcare power of attorney: A document that allows a designated representative, called an agent, to make mental healthcare treatment decisions for an individual who is incapacitated. The authority of the agent becomes effective when a psychiatrist or psychologist determines the author to be incapacitated.

Milieu: The overall setting in which a person with advanced dementia lives. It includes the physical environment and its ambience, as well as the social, psychological, and cultural qualities of that setting.

Nursing facility: A multioccupant facility that provides primary caregiver services.

Nursing care institution: A healthcare institution providing inpatient beds or resident beds and nursing services to persons who need nursing services on a continuing basis but who do not require hospital care or direct daily care from a physician.

Pain: An unpleasant physical or mental experience causing undue distress and discomfort.

Palliative care: The World Health Organization defines palliative care as "the active total care of persons whose disease is not responsive to curative treatment." Control of pain, of other symptoms, and of psychological, social, and spiritual problems is paramount. The goal of palliative care is achievement of the best possible quality of life for persons and their families. With advanced dementia, it is holistic comfort care and includes interventions to address symptom control, psychological needs of patients and families, quality of life, dignity, safety, respect for personhood, emphasis on the use of intact patient abilities, and manipulation of the environment.

Palliative care programming for advanced dementia: A care program involving the interdisciplinary team that focuses on physiological, psychological, social, and spiritual well-being as they relate to quality of life. Addresses comfort needs in a respectful and dignified manner.

Person: Within the context of this guidebook, an individual with advanced dementia.

Personal surroundings: Those aspects of the environment in a person's living space that are either intentionally or unintentionally experienced by the person.

Personhood: The state of being human. The term encompasses the belief that each person has value, status, integrity, self-esteem, and self-identity.

Plan of care: Written program of action for each person's care, based on an assessment of his or her physical, nutritional, psychosocial, economic, and environmental strengths and needs. Includes short- and long-term goals; also called the *care plan*.

Primary care provider: Individual who has expertise in providing healthcare services and supervision to persons with advanced dementia. In this guidebook, refers to physicians and nurse practitioners who are part of the interdisciplinary team.

Prognosis: The probable course of a disease process as predicted by a physician.

Restraint: Any chemical or physical method of restricting a person's freedom of movement, physical activity, or access to his or her own body.

Self-determination: An individual's right to choose one's own path in life.

Sensory stimulation: Intentional process of heightening a person's sensory receptors through the use of items that arouse sense of smell, taste, touch, sound, and sight.

Shared surroundings: Those aspects of the environment in public living areas that are either intentionally or unintentionally experienced by persons who share that space.

Significant change in condition: A sudden and profound change in a person's physical or mental condition that necessitates an update and appropriate intervention in the person's care plan.

Soft and sweet food: Foods with soft texture and sweet taste, such as ice cream and pudding, that people with advanced dementia will eat when they refuse other foods.

Standard: A norm that represents a minimum level of practice and is an agreed-upon criterion for measuring quality in advanced-dementia care services.

Substitute judgment: The process of making healthcare decisions for a person who has lost the ability to make the decisions himself or herself. These decisions are based on knowledge of the person's values and reflect what the person would want if able to express his or her wishes.

Surrogate: A person authorized to make decisions for someone who cannot make or communicate his or her healthcare treatment choices. A surrogate is authorized by a power of attorney document or by court order.

Surroundings: Those aspects of the environment that surround or touch the person and are part of his or her immediate primary sensory experience. Includes both personal and shared surroundings.

Terminally ill: Medical diagnosis by a physician that an individual has a specific, progressive, and normally irreversible disease that will cause the individual's death in 6 months or less.

Training or in-service education: Organized instruction or information provided to healthcare facility personnel or volunteers.

Volunteer: A person, not a family member, who provides services without compensation.

Weight loss: In terms of Alzheimer's care, an unintended loss of body fat or muscle mass because of inadequate nutritional intake to offset metabolic needs.

■ REFERENCES

Alzheimer's Association. (2005b). *Providing culturally sensitive dementia care.* Retrieved June 12, 2005, from http://www.alz.org/Resources/Diversity/downloads/ABOUT_CulturallySensitive DementiaCare.pdf

Arizona Administrative Code, Title 9. Health services definitions. Retrieved January 2006, from http://www.azsos.gov/public_services/Table_of_Contents.htm

Kovach, C. R., Wilson, S. A., & Noonan, P. E. (1996). Effects of hospice interventions on behaviors, discomfort, and physical complications of end-stage nursing home residents. *American Journal of Alzheimer's Disease, 11*(4), 7–10.

Purnell, L. D., & Paulanka, B. J. (2003). The Purnell model of cultural competence. In L. D. Purnell & B. J. Paulanka (Eds.), *Transcultural healthcare: A culturally competent approach* (pp. 8–39). Philadelphia: F. A. Davis.

Spector, R. (2004). *Cultural diversity in health and illness* (6th ed.). Upper Saddle River, NJ: Pearson Prentice Hall.

World Health Organization. (1990). *Cancer pain relief and palliative care*. Geneva, Switzerland: Author.

ADDITIONAL RESOURCES

The *Palliative Care for Advanced Dementia: Guidelines and Standards for Evidence-Based Care* guidebook is part of a larger and more comprehensive set of documents reflecting other key training principles, guidelines, and standards for advanced-dementia care. Additional resources include the following:

Alzheimer's Association, Desert Southwest Chapter. (2004). *Palliative care for advanced dementia: A self-instructional seven-part teaching program* (VHS and DVD). Phoenix, AZ: Sheri Brown Productions.

Long, C. O. (Ed.). (2004). *Palliative care for advanced dementia. Train-the-trainer manual*. Phoenix, AZ: Alzheimer's Association, Desert Southwest Chapter.

Long, C. O. (Ed.). (2005). *Palliative care for advanced dementia. Training manual*. Phoenix, AZ: Alzheimer's Association, Desert Southwest Chapter.

Long, C. O. (Ed.). (2005). *Palliative care for advanced dementia: Uniform assessment tool/guidelines and work statement*. Phoenix, AZ: Alzheimer's Association, Desert Southwest Chapter.

APPENDIX A:
PROFESSIONAL AND CAREGIVER
RESOURCES FOR ADVANCED DEMENTIA

Dan Lawler, Marwan Sabbagh, and Deborah Schaus

▦ OVERVIEW OF THE ALZHEIMER'S ASSOCIATION SERVICES

The Alzheimer's Association Web site (http://www.alz.org) is an invaluable resource both for professionals and for family caregivers. New fact sheets, informational brochures, and publications are frequently posted on the Web site, most of which are available as free downloads, and printed copies may be available through local Alzheimer's Association chapters.

The Alzheimer's Association staffs a helpline 24 hours a day and 7 days a week. This is staffed by professionals that can assist in times of crisis and can direct callers to resources in the local geographical areas. The phone number is 1-800-272-3900.

The Alzheimer's Association's Benjamin B. Green-Field National Alzheimer's Library and Resource Center includes a virtual library that is accessible through the Alzheimer's Association Web site (http://www.alz.org or http://www.alz.org/we_can_help_library_services.asp). It is the nation's largest library and resource center devoted to Alzheimer's disease and related dementias. Resource lists, which include articles, books, videos, and Web sites, are available online on various topics of interest, including *End-of-Life Planning and Decision Making* (updated April 2009; http://www.alz.org/library/downloads/EndofLifePlanning DecisionMaking2009.pdf).

As of this writing, photocopies of articles and book chapters are available to the public through the Alzheimer's Association's Green-Field Library for minimal fees. Although the library does not lend items from its collection directly to the public, materials can be accessed through local Alzheimer's Association chapters and interlibrary loan programs. The Green-Field Library can be contacted by telephone at 312-335-9602 or 1-800-272-3990, by fax at 1-866-699-1238, postal mail at 225 North Michigan Avenue, Floor 17, Chicago, IL, 60601-7633, or by e-mail at Greenfield@alz.org.

Brief List of Alzheimer's Association Publications

The following is a sample of some of the materials available at the National Alzheimer's Association Web site that may be of interest to the reader. Local chapter offices will likely have materials such as these available, in addition to localized resource lists, publications, and training sessions for professionals.

Alzheimer's Association. (2003, October). *Stages in Alzheimer's disease* (topic sheet). Chicago, IL: Alzheimer's Association National Office.
Available at: http://www.alz.org/national/documents/topicsheet_stages.pdf

Alzheimer's Association. (2007). *Dementia care practice recommendations for assisted-living residences and nursing homes. Phase 3 end-of-life care.* Chicago, IL: Alzheimer's Association National Office. (Contains recommendations for care practices related to decision-making and hospice services.)
Available at: http://www.alz.org/national/documents/brochure_DCPRphase3.pdf

Alzheimer's Association. (2005). *Legal Plans - Assisting the person with dementia in planning for the future* (brochure). Chicago, IL: Alzheimer's Association National Office.
Available at: http://www.alz.org/national/documents/brochure_legalplans.pdf

Alzheimer's Association. (2005). *Personal Care - Assisting the person with dementia with changing daily needs* (brochure). Chicago, IL: Alzheimer's Association National Office.
Available at: http://www.alz.org/national/documents/brochure_personalcare.pdf

Alzheimer's Association. (2006). *End-of-life decisions: Honoring the wishes of the person with Alzheimer's disease* (brochure). Chicago, IL: Alzheimer's Association National Office.
Available at: http://www.alz.org/national/documents/brochure_endoflifedecisions.pdf

Alzheimer's Association. (2007, July). *Planning ahead for long-term care expenses* (topic sheet). Chicago, IL: Alzheimer's Association National Office.
Available at: http://www.alz.org/national/documents/topicsheet_planahead.pdf

Alzheimer's Association. (2007, August). *Quality end-of-life care for individuals with dementia in assisted living and nursing homes and public policy barriers to delivering care.* Chicago, IL: Alzheimer's Association National Office.
Available at: http://www.alz.org/national/documents/End_interviewpaper_III.pdf

Volicer L. (2005). *End-of-life care for people with dementia in residential care settings.* Chicago, IL: Alzheimer's Association National Office. (An analysis of the literature on end-of-life care for nursing home residents.)
Available at: http://www.alz.org/national/documents/endoflifelitreview.pdf

Additional Resources through the Alzheimer's Association, Desert Southwest Chapter

The following items are available through the Alzheimer's Association, Desert Southwest Chapter, 1028 East McDowell Rd., Phoenix, AZ, 85006, by phone: 602-528-0545, or on the Web at: http://www.alz.org/dsw.

▪ Alzheimer's Association, Desert Southwest Chapter. (2004). *Palliative care for advanced dementia: A self-instructional seven-part teaching program* (VHS and DVD). Phoenix, AZ: Sheri Brown Productions.

▪ Arizona Direct Care Workforce Committee. (2008). *Principles of caregiving, Alzheimer's disease and other dementias module.* Phoenix, AZ: Author. (The *Principles of Caregiving* training manuals were created under the guidance of the Arizona Direct Care Workforce Committee in response to recommendations from the Citizens Workgroup on the Long-Term Care Workforce. The Alzheimer's Association, Desert Southwest Chapter developed the Alzheimer's Module. This module provides information to help improve the quality of life for those with Alzheimer's disease and other forms of dementia, and to reduce caregiving stress and increase job satisfaction for both professional and volunteer caregivers. The Alzheimer's Module, along with the complete curriculum, can be found at www.azdirectcare.org/Training_Manuals. This curriculum is a public resource and can be used for self-study and in classes.)

▪ Long, C. O. (Ed.). (2005). *Palliative care for advanced dementia. Training manual.* Phoenix, AZ: Alzheimer's Association, Desert Southwest Chapter.

APPENDIX B:
CULTURAL RESOURCES ON THE WEB

Alzheimer's Association's Diversity Toolbox

http://www.alz.org/Resources/Diversity/overview.asp
The Diversity Toolbox was developed to include various resources for people with dementia, their families and caregivers, and health and social service professionals. The toolbox includes educational materials for Chinese, Korean, and Hispanic groups; assessment tools; and outreach tips.

Alzheimer's Disease International

http://www.alz.co.uk/alzheimers/languages.html
This site is only available in English at present, but on it are links to sites in 29 different languages that offer information about Alzheimer's and other forms of dementia.

Alzheimer's Australia

http://www.alzheimers.org.au/content.cfm?categoryid=14
Alzheimer's Australia offers help sheets in Arabic, Chinese, Greek, Italian, Polish, and Vietnamese.

Center for Cross-Cultural Health

http://www.crosshealth.com
The mission of the Center for Cross-Cultural Health is to integrate the role of culture in improving health. This research and information service is involved in the education and training of health providers and organizations in Minnesota and elsewhere. Through information sharing, training, organizational assessments, and research, the center works to develop culturally competent individuals, organizations, systems, and societies.

Center for Healthy Families and Cultural Diversity (CHFCD), Robert Wood Johnson Medical School

http://rwjms.umdnj.edu/fammed/chfcd/index.htm
According to the Web site, "The CHFCD recognizes that persisting racial and ethnic health disparities are a major clinical, public health, and societal problem. The CHFCD exists to foster justice and equity in health care." The site offers many valuable links to cross-cultural health services.

▦ *The Cross-Cultural Healthcare Program (CCHCP)*

http://www.xculture.org/about.php
Since 1992, the CCHCP has been addressing cultural issues that effect the health
of individuals and families in ethnic minority communities in Seattle and nation-
wide. The site provides information on cultural competency training programs,
interpreter training, research projects, and community coalition building.

▦ *Curriculum in Ethnogeriatrics*

http://www.stanford.edu/group/ethnoger/
This site is designed to help educate healthcare providers who work with elderly
patients from diverse backgrounds. It includes information on the beliefs and
practices of 11 minority groups: African American, American Indian and Alas-
kan Native, Asian Indian, Chinese, Filipino, Hispanic, Japanese, Korean, Native
Hawaiian, Pakistani, and Southeast Asian.

▦ *Diversity Rx*

http://www.diversityrx.org
DiversityRx is a good resource for policymakers, healthcare providers, and consumer representatives to learn more about language and cultural competence in
health care.

▦ *EthnoMed*

http://www.ethnomed.org
The EthnoMed site contains information about cultural beliefs, medical issues,
and other issues pertinent to the health care of recent immigrants to Seattle
or the United States. Many of these immigrants are refugees fleeing from war-
torn places in the world. The site includes information on the following cultures:
Amharic-language speakers (who are from Ethiopia), Cambodian, Chinese,
Eritrean, Ethiopian, Hispanic, Oromo speakers (from Ethiopia and Kenya),
Somali, Tigray people (from Eritrea and Kenya), Vietnamese, and other groups
who have substantial numbers in Seattle (Arab, Lao, Mien, South Asian, Soviet
Jewish, Ukrainian, and Samoan).

▦ *National Center for Cultural Competence*

http://www3.georgetown.edu/research/gucchd/nccc/pa.html
The mission of the National Center for Cultural Competence is to increase the
capacity of physical and mental health programs to design, implement, and evaluate culturally and linguistically competent service delivery systems. The site
contains useful information for families, practitioners, institutions, and facilities.

▦ *National Resource Center on Diversity*

http://www.nrcd.com
The National Resource Center on Diversity in End-of-Life Care is committed to
improving the provision of culturally appropriate care for all individuals with
terminal illnesses. They serve as a national clearinghouse and gathering place for

communities and researchers involved in improving care at the end of life for the almost 100 million Americans who are people of color and other minorities. The site offers important information for both families and professionals.

Office of Minority Health (OMH) Resource Center

http://www.omhrc.gov
The mission of the Office of Minority Health (OMH) is to improve and protect the health of racial and ethnic minority populations through the development of health policies and programs that will eliminate health disparities. OMH advises the Secretary and the Office of Public Health and Science on public health program activities affecting American Indians and Alaska Natives, Asian Americans, African Americans, Hispanics, Native Hawaiians, and other Pacific Islanders. Information is available on campaigns and initiatives, employment, federal clearinghouses, and research.

Transcultural Nursing Society

http://www.tcns.org
This society and Web site aims to provide nurses and other healthcare professionals with the knowledge necessary to ensure cultural competence in practice, education, research, and administrative functions.

University of Washington Medical Center's Culture Clues

http://depts.washington.edu/pfes/CultureClues.htm
The University of Washington Medical Center offers online tip sheets for clinicians about the preferences and beliefs of many minority groups, including Chinese, Hispanic, Korean, deaf and hard of hearing. The tips sheets are available for reprint with permission.

APPENDIX C:
FEDERAL GUIDELINES FOR PROVIDING CULTURALLY SENSITIVE CARE

The following national standards, issued by the U.S. Department of Health and Human Services' Office of Minority Health (OMH), respond to the need to ensure that all people entering the healthcare system receive equitable and effective treatment in a culturally and linguistically appropriate manner. These standards for culturally and linguistically appropriate services (CLAS) are proposed as a means to correct inequities that currently exist in the provision of health services and to make these services more responsive to the individual needs of all patients. The standards are intended to be inclusive of all cultures; however, they are especially designed to address the needs of racial, ethnic, and linguistic population groups that experience unequal access to health services. Ultimately, the aim of the standards is to contribute to the elimination of racial and ethnic health disparities and to improve the health of all Americans.

The CLAS standards are primarily directed at healthcare organizations; however, individual providers are also encouraged to use them to make their practices more culturally and linguistically accessible. The principles and activities of CLAS should be integrated throughout an organization and undertaken in partnership with the communities being served.

The 14 standards are organized by themes: Culturally Competent Care (Standards 1–3), Language Access Services (Standards 4–7), and Organizational Supports for Cultural Competence (Standards 8–14). Within this framework, there are three types of standards of varying stringency: mandates, guidelines, and recommendations as follows:

- CLAS mandates are current Federal requirements for all recipients of Federal funds (Standards 4, 5, 6, and 7).
- CLAS guidelines are activities recommended by OMH for adoption as mandates by federal, state, and national accrediting agencies (Standards 1, 2, 3, 8, 9, 10, 11, 12, and 13).
- CLAS recommendations are suggested by OMH for voluntary adoption by healthcare organizations (Standard 14).

1. Healthcare organizations should ensure that patients or consumers receive from all staff members effective, understandable, and respectful care that is provided in a manner compatible with their cultural health beliefs and practices and preferred language.

2. Healthcare organizations should implement strategies to recruit, retain, and promote at all levels of the organizations a diverse staff and diverse leadership that are representative of the demographic characteristics of the service area.

3. Healthcare organizations should ensure that staff at all levels and across all disciplines receive ongoing education and training in CLAS delivery.

4. Healthcare organizations must offer and provide language assistance services, including bilingual staff and interpreter services, at no cost to each patient or consumer with limited English proficiency at all points of contact in a timely manner during all hours of operation.

5. Healthcare organizations must provide to patients or consumers in their preferred language both verbal offers and written notices informing them of their right to receive language assistance services.

6. Healthcare organizations must ensure the competence of language assistance provided to limited English proficient patients or consumers by interpreters and bilingual staff. Family and friends should not be used to provide interpretation services (except on request by the patient or consumer).

7. Healthcare organizations must make available easily understood patient-related materials and post signage in the languages of the commonly encountered groups and/or groups represented in the service area.

8. Healthcare organizations should develop, implement, and promote a written strategic plan that outlines clear goals, policies, operational plans, and management accountability or oversight mechanisms to provide CLAS.

9. Healthcare organizations should conduct initial and ongoing organizational self-assessment of CLAS-related activities and are encouraged to integrate cultural and linguistic competence-related measures into their internal audits, performance improvement programs, patient satisfaction assessment, and outcomes-based evaluations.

10. Healthcare organizations should ensure that data on the individual patient's or consumer's race, ethnicity, and spoken and written language are collected in health records, integrated into the organization's management information system, and periodically updated.

11. Healthcare organizations should maintain a current demographic, cultural, and epidemiological profile of the community as well as a needs assessment to accurately plan for implementing services that respond to the cultural and linguistic characteristics of the service area.

12. Healthcare organizations should develop participatory, collaborative partnerships with communities and use various formal and informal mechanisms to facilitate community and patient or consumer involvement in designing and implementing CLAS-related activities.

13. Healthcare organizations should ensure that conflict and grievance resolution processes are culturally and linguistically sensitive and capable of identifying, preventing, and resolving cross-cultural conflicts or complaints by patients or consumers.

14. Healthcare organizations are encouraged to regularly make available to the public information about their progress and successful innovation in implementing the CLAS standards and to provide public notice in their communities about the availability of this information.

APPENDIX D: CULTURAL HERITAGE ASSESSMENT FORM

Caregivers can use the following questions to begin to understand a person's ethnic, cultural, or religious heritage in the context of healthcare.

1. Where were your parents and/or grandparents born?

    a. Mother:

    _____

    b. Father:

    _____

    c. Mother's mother:

    _____

    d. Mother's father:

    _____

    e. Father's mother:

    _____

    f. Father's father:

    _____

2. How many brothers _____ and sisters _____ do you have?

3. What setting did you grow up in? Urban _____ Rural _____ Suburban _____

Where?

_____

4. What country did your parents or grandparents grow up in?

    a. Mother:

_____

    b. Father:

_____

    c. Mother's mother:

_____

    d. Mother's father:

_____

    e. Father's mother:

_____

    f. Father's father:

_____

5. How old were you when you came to the United States? _____

6. How old were your parents or grandparents when they came to the United States?

    a. Mother:

_____

    b. Father:

_____

    c. Mother's mother:

_____

    d. Mother's father:

_____

    e. Father's mother:

_____

    f. Father's father:

_____

7. When you were growing up, who lived with you? _____

8. Have you maintained contact with:

     a. Aunts, uncles, cousins? _____ Yes _____ No

     b. Brothers and sisters? _____ Yes _____ No

     c. Parents? _____ Yes _____ No

     d. Your own children? _____ Yes _____ No

9. Does most of your family live near you? _____ Describe: _____

10. Approximately how often did you visit your family members who lived outside

     your home? _____ Daily _____ Weekly _____ Monthly _____ Yearly _____ Never

11. Was your original family name changed? _____ Yes _____ No

12. What is your religious preference? _____ Catholic _____ Jewish

     _____ Protestant _____ Denomination _____ Other _____ None

13. Is your spouse of the same religion? _____ Yes _____ No

14. Is your spouse of the same ethnic background as you? _____ Yes _____ No

15. What kind of school did you go to? _____ Public _____ Private _____ Parochial

16. As an adult, do you live in a neighborhood where the neighbors are the same

     religion and ethnic background as you? _____ Yes _____ No

17. Do you belong to a religious institution? _____ Yes _____ No

18. Would you describe yourself as an active member? _____ Yes _____ No

19. How often do you attend your religious institution?

     _____ More than once a week _____ Weekly _____ Monthly

     _____ Special holidays only _____ Never

20. Do you practice your religion in your home? _____ Yes _____ No

If yes, please specify: _____ Praying _____ Bible reading _____ Diet

_____ Celebrating religious holidays _____ Other

Describe:

_____

21. Do you prepare foods of your ethnic background? _____ Yes _____ No

Describe:

_____

22. Do you participate in ethnic activities? _____ Yes _____ No

If yes, specify: _____ Singing _____ Holiday celebrations _____ Dancing

_____ Costumes _____ Festivals _____ Other

Describe:

_____

23. Are your friends from the same religious background? _____ Yes _____ No

24. Are your friends of the same ethnic background as you? _____ Yes _____ No

25. What is your native language? _____

Do you speak this language? _____ Prefer _____ Occasionally _____ Rarely

26. Do you read in your native language? _____ Prefer _____ Occasionally

_____ Rarely

Source: Reprinted by permission from Rachel E. Spector, *Cultural Diversity in Health and Illness* 6th ed. (Upper Saddle, NJ: Pearson Prentice Hall, 2004), 371–374. © 2004 by Pearson Education.

INDEX

Note: An *f* following a page number indicates a figure, a *t* indicates a table, an *e* indicates an exhibit.